Diet and Metabolic Dysfunction

Volume I:
Evidence From Basic Research

Special Issue Editor
Gaetano Santulli

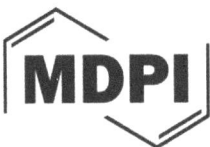

MDPI

Special Issue Editor
Gaetano Santulli
College of Physicians & Surgeons
Columbia University Medical Center
USA

Editorial Office
MDPI AG
St. Alban-Anlage 66
Basel, Switzerland

This edition is a reprint of the Special Issue published online in the open access journal *Nutrients* (ISSN 2072-6643) from 2015–2016 (available at: http://www.mdpi.com/journal/nutrients/special_issues/diet-metabolic-dysfunction).

For citation purposes, cite each article independently as indicated on the article page online and as indicated below:

Author 1; Author 2; Author 3 etc. Article title. *Journal Name.* **Year**. Article number/page range.

ISBN 978-3-03842-320-1 (Pbk) Vol. 1-2
ISBN 978-3-03842-321-8 (PDF) Vol. 1-2

ISBN 978-3-03842-322-5 (Pbk) Vol. 1
ISBN 978-3-03842-323-2 (PDF) Vol. 1

Table of Contents

Section 1: High-fat Diet and Metabolism

Section 2: Diet and Mitochondrial Function

Section 3: Glucose Homeostasis and Dyslipidemia

Section 4: Diet and Obesity

About the Guest Editor

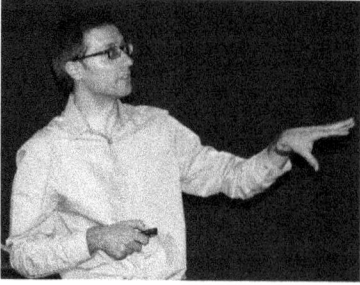

Gaetano Santulli, M.D., Ph.D. is a principal investigator currently working at Columbia University Medical Center. A physician–scientist, he received his M.D. and Ph.D. at the University of Naples "Federico II". Dr. Santulli completed his training at Columbia University in New York City. Dr. Santulli's expertise comprises both clinical—he is a cardiologist—and basic research topics, including hypertension, diabetes, heart failure, arrhythmias, vascular disease, microRNA, and mitochondrial pathophysiology. He serves on the editorial boards of numerous medical journals. He has authored more than 100 peer-reviewed publications and edited several medical books, including "Adrenal Glands: From Pathophysiology to Clinical Evidence" and "microRNA: From Molecular Biology to Clinical Practice".

Preface to "Diet and Metabolic Dysfunction"

The fundamental importance of diet in the pathophysiology of metabolic syndrome is well acknowledged and may be crucial in the determination of cardiovascular risk and the development of cardiovascular complications. The contributions presented here provide an updated systematic overview examining, in detail, the functional role of different diets and dietary components in maintaining glucose homeostasis and preventing long-term complications. The two books encompass 40 peer-reviewed articles, both in the basic research field (*book 1*) and in the clinical scenario (*book 2*), written by worldwide renowned experts. Intriguingly, one of the assets of the present books is in the melting pot of researchers involved in this project, literally working in all continents, with contributions from United States, Canada, Mexico, Argentina, Italy, Ireland, Spain, Sweden, Austria, Liechtenstein, Germany, Japan, Korea, China, Hong Kong, Taiwan, Malaysia, Saudi Arabia, South-Africa, Nigeria, and Australia. These books include both evidence-based original research and state-of-the-art reviews and meta-analyses of the scientific literature. There are articles investigating different dietary regimens and articles focusing on specific nutrients. In particular, studies on the following topics are presented: omega-3 fatty acids, barley, honey, capsaicin, magnesium, selenium, fructose, vanillic acid, glutamine, histidine, isoleucine and valine, quercetin, rutin, naringin, red ginseng, epigallocatechin gallate (a component of green tea), cudrania tricuspidata fruits, aloe vera, and probiotics and prebiotics. This collection of papers shows that the selection of foods should be based on scientific evidence, knowing the properties of each dietary component.

Gaetano Santulli
Guest Editor

Section 1:
High-fat Diet and Metabolism

![nutrients logo] *nutrients*

MDPI

Article

A Moderate Low-Carbohydrate Low-Calorie Diet Improves Lipid Profile, Insulin Sensitivity and Adiponectin Expression in Rats

Jie-Hua Chen [1,†], Caiqun Ouyang [1,†], Qiang Ding [2], Jia Song [1], Wenhong Cao [3] and Limei Mao [1,*]

[1]   Department of Nutrition and Food Hygiene, School of Public Health and Tropical Medicine, Southern Medical University, Guangzhou 510515, Guangdong, China; siyanpijiehua@gmail.com (J.C.); oycq108729@163.com (C.O.); songj_lin@163.com (J.S.)
[2]   Department of Nutrition and Food Hygiene, School of Public Health, Tongji Medical College, Huazhong University of Science and Technology, Wuhan 430030, Hubei, China; dq0306@163.com
[3]   Department of Nutrition, The Gillings School of Global Public Health, The University of North Carolina at Chapel Hill, Chapel Hill, NC 27599, USA; caow@unc.edu
*   Correspondence: mlm912@smu.edu.cn; Tel.: +86-20-6164-8328; Fax: +86-20-6164-8324.
†   These authors contributed equally to this work.

Received: 27 April 2015; Accepted: 2 June 2015; Published: 11 June 2015

Abstract: Calorie restriction (CR) via manipulating dietary carbohydrates has attracted increasing interest in the prevention and treatment of metabolic syndrome. There is little consensus about the extent of carbohydrate restriction to elicit optimal results in controlling metabolic parameters. Our study will identify a better carbohydrate-restricted diet using rat models. Rats were fed with one of the following diets for 12 weeks: Control diet, 80% energy (34% carbohydrate-reduced) and 60% energy (68% carbohydrate-reduced) of the control diet. Changes in metabolic parameters and expressions of adiponectin and peroxisome proliferator activator receptor γ (PPARγ) were identified. Compared to the control diet, 68% carbohydrate-reduced diet led to a decrease in serum triglyceride and increases inlow density lipoprotein-cholesterol (LDL-C), high density lipoprotein-cholesterol (HDL-C) and total cholesterol; a 34% carbohydrate-reduced diet resulted in a decrease in triglycerides and an increase in HDL-cholesterol, no changes however, were shown in LDL-cholesterol and total cholesterol; reductions in HOMA-IR were observed in both CR groups. Gene expressions of adiponectin and PPARγ in adipose tissues were found proportionally elevated with an increased degree of energy restriction. Our study for the first time ever identified that a moderate-carbohydrate restricted diet is not only effective in raising gene expressions of adiponectin and PPARγ which potentially lead to better metabolic conditions but is better at improving lipid profiles than a low-carbohydrate diet in rats.

Keywords: dietary intervention; metabolic syndrome; adiponectin; peroxisome proliferator activator receptor γ; dietary carbohydrate restriction; rats

1. Introduction

Metabolic syndrome (MetS) is a collection of medical conditions that can lead to obesity, diabetes, cardiovascular disease and hypertension. The prevalence of MetS is on a rapid rise due to the shifted paradigm of diet and lifestyle and thus has afflicted many people worldwide. It is well known that calorie restriction (CR) improves some markers of MetS [1–3], such as blood pressure, blood glucose and plasma cholesterol, as demonstrated in a number of animal models, and humans [3,4].

Besides functioning as primary energy storage reservoirs, adipose tissue also acts as an endocrine organ secreting numerous protein hormones into the circulation [5]. It was reported that a reduction in White Adipose Tissue (WAT) via CR is likely to change the levels of its secreted hormones. Among all the WAT depots, Visceral Adipose Tissue (VAT) is closely related in particular to MetS and thus is a pathogenic fat depot [6]. The VAT compartment secretes adipokines and cytokines that are predisposed to the development of metabolic traits [7]. Adiponectin is an adipokine and mainly expressed in adipose tissues. Adiponectin has been shown as an insulin-sensitive hormone that participates in the regulation of glucose and lipid metabolism. It was found that adiponectin levels rise during CR [8].

Several elements are capable of modulating adiponectin gene expression, most notably peroxisome proliferator activator receptor γ (PPAR-γ) [9], which is expressed in adipose tissues. A response element of PPARγ was discovered on the promoter of adiponectin gene [10]. Treatment with PPARγ agonists induced adiponectin synthesis during adiponeogenesis [11–13]. PPARγ can also be upregulated by CR through its antioxidative action [14,15].

The beneficial effect of CR on prevention and treatment of MetS has been widely recognized. The optimal CR diet, however, remains to be identified. Among all the CR diets, CR via manipulating dietary carbohydrate content has attracted increasing interest due to its effectiveness on weight loss, glycemic control, insulin sensitivity and the management of cardiovascular risk factors [16]. However, there is little consensus about the extent of dietary carbohydrate restriction to elicit the optimal result in controlling metabolic parameters. In the present study, 12-week CR by varying dietary carbohydrate content (80% or 60% energy (34% or 68% carbohydrate reduction) of the control diet) was employed in Wistar rats to investigate the changes in metabolic parameters and expressions of adiponectin and PPARγ. The results of the study will provide a new perspective and new scientific evidence for the prevention and treatment of MetS.

2. Experimental Section

2.1. Animals and Diets

Thirty-six male Wistar rats (two months old, body weight 240–260 g) were obtained from a local supplier for laboratory animals (Laboratory Animal Center of Hubei Province; Wuhan, China). Rats were housed individually under laboratory conditions (12 h day and night lighting cycle, 22 °C ± 2 °C, 50% ± 10% humidity). All experimental protocols were reviewed and approved by Tongji Medical College Council of Animal Care Committee. Rats were randomly assigned into three different groups, *ad libitum* group (AL group; n = 12), calorie restriction group 1 (CR1 group; n = 12) and calorie restriction group 2 (CR2 group; n = 12). All rats had *ad libitum* access to drinking water.

Rat chow diets were prepared based on the Association of Official Analytical Chemists (AOAC) and AIN-93G formulas to meet the nutrient and energy requirements for the growth and development of rats [17]. Rats were fed with these diets for 12 weeks. AL group had *ad libitum* access to the feed whereas CR1 and CR2 group were maintained on a CR regimen with daily access to 80% and 60% of the calorie intake of AL group, respectively (Table 1). Starch was the only nutrient reduced from diets to achieve calorie restriction for CR1 and CR2 groups whereas the amount of other nutrients provided were at the same level as those in the AL group to ensure sufficient nutrients were provided to maintain normal growth of rats. As starch constitutes 58.5% (w/w) of the control diet, 80% and 60% CR correspond to 34% and 68% carbohydrate reduction in CR1 and CR2 group, respectively. The amount of feed consumed by each rat was recorded daily and body weights of rats were monitored weekly. At the end of the 12-week study, rats fasted for 10 h overnight and blood samples were collected. Rats were then sacrificed by decapitation. Serum samples were obtained from all blood samples promptly after blood collection and stored at −80 °C. The peri-epididymal and perirenal adipose tissues were obtained, weighed and frozen immediately in liquid nitrogen prior to storage at −80 °C.

Table 1. Composition of rat chow diet *.

Components	AL Group		CR1 Group [a]		CR2 Group [b]	
	g/kg Diet	% Energy	g/0.8 kg Diet	% Energy	g/0.6 kg Diet	% Energy
Casein	200.0	20.2	200.0	25.2	200.0	33.8
Vitamin mix **	10.0	-	10.0	-	10.0	-
Mineral mix **	35.0	-	35.0	-	35.0	-
Sucrose	50.0	5.0	50.0	6.3	50.0	8.4
Corn starch	585.0	58.9	385.0	48.6	185.0	31.2
Fiber	50.0	-	50.0	-	50.0	-
Lipid	70.0	15.9	70.0	19.9	70.0	26.6
Total amount (g)	1000.0	100.0	800.0	100.0	600.0	100.0
Total Calorie/kg diet (Kcal)	3970.0		3170.0		2370.0	
Energy ratio (%)						
Protein/Total	20		25		34	
Carbohydrate/Total	64		55		40	
Lipid/Total	16		20		26	

* Abbreviations: AL: *ad libitum*; CR: calorie restriction; ** The composition of vitamin and mineral mix can be referred to AIN-93G; [a] CR1 group was provided with 80% of *ad libitum* intake based on AL group; [b] CR2 group was provided with 60% of *ad libitum* intake based on AL group.

2.2. Biochemical Measurements

Commercial ELISA kit (R & D Systems, Minneapolis, MN, USA) was used to measure serum adiponectin at the baseline and at the end of the study. Fasting blood glucose, fasting serum insulin, serum total cholesterol, fasting triglyceride and serum high density lipoprotein cholesterol (HDL-C) were determined by enzymatic colorimetric analysis using commercialized kits purchased from BioSino Bio-technology and Science Inc., Beijing, China. All the measurements were performed using an automatic enzymatic analyser (BioTek SpectraMax M2, Winooski, VT, USA). Triglyceride level was measured using glycerol-3-phosphate oxidase-p-aminophenazone (GPO-PAP) method. Total cholesterol was determined using cholesterol oxidase-p-aminophenazone (CHOD-PAP) method. After precipitation of very-low-density lipoprotein (VLDL) and low-density lipoprotein cholesterol (LDL-C), HDL-C was measured, as well. Serum LDL-C were then obtained based on Friedewald equation, in which, LDL-C = Total Cholesterol − (Triglyceride/5 + HDL-C) [18]. Blood glucose level was determined by glucose oxidase method. Insulin level was determined with a commercialized radioimmunoassay kit. Homeostasis Model Assessment of Insulin Resistance (HOMA-IR) was calculated based on the relationship between fasting plasma glucose and insulin: HOMA-IR = fasting plasma glucose (mmol/L) × insulin (mIU/L)/22.5 [19].

2.3. Semiquantitative Reverse Transcriptase Polymerase Chain Reaction

Total RNA of the epididymal adipose tissue was extracted using Trizol reagent (Promega, Madison, WI, USA). The concentration of RNA was determined using nucleic acid analyser (Eppendorf, Germany). RNA (3 µg) was reverse transcribed in a 25 µL reaction system into complementary DNA which was then amplified using polymerase chain reaction (PCR). The following primers were used for PCR: 5′-TCCCTCCACCCAAGGAAACT-3′ (sense) and 5′-TTGCCAGTGCTGCCGTGATA-3′ (antisense) for adiponectin; 5′-CATCACTATCGGCAATGAGC-3′ (sense) and 5′-GACAGCACTG TGTTGGCATA-3′ (antisense) for β-actin; 5′-TCCGTGATGGAAGACCACTC-3′ (sense) and 5′-CCCTTGCATCCTTCACAAGC-3′ for PPARγ. β-actin served as a loading control.

All PCR reactions contained 0.2 mmol/L dNTP (deoxyribonucleotide triphosphate), 1.5 µL complementary DNA, 0.25 µmol/L of each primer, 1 × PCR buffer, and 0.8 µL Taq polymerase. The following cycling profile was used for PCR reactions: 5 min of denaturation at 95 °C followed by 30 cycles with 1 min at 94 °C, 45 s at 58 °C and 1 min at 72 °C for adiponectin or 35 cycles with 1 min at 94 °C, 40 s at 56 °C and 1 min at 72 °C for PPARγ or 35 cycles with 1 min at 94 °C, 45 s at 59 °C and 1 min at 72 °C for β-actin and the final extension step of 10 min at 72 °C in a PCR Thermocycler (Biometra, Göttingen, Germany).

PCR products were subjected to electrophoresis in 1.5% agarose gels and the results were analyszed by gel imaging and analysis system (Biometra, Göttingen, Germany). The expression levels of adiponectin mRNA and PPARγ mRNA were shown using the absorbance ratio of target mRNA and β-actin mRNA.

2.4. Statistical Analysis

All the data were analysed using one-way ANOVA followed by Least Significant Difference (LSD)-test with SPSS version 12 software (SPSS Inc., Chicago, IL, USA). Transformation was applied to correct for unequal variances. Pearson correlation coefficient was used to analyze the linear relationship between adiponectin mRNA level and different parameters, *i.e.*, body weight, blood glucose, total cholesterol, triglyceride, HDL-C and insulin. Similar tests were applied to analyze the linear relationship between PPARγ mRNA level and those parameters. In all tests, a value of $p \leq 0.05$ was considered statistically significant.

3. Results

3.1. Calorie Intake and Body Weight

Average calorie intakes of all three groups demonstrated a similar decreasing trend over the 12-week feeding period due to decreased growth rates of rats with maturation (Figure 1). In good agreement with the study design, the ratio of total calorie intake of AL, CR1 and CR2 groups during the feeding period was calculated as 100:81:61.

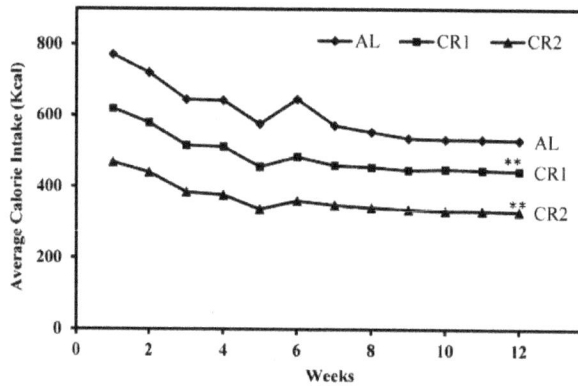

Figure 1. Weekly average calorie intakes of three groups over the 12-week feeding period. Average calorie intake of rats across all groups was shown to be higher at the beginning of the study when rats were fast-growing and then slowly decreased to a plateau with decreasing growth rates of rats. One-way ANOVA followed by LSD-test was used to detect significant differences of the means of the body weights at the end of the study ** $p < 0.001$.

The effect of CR on body weights of rats was found to be significant (Figure 2). Compared to the control group AL, growth rates of rats in CR1 and CR2 group were much slower. Our results indicated that significant differences of body weights of rats among groups were detected in Week 4 ($p < 0.05$) and the differences were greater towards the end of the study ($p < 0.001$).

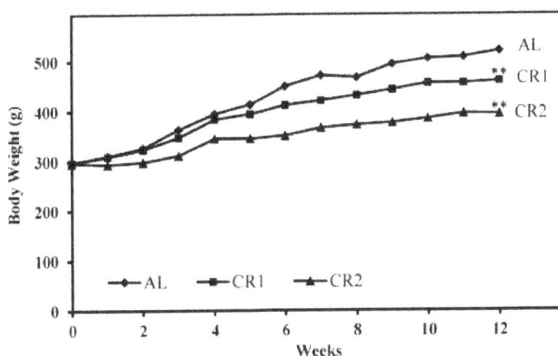

Figure 2. Change of body weights of rats from three groups over the 12-week feeding period. One-way ANOVA followed by LSD-test was used to detect significant differences of the means of the body weights at the end of the study ** $p < 0.001$.

3.2. Changes in Metabolic Parameters

Both 80% (CR1) and 60% (CR2) calorie-restricted diets led to a significant decrease in triglyceride as compared to control diet (AL) ($p < 0.05$; Table 2). However, total cholesterol was found increased in CR2 group ($p < 0.05$) whereas no change was observed in CR1 when compared to AL group ($p > 0.05$; Table 2). Though HDL-C in CR1 and CR2 groups were higher than those in AL group ($p < 0.05$), no significant differences were observed in the ratios of total cholesterol to HDL-C among all the groups ($p > 0.05$). The effect of CR on LDL-C resembled that on total cholesterol which LDL-C increased only in CR2 group ($p < 0.05$).

Table 2. Fasting blood lipid, metabolic and insulin responses in rats of different levels of calorie restriction [†,*].

Group	mmol/L							
	Triglyceride	Total Cholesterol	HDL-C	LDL-C	Total Cholesterol/HDL-C	Glucose	Insulin (IU/mL)	HOMA-IR [#]
AL	1.55 ± 0.59	1.47 ± 0.40	0.69 ± 0.16	0.47 ± 0.39	2.14 ± 0.53	5.54 ± 0.98	23.92 ± 8.76	5.59 ± 0.41
CR1	1.19 ± 0.32 [a]	1.58 ± 0.39	0.82 ± 0.19 [a]	0.52 ± 0.47	1.95 ± 0.39	5.46 ± 0.67	16.02 ± 9.43	3.88 ± 0.63 [a]
CR2	0.92 ± 0.13 [a]	2.09 ± 0.71 [a]	0.92 ± 0.22 [a]	0.99 ± 0.61 [a]	2.25 ± 0.36	5.97 ± 0.98	10.53 ± 7.59 [a]	2.79 ± 0.58 [a,b]

[†] Abbreviations: AL: *ad libitum*; CR: calorie restriction; HDL-C: high density lipoprotein cholesterol; LDL-C: low density lipoprotein cholesterol; * Blood samples were collected at the end of the study; Data was presented as arithmetic mean $\pm$ 1 SD ($n = 12$ for each group); [#] HOMA-IR (Homeostasis Model Assessment of Insulin Resistance) = Fasting Blood Glucose (mmol/L) × Fasting Insulin (mIU/L)/22.5 [19]; [a] $p < 0.05$ *versus* AL group; [b] $p < 0.05$ *versus* CR1 group.

No significant difference was detected in blood glucose among all groups (Table 2). Insulin levels decreased by CR which was significant in CR2 compared to AL ($p < 0.05$). Insulin resistance, as presented as HOMA-IR, significantly decreased with increased levels of CR ($p < 0.05$).

All groups demonstrated a similar level of serum adiponectin at the beginning of the study (Figure 3). At the end of the study, serum adiponectin was only significantly increased in CR2 group but not in AL and CR1 groups.

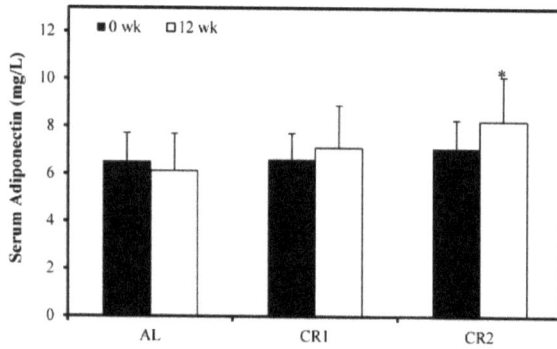

Figure 3. The effect of calorie restriction on serum adiponectin. Serum adiponectin showed no significant difference among all three groups at the beginning of the study. During the 12-week period, only CR2 group demonstrated a significant increase in serum adiponectin level as compared to the baseline. One-way ANOVA followed by LSD-test was used to detect significant differences of the means, * $p < 0.05$.

CR also led to a decrease in mass of visceral adipose tissue (Table 3). At the end of the 12-week study, wet weights of VAT and its percentage to the total body weight in CR groups were significantly lower than those in AL group ($p < 0.05$). As compared to CR1 group, further calorie restriction in CR2 group resulted in a significantly lower visceral fat mass ($p < 0.05$).

Table 3. Effect of calorie restriction on visceral adipose tissue [†].

Group	Visceral Fat Mass [g] [#,*]	Visceral Fat Mass [%] [*,Δ]
AL	16.47 ± 3.76	3.29 ± 0.48
CR1	12.08 ± 3.71 [a]	2.51 ± 0.68 [a]
CR2	6.72 ± 2.61 [a,b]	1.79 ± 0.69 [a,b]

[†] Abbreviations: AL: *ad libitum*; CR: calorie restriction; * Data was presented as arithmetic mean ± 1 S.D. $n = 12$ for each group; [#] Visceral Fat Mass [g] = total perirenal adipose tissue [g] + total peri-epididymal adipose tissue [g] [20]; [Δ] Visceral fat mass [%] = Visceral fat mass/Body weight × 100; [a] $p < 0.05$ *versus* AL group; [b] $p < 0.05$ *versus* CR1 group.

3.3. Gene Expression

Results obtained from RT-PCR indicated that the expression levels of adiponectin mRNA and PPARγ mRNA in CR groups were significantly higher than those in AL group (Figure 4). Within two CR groups, adiponectin and PPARγ mRNA levels in CR2 group were significantly higher than those in CR1 group (Figure 4(A2,B2)).

3.4. Correlation Analysis

Pearson correlation analysis was performed for mRNA levels of adiponectin, PPARγ with different serum parameters (Table 4). Results showed that no correlation was detected between adiponectin, PPARγ mRNA levels, total cholesterol ($p > 0.05$), and fasting glucose ($p > 0.05$). However, adiponectin, and PPARγ mRNA levels were positively associated with HDL-C ($p < 0.05$) and inversely correlated with body weight ($p < 0.05$), triglyceride ($p < 0.05$) and fasting insulin ($p < 0.05$).

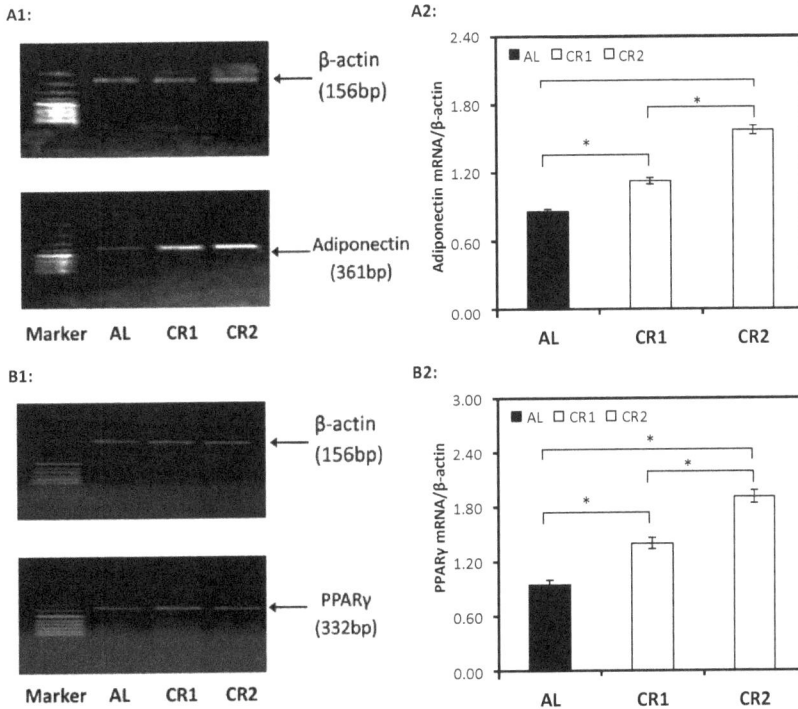

Figure 4. The effect of calorie restriction on the expressions of adiponectin and PPARγ in adipose tissues. (**A1, B1**) demonstrate the expression levels of mRNA of β-actin, adiponectin and PPARγ, respectively, quantified by RT-PCR. The expression levels (absorbance) of mRNA of adiponectin and PPARγ were then normalized against those of β-actin (served as loading control) (**A2, B2**). One-way ANOVA followed by LSD-test was used to detect significant differences of the means, * $p < 0.05$.

Table 4. Correlation analysis of adiponectin mRNA, PPARγ [†] mRNA with different serum parameters.

Independent Variables	Adiponectin		PPARγ	
	r	p	r	p
Body weight	−0.389	0.001	−0.425	0.005
Triglyceride	−0.345	0.042	−0.532	0.032
Total Cholesterol	0.47	0.624	0.673	0.431
HDL-C [†]	0.376	0.026	0.354	0.032
Glucose	0.530	0.231	0.492	0.485
Insulin	−0.411	0.003	−0.537	0.013

[†] Abbreviations: PPAR-γ: peroxisome proliferator activator receptor γ; HDL-C: High density lipoprotein cholesterol.

4. Discussion and Conclusions

MetS represents a cluster of conditions including glucose intolerance, hypertension, dyslipidemia, and insulin resistance. CR via carbohydrate reduction has elicited a great deal of interest among nutritionists because studies have shown that carbohydrate restriction can improve biological markers that define MetS. In the present study, we conducted a 12-week CR with different levels of carbohydrate reduction in healthy Wistar rats to investigate the changes in MetS-associated biomarkers as well as the expressions of insulin-sensitive adiponectin and its regulator PPARγ.

Body weight and peripheral adipose tissues (Table 3) in CR groups were significantly lower than the AL group and the change of these parameters were inversely associated with the degree of CR. VAT is associated with the development of insulin resistance, glucose intolerance, dyslipidemia and hypertension, whereas subcutaneous adipose tissue is not [21–24]. The study conducted by Gerbaix *et al.* has validated that removing perirenal and peri-epididymal adipose tissue in rats appears to be more representative of visceral fat mass as dissection of mesenteric and subcutaneous fat is challenging [20]. Hence, in the present study, visceral fat mass was evaluated as the total weight of perirenal and peri-epididymal adipose tissue (Table 3). Our result indicated that CR via carbohydrate reduction lowered visceral fat mass markedly, even when presented as visceral fat mass %, suggesting the potential beneficial effect of CR via carbohydrate reduction on fat distribution and insulin sensitivity in Wistar rats.

Consistent with the results obtained by previous studies involving carbohydrate restriction [25,26], a 68% carbohydrate reduction in CR2 group led to a significant decrease in serum triglyceride and significant increases in LDL-C, HDL-C and total cholesterol as compared to AL group. Our result suggested that in contrast to traditional carbohydrate restriction diets with a low percentage of carbohydrate or even ketogenic diets, our CR diet with 34% carbohydrate reduction was better at improving lipid profiles, as it not only resulted in an increase in HDL-C and a reduction in triglyceride, but also maintained LDL-C at the same level as those fed with control diets, thereby maintaining the total cholesterol at the same level. Decreases in plasma triglyceride by carbohydrate-restricted diet might be the result of downregulation of hepatic de novo lipogenesis [16,26,27]. In addition, carbohydrate restriction might increase muscle lipoprotein Lipase (LPL), thus enhance triglyceride clearance. Increased tissue expression and activity of LPL may partially explain increases in HDL-C in our experimental groups. Increased LPL-mediated catabolism of triglyceride-rich lipoproteins resulted in transfer of unesterified cholesterol, apoprotein and phospholipid to form mature HDL-C [16,26,27].

It is reported that long-term CR leads to an alteration of glucose homeostasis in humans [16] and rats [15,28,29], resulting in decreased glycemia and insulinemia. Nevertheless, our results demonstrated unchanged plasma glucose in CR groups as compared to the AL group. This finding may be owing to the relatively short experimental period (12-week) and the moderate CR in the present study. When the ingested carbohydrates fail to meet the energy needs of the body, the body starts to mobilize glucose from glycogen storage pools for energy supply, and continues to maintain blood glucose level via gluconeogenesis. The low glycogen storage stimulates insulin action in the body. In good agreement with previous studies [15,28,29], fasting insulin level in the present study demonstrated a decreasing trend with CR but only showed marked reduction in CR2 group. HOMA-IR also manifested a decreasing trend and significant reduction in HOMA-IR was observed in both CR1 and CR2 groups. Maintaining relatively low levels of fasting insulin and HOMA-IR is shown to be beneficial for the prevention and treatment of diabetes.

Adiponectin is considered to have antiatherogenic and antidiabetic effects [30]. In accordance with the findings obtained by Zhu *et al.* [31] and Sung *et al.* [14], our results suggest that though serum adiponectin level was only significantly elevated by 60% calorie-restricted diet, gene expression levels of adiponectin and PPARγ in adipose tissues were proportionally elevated with increased degree of energy restriction (Figures 3 and 4)-lower energy intakes led to higher expression levels. A high level of adiponectin predicts good insulin sensitivity and improves lipid and glucose metabolism [32,33]. Activation of PPARγ can induce the synthesis and secretion of adiponectin as a response element of PPARγ was discovered on the promoter of adiponectin gene [10]. CR might activate PPARγ and thus up-regulate the gene expression of adiponectin. Our result indicated that decreased insulin and HOMA-IR achieved by CR might be a result of increased adiponectin. Consistent with previous findings [7,34], our results demonstrated a significant inverse relationship of VAT adiponectin mRNA level and triglyceride and a significant positive relationship of adiponectin mRNA and HDL-C (Table 4). The present study additionally showed a significant association of PPARγ mRNA with triglyceride and HDL-C. Our correlation analysis suggested that elevated gene expression of adiponectin and PPARγ might lead to elevated level of HDL-C and reduced level of serum triglyceride.

Both low-carbohydrate CR diet [16,35] and low-fat, high-carbohydrate diet [36] have been proposed for the prevention of MetS. Despite the fact that a low-fat, high-carbohydrate diet has been advocated for controlling weight [37], a low-carbohydrate CR diet has gained in popularity. Although the low-fat, high carbohydrate diet was better at reducing total cholesterol and LDL-C [26], it is controversial [38], because it raises plasma triglycerides [39] and may adversely affect LDL composition [40,41]. The greater the amount of carbohydrates that are substituted for fat, the greater the increase in triglycerides [42]. Increasing evidence has pointed to the role of triglycerides in atherogenic risk [43]. Consumption of a low-carbohydrate CR diet, however, as shown in our present study and numerous previous studies, resulted in a reduction in triglycerides due to lack of substrates for triglyceride synthesis in liver. In addition, elevated levels of HDL-C were observed in subjects on low-carbohydrate CR diets [16,44], whereas HDL-C declined in subjects on low fat, high-carbohydrate diets [45]. The elevated HDL-C and reduced triglycerides in plasma are the advantages of a carbohydrate restricted diet over a high carbohydrate diet [24].

The long-term low-carbohydrate CR diet, however, is difficult for patients to comply with. Studies have shown the efficacy of a moderate-carbohydrate CR diet in weight management and improvement of serum lipid profiles [46]. In addition, a moderate-carbohydrate CR diet is more acceptable to people for the prevention and treatment of type 2 diabetes, as a strict carbohydrate restricted diet is not required [47,48]. In the present study, for the first time ever, we identified that a moderate-carbohydrate diet (34% carbohydrate reduction) is not only effective in raising gene expressions of adiponectin and PPARγ that potentially lead to better metabolic conditions but is also better in improving lipid profiles than a low-carbohydrate diet in rats. Our results suggest that a moderate-carbohydrate CR diet can be a new dietary intervention strategy for prevention and treatment of MetS.

There are certainly some limitations in this study. First, the investigation period (12 weeks) may be too short to predict long-term effects of CR on expression of adiponectin, PPARγ and serum parameters. Second, RT-PCR is a semiquantitative technique. Although our conclusions were based on the results of the adiponectin, PPARγ expression and other serum parameters, more quantitative techniques such as real-time PCR for mRNA or Western blotting for protein expression of adiponectin should be used in a future study. Finally, whether the conclusion drawn from rats in the present study can be extrapolated to other organisms, such as humans, remains to be determined.

Acknowledgments: This project was supported by grants from the National Natural Science Foundation of China (Grant No. 81273072, 2012; Grant No.30571561, 2006).

Author Contributions: Jie-Hua Chen and Limei Mao were involved in study design, data collection and analysis and have contributed to manuscript writing. Qiang Ding, Jia Song and Caiqun Ouyang carried out data collection and analysis. Wenhong Cao was involved in data analysis.

Conflicts of Interest: The authors declare no conflict of interest.

References

1. Verdery, R.B.; Walford, R.L. Changes in plasma lipids and lipoproteins in humans during a 2-year period of dietary restriction in biosphere 2. *Arch. Intern. Med.* **1998**, *158*, 900–906. [CrossRef] [PubMed]
2. Walford, R.L.; Mock, D.; Verdery, R.; MacCallum, T. Calorie restriction in biosphere 2: Alterations in physiologic, hematologic, hormonal, and biochemical parameters in humans restricted for a 2-year period. *J. Gerontol. A Biol. Sci. Med. Sci.* **2002**, *57*, B211–B224. [CrossRef] [PubMed]
3. Bordone, L.; Guarente, L. Calorie restriction, sirt1 and metabolism: Understanding longevity. *Nat. Rev. Mol. Cell Biol.* **2005**, *6*, 298–305. [CrossRef] [PubMed]
4. Takahashi, S.; Masuda, J.; Shimagami, H.; Ohta, Y.; Kanda, T.; Saito, K.; Kato, H. Mild caloric restriction up-regulates the expression of prohibitin: A proteome study. *Biochem. Biophys. Res. Commun.* **2011**, *405*, 462–467. [CrossRef] [PubMed]

5. Oana, F.; Takeda, H.; Matsuzawa, A.; Akahane, S.; Isaji, M.; Akahane, M. Adiponectin receptor 2 expression in liver and insulin resistance in db/db mice given a beta3-adrenoceptor agonist. *Eur. J. Pharmacol.* **2005**, *518*, 71–76. [CrossRef] [PubMed]

6. Bjorndal, B.; Burri, L.; Staalesen, V.; Skorve, J.; Berge, R.K. Different adipose depots: Their role in the development of metabolic syndrome and mitochondrial response to hypolipidemic agents. *J. Obes.* **2011**, *2011*, 490650. [CrossRef] [PubMed]

7. Sadashiv; Tiwari, S.; Paul, B.N.; Kumar, S.; Chandra, A.; Dhananjai, S.; Negi, M.P. Adiponectin mrna in adipose tissue and its association with metabolic risk factors in postmenopausal obese women. *Hormones (Athens)* **2013**, *12*, 119–127. [PubMed]

8. Combs, T.P.; Berg, A.H.; Rajala, M.W.; Klebanov, S.; Iyengar, P.; Jimenez-Chillaron, J.C.; Patti, M.E.; Klein, S.L.; Weinstein, R.S.; Scherer, P.E. Sexual differentiation, pregnancy, calorie restriction, and aging affect the adipocyte-specific secretory protein adiponectin. *Diabetes* **2003**, *52*, 268–276. [CrossRef] [PubMed]

9. Vaiopoulos, A.G.; Marinou, K.; Christodoulides, C.; Koutsilieris, M. The role of adiponectin in human vascular physiology. *Int. J. Cardiol.* **2012**, *155*, 188–193. [CrossRef] [PubMed]

10. Iwaki, M.; Matsuda, M.; Maeda, N.; Funahashi, T.; Matsuzawa, Y.; Makishima, M.; Shimomura, I. Induction of adiponectin, a fat-derived antidiabetic and antiatherogenic factor, by nuclear receptors. *Diabetes* **2003**, *52*, 1655–1663. [CrossRef] [PubMed]

11. Combs, T.P.; Wagner, J.A.; Berger, J.; Doebber, T.; Wang, W.J.; Zhang, B.B.; Tanen, M.; Berg, A.H.; O'Rahilly, S.; Savage, D.B.; *et al.* Induction of adipocyte complement-related protein of 30 kilodaltons by ppargamma agonists: A potential mechanism of insulin sensitization. *Endocrinology* **2002**, *143*, 998–1007. [PubMed]

12. Maeda, N.; Takahashi, M.; Funahashi, T.; Kihara, S.; Nishizawa, H.; Kishida, K.; Nagaretani, H.; Matsuda, M.; Komuro, R.; Ouchi, N.; *et al.* Ppargamma ligands increase expression and plasma concentrations of adiponectin, an adipose-derived protein. *Diabetes* **2001**, *50*, 2094–2099. [CrossRef] [PubMed]

13. Yang, W.S.; Jeng, C.Y.; Wu, T.J.; Tanaka, S.; Funahashi, T.; Matsuzawa, Y.; Wang, J.P.; Chen, C.L.; Tai, T.Y.; Chuang, L.M. Synthetic peroxisome proliferator-activated receptor-gamma agonist, rosiglitazone, increases plasma levels of adiponectin in type 2 diabetic patients. *Diabetes Care* **2002**, *25*, 376–380. [CrossRef] [PubMed]

14. Sung, B.; Park, S.; Yu, B.P.; Chung, H.Y. Modulation of ppar in aging, inflammation, and calorie restriction. *J. Gerontol. A Biol. Sci. Med. Sci.* **2004**, *59*, 997–1006. [CrossRef] [PubMed]

15. Zhu, M.; Miura, J.; Lu, L.X.; Bernier, M.; DeCabo, R.; Lane, M.A.; Roth, G.S.; Ingram, D.K. Circulating adiponectin levels increase in rats on caloric restriction: The potential for insulin sensitization. *Exp. Gerontol.* **2004**, *39*, 1049–1059. [CrossRef] [PubMed]

16. Volek, J.S.; Fernandez, M.L.; Feinman, R.D.; Phinney, S.D. Dietary carbohydrate restriction induces a unique metabolic state positively affecting atherogenic dyslipidemia, fatty acid partitioning, and metabolic syndrome. *Prog. Lipid Res.* **2008**, *47*, 307–318. [CrossRef] [PubMed]

17. Reeves, P.G.; Nielsen, F.H.; Fahey, G.C., Jr. AIN-93 purified diets for laboratory rodents: Final report of the american institute of nutrition ad hoc writing committee on the reformulation of the AIN-76A rodent diet. *J. Nutr.* **1993**, *123*, 1939–1951. [PubMed]

18. Tanno, K.; Okamura, T.; Ohsawa, M.; Onoda, T.; Itai, K.; Sakata, K.; Nakamura, M.; Ogawa, A.; Kawamura, K.; Okayama, A. Comparison of low-density lipoprotein cholesterol concentrations measured by a direct homogeneous assay and by the friedewald formula in a large community population. *Clin. Chim. Acta* **2010**, *411*, 1774–1780. [CrossRef] [PubMed]

19. Matthews, D.R.; Hosker, J.P.; Rudenski, A.S.; Naylor, B.A.; Treacher, D.F.; Turner, R.C. Homeostasis model assessment: Insulin resistance and beta-cell function from fasting plasma glucose and insulin concentrations in man. *Diabetologia* **1985**, *28*, 412–419. [CrossRef] [PubMed]

20. Gerbaix, M.; Metz, L.; Ringot, E.; Courteix, D. Visceral fat mass determination in rodent: Validation of dual-energy X-ray absorptiometry and anthropometric techniques in fat and lean rats. *Lipids Health Dis.* **2010**, *9*, 140. [CrossRef] [PubMed]

21. Fox, C.S.; Massaro, J.M.; Hoffmann, U.; Pou, K.M.; Maurovich-Horvat, P.; Liu, C.Y.; Vasan, R.S.; Murabito, J.M.; Meigs, J.B.; Cupples, L.A.; *et al.* Abdominal visceral and subcutaneous adipose tissue compartments: Association with metabolic risk factors in the framingham heart study. *Circulation* **2007**, *116*, 39–48. [CrossRef] [PubMed]

22. Freedland, E.S. Role of a critical visceral adipose tissue threshold (CVATT) in metabolic syndrome: Implications for controlling dietary carbohydrates: A review. *Nutr. Metab. (Lond.)* **2004**, *1*, 12. [CrossRef] [PubMed]

23. Wajchenberg, B.L. Subcutaneous and visceral adipose tissue: Their relation to the metabolic syndrome. *Endocr. Rev.* **2000**, *21*, 697–738. [CrossRef] [PubMed]

24. Sasakabe, T.; Haimoto, H.; Umegaki, H.; Wakai, K. Effects of a moderate low-carbohydrate diet on preferential abdominal fat loss and cardiovascular risk factors in patients with type 2 diabetes. *Diabetes Metab. Syndr. Obes.* **2011**, *4*, 167–174. [CrossRef] [PubMed]

25. Sharman, M.J.; Kraemer, W.J.; Love, D.M.; Avery, N.G.; Gomez, A.L.; Scheett, T.P.; Volek, J.S. A ketogenic diet favorably affects serum biomarkers for cardiovascular disease in normal-weight men. *J. Nutr.* **2002**, *132*, 1879–1885. [PubMed]

26. Volek, J.S.; Sharman, M.J.; Forsythe, C.E. Modification of lipoproteins by very low-carbohydrate diets. *J. Nutr.* **2005**, *135*, 1339–1342. [PubMed]

27. Volek, J.S.; Sharman, M.J.; Gomez, A.L.; Scheett, T.P.; Kraemer, W.J. An isoenergetic very low carbohydrate diet improves serum HDL cholesterol and triacylglycerol concentrations, the total cholesterol to HDL cholesterol ratio and postprandial pipemic responses compared with a low fat diet in normal weight, normolipidemic women. *J. Nutr.* **2003**, *133*, 2756–2761. [PubMed]

28. Masoro, E.J.; McCarter, R.J.; Katz, M.S.; McMahan, C.A. Dietary restriction alters characteristics of glucose fuel use. *J. Gerontol.* **1992**, *47*, B202–B208. [CrossRef] [PubMed]

29. Wetter, T.J.; Gazdag, A.C.; Dean, D.J.; Cartee, G.D. Effect of calorie restriction on *in vivo* glucose metabolism by individual tissues in rats. *Am. J. Physiol.* **1999**, *276*, E728–E738. [PubMed]

30. Yang, X.; Zhang, Y.; Lin, J.; Pen, A.; Ying, C.; Cao, W.; Mao, L. A lower proportion of dietary saturated/monounsaturated/polyunsaturated fatty acids reduces the expression of adiponectin in rats fed a high-fat diet. *Nutr. Res.* **2012**, *32*, 285–291. [CrossRef] [PubMed]

31. Zhu, M.; Lee, G.D.; Ding, L.; Hu, J.; Qiu, G.; de Cabo, R.; Bernier, M.; Ingram, D.K.; Zou, S. Adipogenic signaling in rat white adipose tissue: Modulation by aging and calorie restriction. *Exp. Gerontol.* **2007**, *42*, 733–744. [CrossRef] [PubMed]

32. Saltiel, A.R.; Kahn, C.R. Insulin signalling and the regulation of glucose and lipid metabolism. *Nature* **2001**, *414*, 799–806. [CrossRef] [PubMed]

33. Tschritter, O.; Fritsche, A.; Thamer, C.; Haap, M.; Shirkavand, F.; Rahe, S.; Staiger, H.; Maerker, E.; Haring, H.; Stumvoll, M. Plasma adiponectin concentrations predict insulin sensitivity of both glucose and lipid metabolism. *Diabetes* **2003**, *52*, 239–243. [CrossRef] [PubMed]

34. Yang, W.S.; Chen, M.H.; Lee, W.J.; Lee, K.C.; Chao, C.L.; Huang, K.C.; Chen, C.L.; Tai, T.Y.; Chuang, L.M. Adiponectin mRNA levels in the abdominal adipose depots of nondiabetic women. *Int. J. Obes. Relat. Metab. Disord.* **2003**, *27*, 896–900. [CrossRef] [PubMed]

35. Accurso, A.; Bernstein, R.K.; Dahlqvist, A.; Draznin, B.; Feinman, R.D.; Fine, E.J.; Gleed, A.; Jacobs, D.B.; Larson, G.; Lustig, R.H.; *et al.* Dietary carbohydrate restriction in type 2 diabetes mellitus and metabolic syndrome: Time for a critical appraisal. *Nutr. Metab. (Lond.)* **2008**, *5*, 9. [CrossRef] [PubMed]

36. Krauss, R.M.; Deckelbaum, R.J.; Ernst, N.; Fisher, E.; Howard, B.V.; Knopp, R.H.; Kotchen, T.; Lichtenstein, A.H.; McGill, H.C.; Pearson, T.A.; *et al.* Dietary guidelines for healthy american adults: A statement for health professionals from the nutrition committee, American heart association. *Circulation* **1996**, *94*, 1795–1800. [CrossRef] [PubMed]

37. Halton, T.L.; Willett, W.C.; Liu, S.; Manson, J.E.; Albert, C.M.; Rexrode, K.; Hu, F.B. Low-carbohydrate-diet score and the risk of coronary heart disease in women. *N. Engl. J. Med.* **2006**, *355*, 1991–2002. [CrossRef] [PubMed]

38. Schneeman, B.O. Carbohydrate: Friend or foe? Summary of research needs. *J. Nutr.* **2001**, *131*, 2764S–2765S. [PubMed]

39. Parks, E.J.; Hellerstein, M.K. Carbohydrate-induced hypertriacylglycerolemia: Historical perspective and review of biological mechanisms. *Am. J. Clin. Nutr.* **2000**, *71*, 412–433. [PubMed]

40. Dreon, D.M.; Fernstrom, H.A.; Miller, B.; Krauss, R.M. Low-density lipoprotein subclass patterns and lipoprotein response to a reduced-fat diet in men. *FASEB J.* **1994**, *8*, 121–126. [PubMed]

41.	Dreon, D.M.; Fernstrom, H.A.; Williams, P.T.; Krauss, R.M. A very low-fat diet is not associated with improved lipoprotein profiles in men with a predominance of large, low-density lipoproteins. *Am. J. Clin. Nutr.* **1999**, *69*, 411–418. [PubMed]

42.	Retzlaff, B.M.; Walden, C.E.; Dowdy, A.A.; McCann, B.S.; Anderson, K.V.; Knopp, R.H. Changes in plasma triacylglycerol concentrations among free-living hyperlipidemic men adopting different carbohydrate intakes over 2 y: The dietary alternatives study. *Am. J. Clin. Nutr.* **1995**, *62*, 988–995. [PubMed]

43.	Yuan, G.; Al-Shali, K.Z.; Hegele, R.A. Hypertriglyceridemia: Its etiology, effects and treatment. *CMAJ* **2007**, *176*, 1113–1120. [CrossRef] [PubMed]

44.	Fontana, L.; Meyer, T.E.; Klein, S.; Holloszy, J.O. Long-term calorie restriction is highly effective in reducing the risk for atherosclerosis in humans. *Proc. Natl. Acad. Sci. USA* **2004**, *101*, 6659–6663. [CrossRef] [PubMed]

45.	Turley, M.L.; Skeaff, C.M.; Mann, J.I.; Cox, B. The effect of a low-fat, high-carbohydrate diet on serum high density lipoprotein cholesterol and triglyceride. *Eur. J. Clin. Nutr.* **1998**, *52*, 728–732. [CrossRef] [PubMed]

46.	Johnston, C.S.; Tjonn, S.L.; Swan, P.D.; White, A.; Hutchins, H.; Sears, B. Ketogenic low-carbohydrate diets have no metabolic advantage over nonketogenic low-carbohydrate diets. *Am. J. Clin. Nutr.* **2006**, *83*, 1055–1061. [PubMed]

47.	Daly, M.E.; Paisey, R.; Paisey, R.; Millward, B.A.; Eccles, C.; Williams, K.; Hammersley, S.; MacLeod, K.M.; Gale, T.J. Short-term effects of severe dietary carbohydrate-restriction advice in type 2 diabetes—A randomized controlled trial. *Diabet. Med.* **2006**, *23*, 15–20. [CrossRef] [PubMed]

48.	Haimoto, H.; Iwata, M.; Wakai, K.; Umegaki, H. Long-term effects of a diet loosely restricting carbohydrates on HbA1c levels, BMI and tapering of sulfonylureas in type 2 diabetes: A 2-year follow-up study. *Diabetes Res. Clin. Pract.* **2008**, *79*, 350–356. [CrossRef] [PubMed]

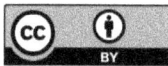

nutrients

MDPI

Article

High Fat Diet Exposure during Fetal Life Enhances Plasma and Hepatic Omega-6 Fatty Acid Profiles in Fetal Wistar Rats

Marlon E. Cerf [1],*, Johan Louw [1] and Emilio Herrera [2]

[1] Diabetes Discovery Platform, South African Medical Research Council, P.O. Box 19070, Tygerberg,
    Cape Town 7505, South Africa; johan.louw@mrc.ac.za
[2] Department of Chemistry and Biochemistry, University of San Pablo-CEU, Ctra. Boadilla del Monte km 5.3,
    Madrid 28668, Spain; eherrera@ceu.es
* Correspondence: marlon.cerf@mrc.ac.za; Tel.: +27-21-938-0818; Fax: +27-21-938-0456.

Received: 24 March 2015; Accepted: 30 June 2015; Published: 28 August 2015

Abstract: Pregnant rats were fed a high fat diet (HFD) for the first (HF1), second (HF2), third (HF3) or all three weeks (HFG) of gestation. Maintenance on a HFD during specific periods of gestation was hypothesized to alter fetal glycemia, insulinemia, induce insulin resistance; and alter fetal plasma and hepatic fatty acid (FA) profiles. At day 20 of gestation, fetal plasma and hepatic FA profiles were determined by gas chromatography; body weight, fasting glycemia, insulinemia and the Homeostasis Model Assessment (HOMA-insulin resistance) were also determined. HF3 fetuses were heaviest concomitant with elevated glycemia and insulin resistance ($p < 0.05$). HFG fetuses had elevated plasma linoleic (18:2 n-6) and arachidonic (20:4 n-6) acid proportions ($p < 0.05$). In the liver, HF3 fetuses displayed elevated linoleic, eicosatrienoic (20:3 n-6) and arachidonic acid proportions ($p < 0.05$). HFG fetuses had reduced hepatic docosatrienoic acid (22:5 n-3) proportions ($p < 0.05$). High fat maintenance during the final week of fetal life enhances hepatic omega-6 FA profiles in fetuses concomitant with hyperglycemia and insulin resistance thereby presenting a metabolically compromised phenotype.

Keywords: fatty acid analysis; fetal programming; metabolic disease

---

1. Introduction

Fetal metabolism, and consequently fetal growth, directly depends on the nutrients crossing the placenta, and therefore the mother adapts her metabolism to support this continuous draining of substrates [1].

Fatty acids (FAs) are important for fetal growth and development. Specifically, linoleic acid (18:2 n-6) and α-linolenic acid (ALA, 18:3 n-3) are the essential fatty acids (EFAs), which together with their long-chain polyunsaturated FA (LCPUFA) derivatives are essential for fetal and postnatal development. The fetus obtains both EFAs and LCPUFAs from maternal circulation by transfer across the placenta [2,3].

High intakes of n-3 FAs solely during early pregnancy in rats have beneficial long-term consequences in their offspring, reducing the age-related decline in insulin sensitivity in male offspring [4].

A high fat diet (HFD) was shown to contribute to the development of obesity, insulin resistance, type 2 diabetes and the impairment of the glucose signaling system in the beta cells [5–8]; in neonates, these effects were dependent on the period of fetal life when the HFD was administered [5]. In the present study, we investigated, in fetal rats, how exposure to a HFD during specific weeks of fetal life influences plasma and hepatic FA profiles, glycemia, insulinemia and insulin resistance.

2. Experimental Section

Institutional ethical approval was obtained before the experiments commenced. Wistar rats were maintained as previously described [5]. Briefly, pregnant mothers were fed a HFD during specific periods of gestation. The experimental groups are displayed in Figure 1. Although the HFD was administered to the mothers, their fetal offspring were subsequently maintained on the respective gestational diets. In the present study, 20-day-old fetuses maintained on a HFD for the first (HF1), second (HF2), third (HF3) or all three (HFG) weeks of fetal life were studied. Specifically, HF1 fetuses were maintained on a HFD from embryonic day (e) 0–7, HF2 fetuses from e8–14, HF3 fetuses from e15–20 and HFG fetuses from e0–20. When HF1, HF2 and HF3 fetuses were not maintained on a HFD, they were instead maintained on a standard laboratory diet for the remainder of fetal life, e.g., HF1 fetuses were maintained on a HFD for the first week of fetal life and a control diet for weeks 2 and 3 of fetal life (Figure 1). Fetuses maintained on a standard laboratory diet throughout represented the control group. The standard laboratory diet (control) (Epol, South Africa) comprised 10% fat, 15% protein and 75% carbohydrate (2.6 kcal/g). The HFD contained 40% fat, 14% protein and 46% carbohydrate (2.06 kcal/g). The HFD predominantly comprised saturated FAs (myristic, palmitic and stearic acid) and the mono-unsaturated FA, oleic acid, derived from animal fat with carbohydrates mainly derived from starch to mimic a westernized diet. The control diet was a standard commercial rodent laboratory diet.

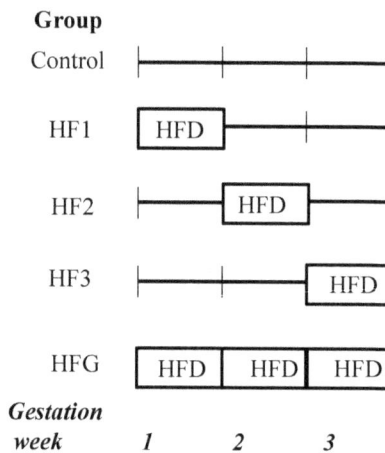

Figure 1. Experimental groups. The fetuses were maintained (through their mothers' nutrition) on a high fat diet (HFD) for either the first week (HF1), second week (HF2), third week (HF3) or all 3 weeks (HFG) of fetal life.

Mothers were maintained on a HFD for specific periods of gestation and their 20-day-old fetal offspring were studied. Therefore fetuses were maintained (through their mothers' nutrition) on HFD for either the first (HF1), second (HF2), third (HF3) or all 3 weeks (HFG) of fetal life. Control fetuses were maintained on a standard commercial rodent laboratory diet.

At day 20 of pregnancy, mothers were euthanized after a 3 h fast. After removal from the uterus, fetuses were weighed and decapitated and the trunk blood was used for FA analysis. Whole liver was collected, weighed and stored at −80 °C until analysis. Blood was collected on ice-chilled tubes containing 1 g/L of Na$_2$-EDTA and pooled per litter from each mother. The pooled fetal blood was centrifuged and plasma aliquots were stored at −20 °C until analysis.

Blood glucose (glucometer, Precision QID, MediSense, Oxfordshire, UK) and serum insulin (rat insulin radio-immunoassay (RIA) kit, Linco Research, St. Charles, MO, USA) concentrations were measured. The Homeostasis Model Assessment (HOMA-insulin resistance) was calculated (fasting plasma glucose (mmol/L) × fasting serum insulin (mU/L)/22.5)).

For FA analysis, nonadecenoic acid (19:1; Sigma-Aldrich, Madrid, Spain) was added as the internal standard to fresh aliquots of frozen plasma and liver which were used for lipid extraction and purification [9]. The final lipid extract was evaporated under vacuum and the residue suspended in methanol/toluene followed by methanolysis in the presence of acetyl chloride at $-80°C$ for 2.5 h as previously described [10]. FA methyl esters were separated and quantified on a gas chromatograph (Autosystem, Perkin-Elmer, Madrid, Spain) with a flame ionization detector and a 20 m Omegawax capillary column (internal diameter 0.25 mm). Nitrogen was used as carrier gas and the FA methyl esters were compared to purified standards (Sigma-Aldrich). Quantification of the FAs in the samples was performed as a function of the corresponding peak areas and compared to the internal standard.

One-way analysis of variance (ANOVA) and Bonferroni's post-test were applied with data reported as means ± standard error of the means (SEM) and significance established at $p < 0.05$.

3. Results

3.1. Anthropometry

As shown in Table 1, the HF3 fetuses had higher body weights relative to the other fetuses. HF2 fetuses had lower liver weights compared to the control, HF3 and HFG fetuses; after adjustment for body weight, lower HF2 fetal liver weights persisted relative to all the groups (Table 1).

Table 1. Fetal anthropometry and metabolic parameters of 20-day-old rat fetuses.

	Control	HF1	HF2	HF3	HFG
Weight (g)	3.19 ± 0.06	3.23 ± 0.07	3.22 ± 0.05	3.79 ± 0.11 *,†,‡,∧	3.20 ± 0.07
Liver weight (mg)	246.7 ± 12.69	196.0 ± 11.47	144.0 ± 16.85 *,§,∧	253.7 ± 20.03	218.7 ± 10.81
Adjusted liver weight (mg/100 g)	7.26 ± 0.24	6.23 ± 0.38	4.31 ± 0.50 *,†,§,∧	6.67 ± 0.43	6.95 ± 0.25
Blood glucose (mmol/L)	2.54 ± 0.12	3.16 ± 0.16	2.97 ± 0.23	4.99 ± 0.56 *,†,‡,∧	3.06 ± 0.20
Serum insulin (pM)	48.24 ± 13.57	66.59 ± 11.50	62.68 ± 13.33	86.10 ± 22.96	75.72 ± 16.54
HOMA-insulin resistance	1.09 ± 0.26	1.84 ± 0.30	1.68 ± 0.42	3.59 ± 0.13*	2.42 ± 0.92

The fetuses were maintained (through their mothers' nutrition) on a high fat diet (HFD) for either the first week (HF1), second week (HF2), third week (HF3) or all 3 weeks (HFG) of fetal life. Values are means ± standard error of the means (SEM). $n = 31$–59 per group, but $n = 3$–6 for serum insulin and Homeostasis Model Assessment (HOMA)-insulin resistance (due to pooling). Bonferroni's test was used to determine differences between groups after ANOVA. HF = high fat. Numerals refer to the week of maintenance on a high fat diet. * $p < 0.05$ vs. control, † $p < 0.05$ vs. HF1, ‡ $p < 0.05$ vs. HF2, § $p < 0.05$ vs. HF3, ∧ $p < 0.05$ vs. HFG.

3.2. Metabolic Parameters

The HF3 fetuses had higher glucose concentrations relative to the other fetuses (Table 1). However, insulin concentrations did not differ amongst the groups (Table 1). Further, the HF3 fetuses were also insulin resistant evident by their higher HOMA-insulin resistance values compared to the control fetuses (Table 1).

3.3. Plasma and Hepatic FA Profiles

Changes in the FA profile in the maternal diet may affect the availability of certain FAs in fetal plasma. HFG fetuses had enhanced plasma omega-6 FA profiles. Specifically, plasma linoleic acid was higher in HFG fetuses relative to control, HF1 and HF2 fetuses (Table 2). Further, plasma dihomo-gamma-linolenic acid (DGLA; 20:3 *n*-6) was higher in HFG fetuses compared to HF1 fetuses.

In addition, plasma arachidonic acid (20:4 n-6) was higher in HFG fetuses compared to control and HF1 fetuses (Table 2).

Table 2. Plasma fatty acid profiles (%) of 20-day-old rat fetuses maintained on a high fat diet.

Fatty Acid	Control	HF1	HF2	HFG
Saturated				
14:0	1.59 ± 0.17	2.47 ± 0.40	1.86 ± 0.17	2.20 ± 0.17
16:0	27.47 ± 0.57	32.34 ± 3.59	31.77 ± 0.99	25.90 ± 0.54
18:0	11.43 ± 0.60	12.49 ± 0.58	11.83 ± 0.49	11.20 ± 0.60
22:0	0.84 ± 0.09	0.81 ± 0.19	0.82 ± 0.05	0.75 ± 0.11
24:0	0.84 ± 0.14	0.72 ± 0.01	0.65 ± 0.09	0.71 ± 0.18
Monounsaturated				
14:1	0.62 ± 0.28	0.71 ± 0.08	1.29 ± 0.30	0.96 ± 0.22
16:1 (n-7)	5.42 ± 0.52	5.00 ± 0.52	5.61 ± 0.41	5.27 ± 0.42
18:1 (n-9)	25.55 ± 1.23	25.23 ± 0.39	23.65 ± 0.49	26.15 ± 0.90
Omega-3				
20:5 (n-3)	1.34 ± 0.45	2.03 ± 1.39	1.08 ± 0.37	1.05 ± 0.63
22:5 (n-3)	0.58 ± 0.27	-	0.13 ± 0.05	0.69 ± 0.35
22:6 (n-3)	8.99 ± 0.68	5.44 ± 1.15	7.19 ± 1.10	5.57 ± 0.98
Omega-6				
18:2 (n-6)	8.10 ± 0.35	6.54 ± 0.47	7.23 ± 0.42	9.87 ± 0.29 [*,†,‡]
18:3 (n-6)	0.38 ± 0.03	0.32 ± 0.04	0.41 ± 0.03	0.48 ± 0.04
20:3 (n-6)	0.45 ± 0.10	0.38 ± 0.12	0.50 ± 0.04	0.76 ± 0.03 [†]
20:4 (n-6)	5.84 ± 0.39	5.05 ± 0.94	5.97 ± 0.62	8.41 ± 0.32 [*,†]

The fetuses were maintained (through their mothers' nutrition) on a high fat diet (HFD) for either the first (HF1), second (HF2), third (HF3) or all 3 weeks (HFG) of fetal life. Values are means ± standard error of the means (SEM). n = 3–4 per group. n = 2 for HF3 which was excluded from analyses. Bonferroni's test was used to determine differences between groups after one-way analysis of variance (ANOVA). HF = high fat; Numerals refer to the week of maintenance on a high fat diet. * $p < 0.05$ *vs.* control, † $p < 0.05$ *vs.* HF1, ‡ $p < 0.05$ *vs.* HF2 − n = 2 for HF1.

As shown in Table 3, the proportion of different FAs in fetal liver remained relatively constant. However, specific omega-6 FAs were elevated in HF3 fetuses: linoleic (compared to control and HF2 fetuses), eicosatrienoic (compared to HF1 fetuses) and arachidonic acid (compared to control fetuses; Table 3). Further, hepatic docosapentaenoic acid (DPA; 22:5 n-3) was lower in HFG fetuses compared to control and HF3 fetuses (Table 3).

Table 3. Hepatic fatty acid profiles (%) of 20-day-old rat fetuses exposed to a maternal high fat diet.

Fatty Acid	Control	HF1	HF2	HF3	HFG
Saturated					
14:0	1.03 ± 0.20	0.93 ± 0.09	1.00 ± 0.07	1.39 ± 0.16	1.22 ± 0.15
16:0	24.46 ± 0.92	23.15 ± 0.43	23.62 ± 0.59	24.20 ± 0.90	23.75 ± 0.50
18:0	15.40 ± 0.40	15.57 ± 0.37	14.85 ± 0.17	15.20 ± 0.43	14.55 ± 0.21
20:0	0.31 ± 0.05	0.30 ± 0.04	0.26 ± 0.01	0.28 ± 0.02	0.32 ± 0.04
Monounsaturated					
15:1	0.49 ± 0.05	0.33 ± 0.09	0.34 ± 0.07	0.36 ± 0.06	0.36 ± 0.06
16:1 (*n*-7)	4.20 ± 0.37	3.82 ± 0.31	3.93 ± 0.13	3.43 ± 0.23	4.03 ± 0.11
18:1 (*n*-9)	21.01 ± 0.70	20.09 ± 0.77	21.35 ± 0.79	19.03 ± 1.31	22.44 ± 0.67
20:1 (*n*-9)	0.21 ± 0.07	0.24 ± 0.03	0.24 ± 0.01	0.23 ± 0.03	0.23 ± 0.03
Omega-3					
20:5 (*n*-3)	0.83 ± 0.10	0.70 ± 0.08	0.57 ± 0.03	0.65 ± 0.09	0.69 ± 0.10
22:5 (*n*-3)	0.40 ± 0.03	0.37 ± 0.06	0.34 ± 0.03	0.41 ± 0.04	0.24 ± 0.01 *,§
22:6 (*n*-3)	12.64 ± 0.91	13.00 ± 0.96	12.01 ± 0.56	9.99 ± 1.21	8.81 ± 0.51
Omega-6					
18:2 (*n*-6)	7.24 ± 0.30	7.86 ± 0.53	8.06 ± 0.25	10.16 ± 0.79 *,‡	8.79 ± 0.30
20:2 (*n*-6)	0.22 ± 0.03	0.25 ± 0.05	0.24 ± 0.02	0.25 ± 0.01	0.23 ± 0.02
20:3 (*n*-6)	0.83 ± 0.03	0.79 ± 0.03	0.87 ± 0.06	1.03 ± 0.03 †	0.99 ± 0.05
20:4 (*n*-6)	8.68 ± 0.33	10.53 ± 0.46	10.21 ± 0.26	10.95 ± 0.52*	10.65 ± 0.72
22:4 (*n*-6)	0.40 ± 0.01	0.43 ± 0.01	0.47 ± 0.02	0.50 ± 0.05	0.48 ± 0.04

The fetuses were maintained (through their mothers' nutrition) on a high fat diet (HFD) for either the first week (HF1), second week (HF2), third week (HF3) or all 3 weeks (HFG) of fetal life. Values are means ± standard error of the means (SEM). n = 3–5 per group. Bonferroni's test was used to determine differences between groups after one-way analysis of variance (ANOVA). HF = high fat. Numerals refer to the week of maintenance on a high fat diet. * $p < 0.05$ *vs.* control, † $p < 0.05$ *vs.* HF1, ‡ $p < 0.05$ *vs.* HF2, § $p < 0.05$ *vs.* HF3.

4. Discussion

The hyperglycemia and insulin resistance in fetuses maintained on a HFD for the final week of fetal life concomitant with increased hepatic omega-6 FA proportions were the main findings. During the final week of fetal life the endocrine pancreas differentiates into functional islet cells specialized for the maintenance of glucose homeostasis. Fetal programming refers to intrauterine stimuli or insults (such as the insult of maintenance on a HFD) that have immediate, transient or durable effects. With the fetal high fat programming insult during this critical developmental window, viz., late fetal life, islet cell, and specifically beta cell, development coincides with the HFD insult. We have previously shown that neonates maintained on a HFD throughout fetal life had compromised beta cell development and function [5,11]. Fetal high fat programming may therefore contribute to the hyperglycemia and insulin resistance in fetuses maintained on a HFD for the final week of fetal life.

In Westernized society, diets contain omega-6 to omega-3 ratios that far exceed the recommended ratio of 1:1; this increased ratio is believed to contribute to the global increase in metabolic disease.

In rodents, from e15 up to birth and into postnatal life, the maturation and growth of the liver occurs [12,13] with liver expansion of 84-fold, from e13.5–20.5, evident by the hepatoblasts undergoing 8-doublings [14–16]. Hence this critical hepatic developmental period of rapid and significant expansion overlaps with the administration of the HFD to HF3 neonates (exposed to a HFD from e15–20). With an increase of the precursor, linoleic acid, in the HF3 fetal livers, more substrate was available for conversion into arachidonic acid to help meet the fetal growth demands. FA elongation and desaturation are two key metabolic routes for the synthesis of saturated, monounsaturated and polyunsaturated FAs [17]. The elevated hepatic eicosatrienoic acid provided further evidence of lipogenesis along the omega-6 pathway. This also suggested activation of delta-6 desaturase, elongase and delta-5 desaturase to facilitate fetal hepatic lipogenesis. However, this requires the application of assays to assess enzymatic activities followed by Western blot analyses. However, enzyme activity and expression should be studied in older progeny due to low elongase and desaturase expression in the fetal liver [18]. The increase in hepatic omega-6 FA in fetuses maintained on a HFD for the final week of fetal life appears to contribute to their compromised metabolic phenotype. The exact role of the elevated hepatic omega-6 FAs in inducing these metabolically compromised fetuses remains to be elucidated.

DPA (22:5 *n*-3) is an elongation metabolite of eicosapentaenoic acid (EPA; 20:5 *n*-3) and an underexplored omega-3 FA. Supplementation of liver cells with DPA down-regulated the expression levels of key genes and proteins involved in FA synthesis [19]. The reduced DPA *n*-3 proportions in the livers of fetuses maintained on a HFD throughout fetal life may therefore result in higher expression profiles of FA synthesis factors.

The elevated omega-6 plasma FAs in HFG fetuses to some extent mimicked the hepatic FA profiles of HF3 fetuses. The EFAs, linoleic and alpha-linoleic acid are supplied by the diet, and their LCPUFA derivatives, play a critical role in fetal development [1]. Linoleic acid's metabolite, arachidonic acid, is essential for neonatal growth and development [20] which suggests that postnatal growth in these HF3 fetuses may be accelerated. Both fetuses and neonates are dependent upon the supply of preformed LCPUFAs from their mothers, which is obtained from maternal circulation [21]. An enhancement in arachidonic acid and docosahexaenoic acid (DHA; 22:6 *n*-3) in fetal circulation is called magnification and infers their effective transfer throughout the placenta [22]. The ratio of the proportions of arachidonic acid to linoleic acid is higher in fetal serum than in maternal serum [23], which suggests the preferential transfer of arachidonic acid through the placenta [24]. In all of the groups, the ratios of arachidonic acid to linoleic acid were elevated in the fetal plasma relative to the maternal plasma (data not shown) reflecting the preferential transfer of arachidonic acid through the placenta [24]. Despite the pooling of fetal litter plasma samples to yield sufficient volumes for analyses, the plasma sample number was too low for HF3 fetuses. Hence no HF3 fetal plasma FA profiles were determined which was a constraint. In summary, fetuses maintained on a HFD throughout fetal life had elevated plasma linoleic and arachidonic acid proportions concomitant with elevated plasma arachidonic acid to linoleic acid ratios in fetuses relative to mothers which suggested preferential placental transfer of arachidonic acid to sustain fetal and postnatal growth.

DGLA (20:3 *n*-6) is metabolized to the anti-inflammatory eicosanoid, prostaglandin (PG) E1, via the cyclooxygenase (COX) pathway [25] and was recently reported to be positively correlated to increased type 2 diabetes risk [26]. Although plasma DGLA proportions were increased in HFG fetuses relative to HF1 fetuses, the increase in this rare FA may not have any biological relevance [26].

Liver mass and its later function are essentially set during fetal development which is regulated by the intrauterine environment [27]. Disease risk is amplified by a greater mismatch between the prenatally predicted and actual adult environments [28]. Epidemiological data imply that hepatic organogenesis is susceptible to nutritional reprogramming and that impaired liver development in utero can result in durable functional consequences on disease risk later in life [27]. From e8–14 hepatic fate is specified, followed by gut tube formation, the liver domain relocating to the mid-gut followed by the liver diverticulum expanding into a liver bud [12,13]. These major liver development processes coincide with the HF2 neonates who had low liver weights. Hence the HFD administration during mid fetal life, i.e., e8–14, appeared to stunt liver development. The reduced liver weights in fetuses maintained on a HFD for the second week of fetal life may render them susceptible to metabolic disease.

Although we found altered fetal plasma and hepatic FA profiles in some offspring, our study has several limitations. Varying FA abundance can affect processes such as inflammation, angiogenesis and insulin sensitivity [29]. Early life hepatic fat accumulation is an early manifestation of non-alcoholic fatty liver disease (NAFLD) and an independent pathophysiological event that potentiates postnatal metabolic liver disease [30]. Therefore hepatic inflammation, steatosis and disrupted insulin signaling potentially contribute to the metabolically compromised phenotype that presented in the HF3 fetuses. Unfortunately FA analyses were conducted on all the frozen fetal liver samples, with no additional

Nutrients **2015**, *7*, 7231–7241

samples available for further investigation to reinforce our findings. Moreover, stratifying the study according to gender would likely have revealed gender-specific differences. The role of the elevated plasma and hepatic omega-6 FAs also remains to be fully elucidated.

5. Conclusions

Fetuses maintained on a HFD solely for the final week of fetal life were hyperglycemic and insulin resistant concomitant with enhanced hepatic omega-6 FA proportions, viz., linoleic, eicosatrienoic and arachidonic acid. These events may reflect enhanced omega-6 lipogenesis in response to the compromised metabolic phenotype.

Acknowledgments: The authors extend their gratitude to Milagros Morante and Christo Muller for their expert technical assistance and the National Research Foundation of South Africa and Fundación Ramón Areces of Spain (CIVP16A1835) for funding.

Author Contributions: Marlon E. Cerf participated in the design of the study, performed statistical analysis and drafted the paper. Johan Louw participated in the design of the study. Emilio Herrera made substantial contributions to conception and design, interpretation of data and final approval of the paper prior to submission.

Conflicts of Interest: The authors declare no conflict of interest.

References

1. Herrera, E. Implications of dietary fatty acids during pregnancy on placental, fetal and postnatal development—A review. *Placenta* **2002**, *23*, S9–S19. [CrossRef] [PubMed]
2. Haggarty, P. Fatty acid supply to the human fetus. *Annu. Rev. Nutr.* **2010**, *30*, 237–255. [CrossRef] [PubMed]
3. Herrera, E.; Lasunción, M.A. Maternal-fetal transfer of lipid metabolites. In *Fetal and Neonatal Physiology*; Polin, R.A., Fox, W.W., Eds.; Elsevier Saunders: Philadelphia, PA, USA, 2011; pp. 441–454.
4. Sardinha, F.L.; Fernandes, F.S.; Tavares do Carmo, M.G.; Herrera, E. Sex-dependent nutritional programming: Fish oil intake during early pregnancy in rats reduces age-dependent insulin resistance in male, but not female, offspring. *Am. J. Physiol. Regul. Integr. Comp. Physiol.* **2013**, *304*, R313–R320. [CrossRef] [PubMed]
5. Cerf, M.E.; Williams, K.; Nkomo, X.I.; Muller, C.J.; Du Toit, D.F.; Louw, J.; Wolfe-Coote, S.A. Islet cell response in the neonatal rat after exposure to a high-fat diet during pregnancy. *Am. J. Physiol. Regul. Integr. Comp. Physiol.* **2005**, *288*, R1122–R1128. [CrossRef] [PubMed]
6. Kim, C.H.; Youn, J.H.; Park, J.Y.; Hong, S.K.; Park, K.S.; Park, S.W.; Suh, K.I.; Lee, K.U. Effects of high-fat diet and exercise training on intracellular glucose metabolism in rats. *Am. J. Physiol. Endocrinol. Metab.* **2000**, *278*, E977–E984. [PubMed]
7. Kim, Y.; Tamura, T.; Iwashita, S.; Tokuyama, K.; Suzuki, M. Effect of high-fat diet on gene expression of GLUT4 and insulin receptor in soleus muscle. *Biochem. Biophys. Res. Commun.* **1994**, *202*, 519–526. [CrossRef] [PubMed]
8. West, D.B.; York, B. Dietary fat, genetic predisposition, and obesity: Lessons from animal models. *Am. J. Clin. Nutr.* **1998**, *67*, 505S–512S. [PubMed]
9. Folch, J.; Lees, M.; Sloane Stanley, G.H. A simple method for the isolation and purification of total lipids from animal tissues. *J. Biol. Chem.* **1957**, *226*, 497–509. [PubMed]
10. Amusquivar, E.; Schiffner, S.; Herrera, E. Evaluation of two methods for plasma fatty acid analysis by GC. *Eur. J. Lipid Sci. Technol.* **2011**, *113*, 711–716. [CrossRef]
11. Cerf, M.E.; Chapman, C.S.; Muller, C.J.; Louw, J. Gestational high-fat programming impairs insulin release and reduces Pdx-1 and glucokinase immunoreactivity in neonatal Wistar rats. *Metabolism* **2009**, *58*, 1787–1792. [CrossRef] [PubMed]
12. Zhao, R.; Duncan, S.A. Embryonic development of the liver. *Hepatology* **2005**, *41*, 956–967. [CrossRef] [PubMed]
13. Zorn, A.M. Liver development. In *StemBook*; The Stem Cell Research Community: Cambridge, MA, USA, 2008.
14. Greengard, O.; Federman, M.; Knox, W.E. Cytomorphometry of developing rat liver and its application to enzymic differentiation. *J. Cell. Biol.* **1972**, *52*, 261–272. [CrossRef] [PubMed]

15. Grisham, J.W.; Thorgeirsson, S.S. Liver stem cells. In *Stem Cells*; Potten, C.S., Ed.; Academic Press: New York, NY, USA, 1997; pp. 233–282.

16. Vassy, J.; Kraemer, M.; Chalumeau, M.T.; Foucrier, J. Development of the fetal rat liver: Ultrastructural and stereological study of hepatocytes. *Cell Differ.* **1988**, *24*, 9–24. [CrossRef]

17. Wang, Y.; Botolin, D.; Xu, J.; Jump, D.B. Regulation of hepatic fatty acid elongase and desaturase expression in diabetes and obesity. *J. Lipid Res.* **2006**, *47*, 2028–2041. [CrossRef] [PubMed]

18. Wang, Y.; Botolin, D.; Christian, B.; Jump, D.B. Tissue-specific, nutritional, and developmental regulation of rat fatty acid elongases. *J. Lipid Res.* **2005**, *46*, 706–715. [CrossRef] [PubMed]

19. Kaur, G.; Sinclair, A.J.; Cameron-Smith, D.; Barr, D.P.; Molero-Navajasa, J.C.; Konstantopoulosa, N. Docosapentaenoic acid (22:5 *n*-3) down-regulates the expression of genes involved in fat synthesis in liver cells. *Prostaglandins Leukot. Essent. Fatty Acids* **2011**, *85*, 155–161. [CrossRef] [PubMed]

20. Innis, S.M.; Sprecher, H.; Hachey, D.; Edmond, J.; Anderson, R.E. Neonatal polyunsaturated fatty acid metabolism. *Lipids* **1999**, *34*, 139–149. [CrossRef] [PubMed]

21. Fernandes, F.S.; Sardinha, F.L.; Badia-Villanueva, M.; Carulla, P.; Herrera, E.; Do Carmo, M.G.T. Dietary lipids during early pregnancy differently influence adipose tissue metabolism and fatty acid composition in pregnant rats with repercussions on pup's development. *Prostaglandins Leukot. Essent. Fatty Acids* **2012**, *86*, 167–174. [CrossRef] [PubMed]

22. Haggarty, P. Placental regulation of fatty acid delivery and its effect on fetal growth—A review. *Placenta* **2002**, *23*, S28–S38. [CrossRef] [PubMed]

23. Satomi, S.; Matsuda, I. Microsomal desaturation of linoleic into γ-linolenic acid in livers of fetal, suckling and pregnant rats. *Biol. Neonate* **1973**, *22*, 1–8. [CrossRef] [PubMed]

24. Pascaud, M.P.R.J. Transfert materno-foetal et captation des acides gras essentiels chez le rat. *Ann. Biol. Anim. Biochem. Biophys.* **1979**, *19*, 251–256. [CrossRef]

25. Fan, Y.Y.; Chapkin, R.S. Mouse peritoneal macrophage prostaglandin E1 synthesis is altered by dietary gamma-linolenic acid. *J. Nutr.* **1992**, *122*, 1600–1606. [PubMed]

26. Alhazmi, A.; Stojanovski, E.; Garg, M.L.; McEvoy, M. Fasting whole blood fatty acid profile and risk of type 2 diabetes in adults: A nested case control study. *PLoS ONE* **2014**, *9*, e97001. [CrossRef] [PubMed]

27. Hyatt, M.A.; Budge, H.; Symonds, M.E. Early developmental influences on hepatic organogenesis. *Organogenesis* **2008**, *4*, 170–175. [CrossRef] [PubMed]

28. Godfrey, K.M.; Lillycrop, K.A.; Burdge, G.C.; Gluckman, P.D.; Hanson, M.A. Epigenetic mechanisms and the mismatch concept of the developmental origins of health and disease. *Pediatr. Res.* **2007**, *61*, 5R–10R. [CrossRef] [PubMed]

29. Shaw, B.; Lambert, S.; Wong, M.H.; Ralston, J.C.; Stryjecki, C.; Mutch, D.M. Individual saturated and monounsaturated fatty acids trigger distinct transcriptional networks in differentiated 3T3-L1 preadipocytes. *J. Nutrigenet Nutrigenomics* **2013**, *6*, 1–15. [CrossRef] [PubMed]

30. Brumbaugh, D.E.; Friedman, J.E. Developmental origins of nonalcoholic fatty liver disease. *Pediatr. Res.* **2014**, *75*, 140–147. [CrossRef] [PubMed]

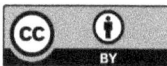

nutrients

MDPI

Article

High Fat Diet Administration during Specific Periods of Pregnancy Alters Maternal Fatty Acid Profiles in the Near-Term Rat

Marlon E. Cerf [1],* and Emilio Herrera [2]

[1] Diabetes Discovery Platform, South African Medical Research Council, PO Box 19070, Tygerberg, Cape Town 7505, South Africa

[2] Department of Chemistry and Biochemistry, University of San Pablo-CEU, Ctra. Boadilla del Monte km 5.3, Madrid 28668, Spain; eherrera@ceu.es

*   Correspondence: marlon.cerf@mrc.ac.za; Tel.: +27-21-938-0818; Fax: +27-21-938-0456

Received: 7 July 2015; Accepted: 18 September 2015; Published: 4 January 2016

Abstract: Excessive fat intake is a global health concern as women of childbearing age increasingly ingest high fat diets (HFDs). We therefore determined the maternal fatty acid (FA) profiles in metabolic organs after HFD administration during specific periods of gestation. Rats were fed a HFD for the first (HF1), second (HF2), or third (HF3) week, or for all three weeks (HFG) of gestation. Total maternal plasma non-esterified fatty acid (NEFA) concentrations were monitored throughout pregnancy. At day 20 of gestation, maternal plasma, liver, adipose tissue, and placenta FA profiles were determined. In HF3 mothers, plasma myristic and stearic acid concentrations were elevated, whereas docosahexaenoic acid (DHA) was reduced in both HF3 and HFG mothers. In HF3 and HFG mothers, hepatic stearic and oleic acid proportions were elevated; conversely, DHA and linoleic acid (LA) proportions were reduced. In adipose tissue, myristic acid was elevated, whereas DHA and LA proportions were reduced in all mothers. Further, adipose tissue stearic acid proportions were elevated in HF2, HF3, and HFG mothers; with oleic acid increased in HF1 and HFG mothers. In HF3 and HFG mothers, placental neutral myristic acid proportions were elevated, whereas DHA was reduced. Further, placental phospholipid DHA proportions were reduced in HF3 and HFG mothers. Maintenance on a diet, high in saturated fat, but low in DHA and LA proportions, during late or throughout gestation, perpetuated reduced DHA across metabolic organs that adapt during pregnancy. Therefore a diet, with normal DHA proportions during gestation, may be important for balancing maternal FA status.

Keywords: docosahexaenoic acid; feto-placental; lipids; ω-3 fatty acids; ω-6 fatty acids; triglycerides

1. Introduction

Fatty acids (FAs) are structural components of organs, energy sources, precursors of bioactive compounds such as eicosanoids, including prostacyclins, prostaglandins, thromboxanes, and leukotrienes. FAs also regulate the expression of transcription factors. All FAs provide energy, whereas polyunsaturated fatty acids (PUFAs) are required for structural and metabolic functions.

The ω-3 and ω-6 PUFA families are synthesized from their essential fatty acids (EFAs), namely α-linolenic acid (αLA, 18:3 ω-3) and linoleic acid (LA, 18:2 ω-6), respectively. αLA and LA cannot be synthesized *de novo* [1] and are, therefore, supplied in the diet [2]. During pregnancy, the EFAs and PUFAs cross the placenta to maintain their supply to the fetus [3]. LA is abundant in the Western dietary pattern and is the precursor of arachidonic acid (AA, 20:4 ω-6) [2]. αLA is abundant in seed oils and is the precursor of eicosapentanoic acid (EPA, 20:5 ω-3) and docosahexaenoic acid (DHA, 22:6 ω-3) [1]. Metabolically important PUFAs during development are AA, EPA, and DHA which are not required from the maternal diet during pregnancy to meet fetal demands since they can be synthesized endogenously from the EFAs. However, the conversion of EFAs to PUFAs by the fetus is very limited and, therefore, the plasma and tissue concentrations of these FAs depend mainly on exogenous supply. Thus, during periods of rapid intrauterine growth, the production of the EPAs, DHA, and AA may be inadequate and considered as EFAs for the fetuses [4]. A sufficient supply of these FAs during pregnancy and the neonatal period is critical for normal fetal growth and proper neurological development and function [5,6].

Maternal dietary FAs, particularly PUFAs, may influence epigenetic gene regulation by inducing or repressing transcription of specific genes during critical ontogenic periods [7,8] with long-term consequences for offspring health. During pregnancy, the mother transitions through different metabolic conditions, shifting from anabolism during the first two thirds of gestation, by accumulating fat depots, to a catabolic state during the last third, when fat depot breakdown is enhanced [9–11]. These metabolic transitions contribute to the development of maternal hyperlipidemia with major implications for fetal growth [12]. Moreover, these adaptations are altered when the maternal diet is unbalanced by a high fat (HF) content with consequences in placental nutrient transport and fetal growth [13]. Specific placental nutrient transporters, namely glucose transporter (GLUT) 1 and sodium-coupled neutral amino acid transporter (SNAT) 2, are up-regulated in response to a high fat diet (HFD) [13].

The ingestion of a HFD during pregnancy influences both maternal and offspring health outcomes as gestational HF feeding are associated with derangements in both their metabolism and physiology that may be immediate, transient or permanent. Whereas most studies focus on developmental programming effects, the present study will investigate the differential FA profiles in maternal metabolic organs near term. With the increasing proportion of women of childbearing age that are overweight or obese and consume unhealthy diets during pregnancy, there is a great need to study dietary patterns as they influence both maternal and offspring health outcomes. Since altered dietary composition during specific periods of pregnancy could differentially affect maternal FA profiles with consequences in their availability to the fetus, this study investigates the effect of a HFD administered to pregnant rats at different stages of pregnancy on lipid profiles in near-term mothers. Maternal plasma, hepatic, adipose tissue, and placenta FA profiles were determined.

2. Experimental Section

2.1. Experimental Design

Ethical approval was obtained by the Animal Ethics Committee of the South African Medical Research Council prior to experimentation. Adult female Wistar rats from our animal facility were maintained at $22 \pm 2\,°C$, $55\% \pm 10\%$ relative humidity and 12 h light/dark cycles and fed the control diet. The female rats fed a control diet were mated with age-matched male rats. After mating was confirmed by the presence of vaginal plug(s), pregnant rats were randomly assigned to the experimental groups, housed singly, and subjected to the experimental design summarized in Table 1. Briefly, pregnant mothers (n = 4–6 per group) were fed a control or HF diet *ad libitum* during specific periods of gestation. The HFD was formulated by in-house dieticians and was constituted by 40% fat, 14% protein, and 46% carbohydrate, whereas the control diet was acquired commercially (Epol, Pietermaritzburg, South Africa) and contained 10% fat, 15% protein, and 75% carbohydrate (Table S1). As summarized in Table 1, the groups were mothers maintained on a HFD during the first (HF1), second (HF2), or third (HF3) week of gestation, or for all three (HFG) weeks of gestation; for the remainder of gestation, mothers were fed the control diet.

Table 1. Experimental design.

Groups	Gestational Diet		
	Week 1	Week 2	Week 3
Control	Control	Control	Control
HF1	HFD	Control	Control
HF2	Control	HFD	Control
HF3	Control	Control	HFD
HFG	HFD	HFD	HFD

Control mothers ($n = 4$) were maintained on a standard laboratory (control) diet throughout. Experimental mothers ($n = 4$ per group, but $n = 6$ for HF2) were maintained on a high fat diet (HFD) for specific weeks of gestation. HF1, mothers maintained on a HFD for week one; HF2, mothers maintained on a HFD for week two; HF3, mothers maintained on a HFD for week three; HFG, mothers maintained on a HFD for all three weeks of gestation.

2.2. Sample Collection

At days zero (e0, just prior to mating), seven (e7, early pregnancy), 14 (e14, mid pregnancy) and 20 (e20, near-term), blood was collected from the tail after 3 h of fasting. Mothers were anesthetized via an anesthetic machine (Motivus Resuscitator Type AV, Crest Healthcare Technology Ltd., Johannesburg, South Africa) with fluothane (Halothane, AstraZeneca Pharmaceuticals, Johannesburg, South Africa) and 2% oxygen. After the mothers were anesthetized, the tip of the tail was heated with a ultraviolet (UV) lamp to facilitate blood flow then snipped with a surgical blade. Blood was collected in ice-cooled tubes containing 1 mg/ml of Na_2-EDTA. After centrifugation, plasma samples were stored at $-20\,^{\circ}C$ until analysis. After the last blood collection (e20), mothers were maintained under anesthesia and whole liver, lumbar adipose tissue, and placenta were collected and stored at $-80\,^{\circ}C$ until analysis.

2.3. Determination of Blood Glucose and Serum Insulin Concentrations and Lipid Profiles

Blood glucose (glucometer, Precision QID, MediSense, Cambridge, UK) and serum insulin (rat insulin RIA kit, Linco Research, St. Charles, MO, USA) concentrations were measured. Homeostasis model assessment (HOMA)-insulin resistance ((fasting plasma glucose (mmol/L) X fasting serum insulin (mU/L))/22.5)) was calculated. Plasma triglycerides (TAG), cholesterol (Spinreact Reactives, Girona, Spain), and non-esterified fatty acid (NEFA) (Wako Chemicals, Neuss, Germany) were determined enzymatically using commercial kits. For FA profile analyses, nonadecenoic acid (19:1) (Sigma-Aldrich, Madrid, Spain) was added as the internal standard to fresh aliquots of diets and frozen plasma and tissue which were used for lipid extraction and purification [14]. For the placenta, lipid extracts were evaporated to dryness and resuspended in chloroform in the presence of activated silicic acid to extract the neutral lipids whereas the dried chloroform-washed silicic acid fraction was treated with methanol to extract the phospholipids. The final lipid extracts were evaporated under vacuum and the residue suspended in methanol/toluene followed by methanolysis in the presence of acetyl chloride at $-80\,^{\circ}C$ for 2.5 h as previously described [15]. FA methyl esters were separated and quantified on a Perkin-Elmer gas chromatograph (Autosystem, Madrid, Spain) with a flame ionization detector and a 20 m Omegawax capillary column (internal diameter 0.25 mm). Nitrogen was used as the carrier gas and the FA methyl esters were compared to purified standards (Sigma-Aldrich). Quantification of the FAs in the samples was performed as a function of the corresponding peak areas and compared to the internal standard.

2.4. Statistical Analysis

One-way analysis of variance (ANOVA) and Bonferroni's post-test were applied with data reported as means $\pm$ standard error of the mean (SEM) and significance established at $p < 0.05$. However, for dietary FA and fetal-maternal FA analyses, the Student's *t*-test was applied.

3. Results

3.1. Anthropometry

Although HFG mothers consumed more food compared to the other mothers, there were no differences in body weights (Table S2). Despite no differences in placental weight, when adjusted for body weight, placental weights were reduced in HF3 mothers relative to control mothers (Table S2). There were no differences in conceptus weight, litter sizes, or any of the maternal organs that were studied (Table S2).

3.2. Glycemia, Insulinemia and HOMA-Insulin Resistance

There were no differences in glycemia, insulinemia, and HOMA-insulin resistance amongst the groups (Table S3).

3.3. Fatty Acid Profile in the Diets

As shown in Figure 1, the proportion of saturated FAs (namely myristic, palmitic, and stearic acids) and oleic acid were higher in the HFD than in the control diet with lower proportions of αLA, DHA, and LA in the HFD. In the HFD, palmitic and oleic acid were the predominant FAs (57% of total diet), whereas in the control diet LA was most abundant.

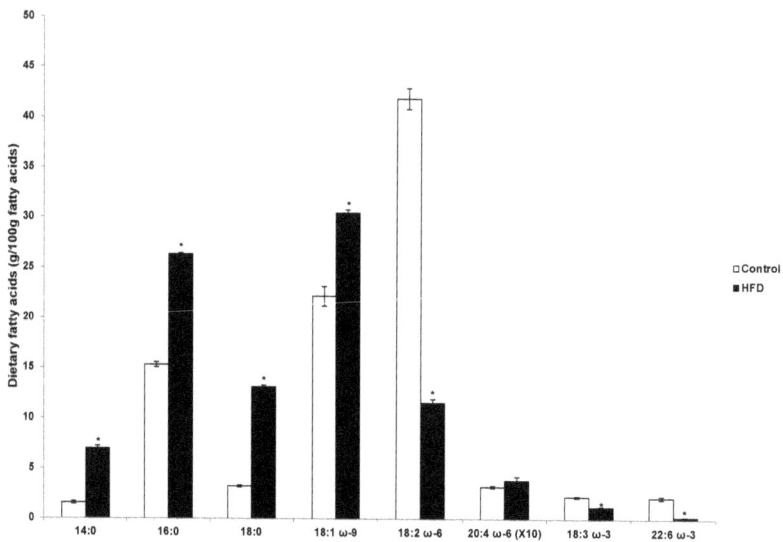

Figure 1. Dietary fatty acids (g/100 g fatty acids). Values are means ± standard error of the mean (SEM). HFD, high fat diet. * $p < 0.0001$.

3.4. Plasma Total Non-Esterified Fatty Acid, Triglyceride, and Cholesterol Concentrations and Individual Fatty Acid Profiles

Near-term (e20) plasma total NEFA concentrations were elevated in control, HF1, HF2, and HF3 mothers compared to pre-gravidity (e0), early (e7), and mid-term (e14); and in HFG mothers at near-term (e20), compared to pre-gravidity (e0) and early term (e7) (Figure 2A).

With reference to the individual FA profiles at e20 in HF3 mothers, myristic (14:0) and stearic acid (18:0) concentrations were elevated compared to control, HF1, HF2, and HFG mothers (Figure 2B). However, DHA concentrations were reduced in HF3 and HFG mothers compared to the control mothers (Figure 2B). Plasma αLA values in all the groups were negligible (data not shown).

Plasma TAG concentrations at mid-term (e14) were elevated in HFG mothers compared to HF1 mothers (Figure 2C). Further, mid-term (e14) TAG concentrations were elevated in HF2 mothers compared to pre-gravidity (e0) and early term (e7) (Figure 2C). Near-term (e20) TAG concentrations were elevated in control and HFG mothers compared to pre-gravidity (e0) and early term (e7); further, near-term (e20) TAG concentrations were elevated in HF1, HF2, and HF3 mothers compared to pre-gravidity (e0), early (e7), and mid-term (e14) (Figure 2C).

Early term (e7) plasma cholesterol concentrations were reduced in HF2 mothers compared to HF1 mothers (Figure 2D). In HF1 mothers, mid-term (e14) cholesterol concentrations were reduced compared to early (e7) and near-term (e20) (Figure 2D). Near-term (e20) cholesterol concentrations were elevated in HF3 mothers compared to HF2 mothers (Figure 2D). In HF1 mothers, near-term (e20) cholesterol concentrations were elevated compared to pre-gravidity (e0) and mid-term (e14); and in HF2 mothers only relative to mid-term (e14) (Figure 2D). In both HF3 and HFG mothers, near-term (e20) cholesterol concentrations were elevated compared to pre-gravidity (e0), early (e7), and mid-term (e14) (Figure 2D).

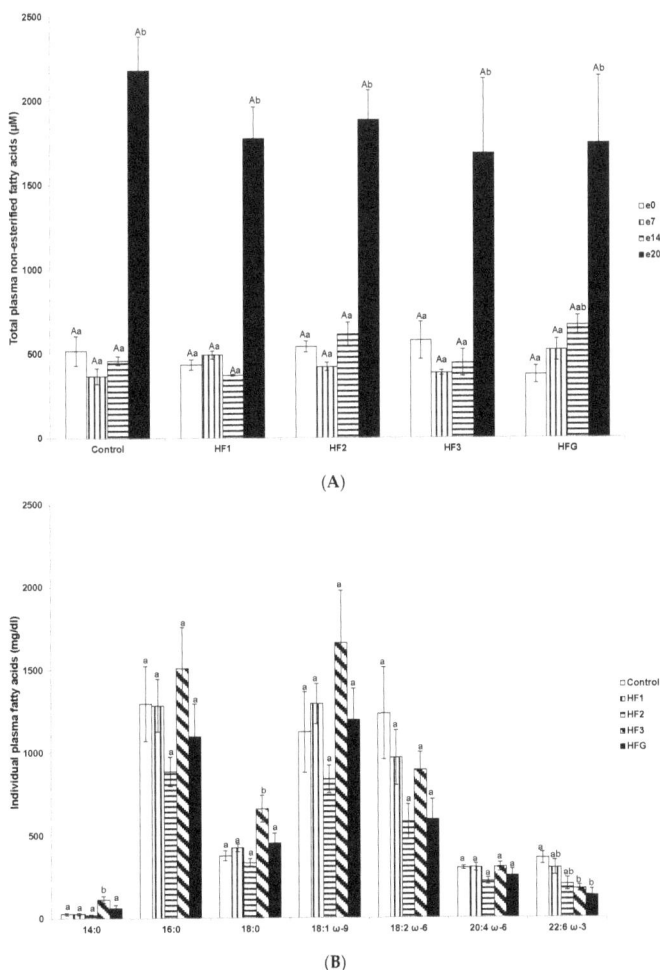

(A)

(B)

Figure 2. *Cont.*

(C)

(D)

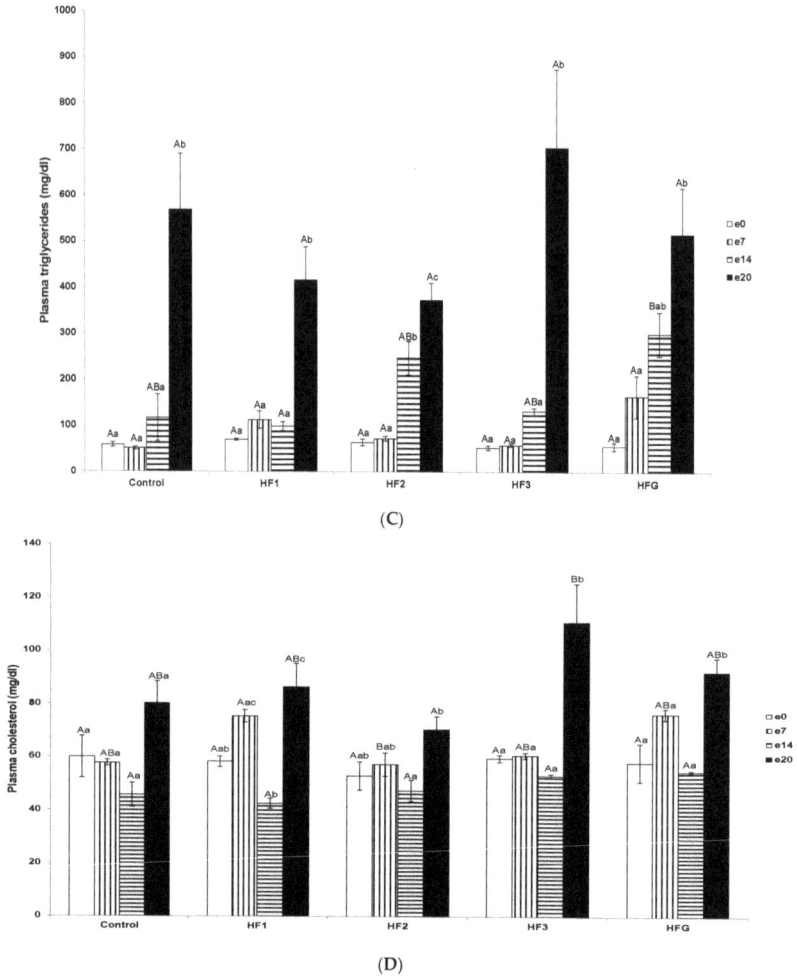

Figure 2. Lipid profiles during gestation. (**A**) Plasma non-esterified fatty acid concentrations (μM); (**B**) individual plasma fatty acid concentrations (mg/dL); (**C**) plasma triglyceride concentrations (mg/dL); and (**D**) plasma cholesterol concentrations (mg/dL). Numerals refer to the specific week of gestational high fat (HF) maintenance. G, gestation refers to HF maintenance throughout gestation. Values are means ± standard error of the mean (SEM). Capital letters refer to inter-groups. Lower case letters refer to intra-groups. Different letters reflect significant changes.

3.5. Placental Neutral Lipids and Phospholipid Fatty Acids Near Term (e20)

In HF3 mothers, placental neutral lipid myristic acid was increased compared to the control, HF1 and HF2 mothers (Figure 3A). In both HF3 and HFG mothers, DHA was reduced compared to control and HF2 mothers (Figure 3A).

Similarly in HF3 and HFG mothers, placental phospholipid DHA was reduced compared to control, HF1 and HF2 mothers (Figure 3B). Placental phospholipid myristic acid was elevated in HF3 mothers compared to HF2 mothers (Figure 3B).

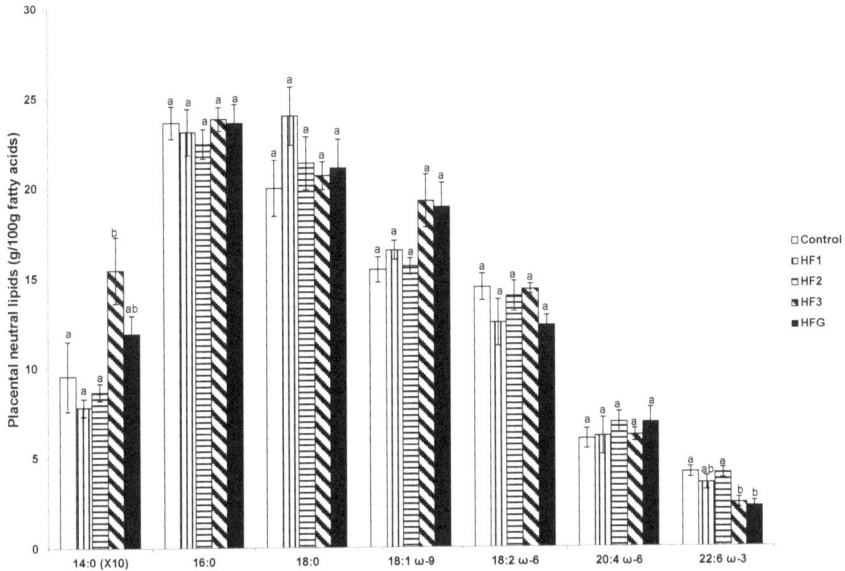

(A)

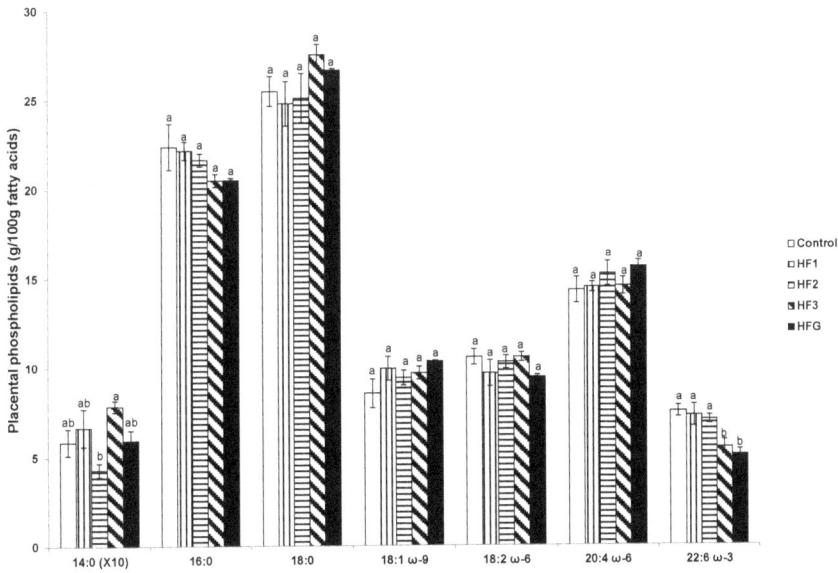

(B)

Figure 3. Placental fatty acids. (**A**) Placental neutral fatty acids (g/100 g fatty acids); and (**B**) placental phospholipid fatty acids (g/100 g fatty acids). Numerals refer to the specific week of gestational high fat (HF) maintenance. G, gestation refers to HF maintenance throughout gestation. Values are means ± standard error of the mean (SEM). Different letters reflect significant changes.

3.6. Plasma Fetal: Maternal Fatty Acids and Fetal and Maternal AA:LA Ratios

Although we recently reported the FA profiles in fetal plasma [16], we subsequently determined the plasma fetal:maternal ratios of individual FAs. As shown in Figure 4, the fetal:maternal plasma ratio of stearic acid was reduced in HF2, HF3, and HFG mothers compared to control mothers. The fetal:maternal plasma oleic acid ratio in HF3 and HFG mothers was reduced, whereas the LA ratio was elevated relative to control mothers (Figure 4). Fetal:maternal plasma LA ratio was also elevated in HF3 mothers relative to HF1 mothers (Figure 4). Fetal:maternal plasma palmitic acid ratio was reduced in HFG mothers compared to HF1 and HF2 mothers (Figure 4).

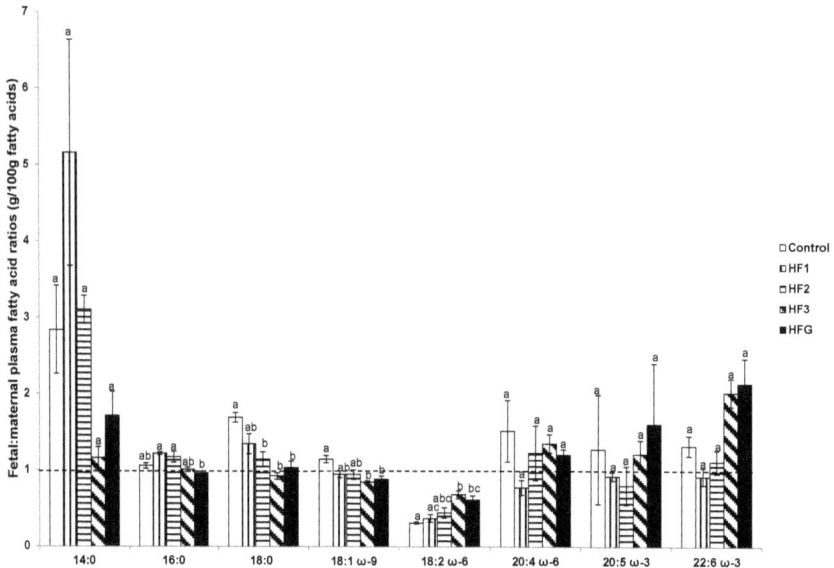

Figure 4. Fetal: maternal ratio of plasma fatty acids (g/100 g fatty acids). Numerals refer to the specific week of gestational high fat (HF) maintenance. G, gestation refers to HF maintenance throughout gestation. Values are means ± standard error of the mean (SEM). Different letters reflect significant changes.

Although the fetal:maternal ratio of most FAs did not exceed 1, the DHA ratios in the HF3 and HFG groups were increased ~two-fold, albeit non-significant. The plasma AA:LA ratio in either the fetuses or the mothers did not differ between the different groups, but values were consistently higher in fetuses than in mothers in all groups (Table S4).

3.7. Hepatic Fatty Acids

Hepatic stearic and oleic acid were elevated in HF3 and HFG mothers whereas LA and DHA were reduced relative to control mothers (Figure 5). Hepatic LA proportions were also reduced in HF2 mothers compared to control mothers (Figure 5).

3.8. Adipose Tissue Fatty Acids

The proportion of adipose tissue myristic acid was elevated whereas LA and DHA were reduced in HF1, HF2, HF3, and HFG mothers compared to controls (Figure 6). Further, adipose tissue LA was reduced in HFG mothers compared to HF1, HF2, and HF3 mothers (Figure 6). In addition, adipose tissue stearic acid was elevated in HF2, HF3, and HFG mothers relative to control mothers, and in HFG mothers compared to HF1 mothers (Figure 6). Adipose tissue oleic acid was elevated in HF1 and HFG mothers compared to control mothers (Figure 6). Further, adipose tissue palmitic acid was elevated in HF3 relative to HF1 mothers (Figure 6).

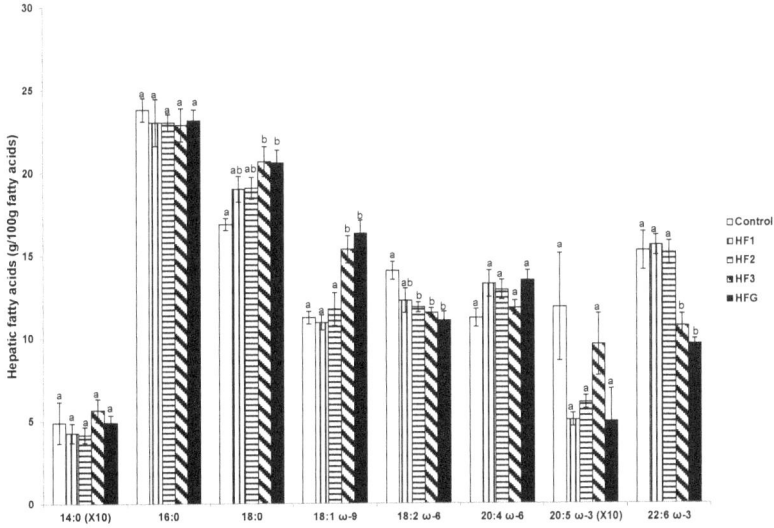

Figure 5. Hepatic fatty acids (g/100 g fatty acids). Numerals refer to the specific week of gestational high fat (HF) maintenance. G, gestation refers to HF maintenance throughout gestation. Values are means ± standard error of the mean (SEM). Different letters reflect significant changes.

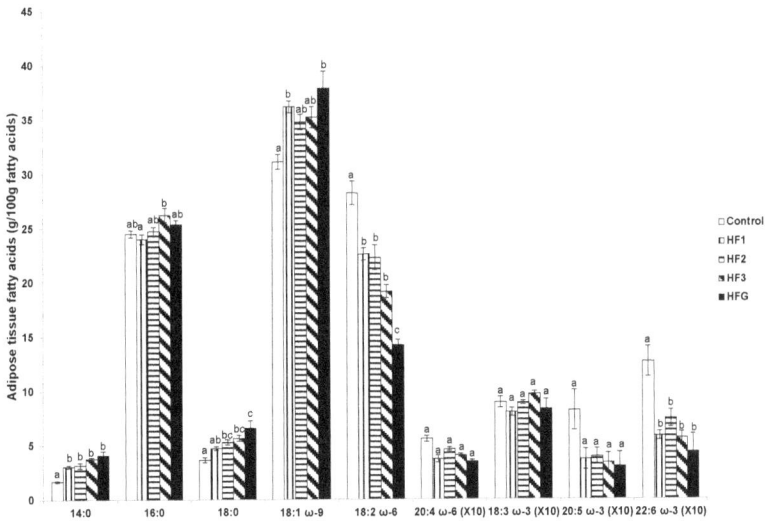

Figure 6. Adipose tissue fatty acids (g/100 g fatty acids). Numerals refer to the specific week of gestational high fat (HF) maintenance. G, gestation refers to HF maintenance throughout gestation. Values are means ± standard error of the mean (SEM). Different letters reflect significant changes.

4. Discussion

The present rodent study sought to determine the effects of HFD administration during specific periods of gestation on maternal lipid profiles, since we recently described its consequences on the availability of FAs to the fetus [16]. The HFD administered was rich in saturated and oleic acids but depleted in LA and DHA relative to the control diet with negligible amounts of αLA. One of the key findings was that the intake of the HFD during the first, second, or third week of gestation or throughout gestation did not modify the intense increase in plasma NEFA that occurs physiologically near-term (in control rats). This observation may reflect an index of adipose tissue lipolysis and, therefore, our data suggest that this pathway is highly augmented during late pregnancy as expected [10]. The main fate of plasma NEFA is the liver [17,18] for partial re-esterification in the synthesis of TAG which are released back into the circulation, and this pathway is also known to be enhanced in late pregnancy in the rat [19,20]. Bearing this in mind, we found that plasma TAG was also greatly increased in all pregnant rats close to term, although the increase seemed to be gradual as it was also evident at the end of mid pregnancy (day 14 of gestation) in those rats maintained on the HFD solely for the second week of pregnancy (HF2) or throughout pregnancy (HFG). This occurred despite unaltered plasma NEFA until near-term in all the groups suggesting that the HFD may increase TAG release from the liver already from mid pregnancy.

The profile of individual FAs in plasma and in the various organs provides insight into the metabolic changes taking place due to the HFD administration during gestation. In agreement with the known direct relationship between FA composition in the diet and maternal adipose tissue in pregnant rats fed different diets [21], the profile of FAs in the adipose tissue of the mothers maintained on the HFD for the different weeks of gestation closely reflected those of the diet. Moreover, there were higher proportions of saturated FAs and oleic acid but lower LA and DHA proportions. However, only the plasma had a decline in DHA in rats fed the HFD for the third week of gestation or throughout gestation suggesting that other organs may compensate for the altered dietary FA profile. This seems to be the case in the liver where an increase in stearic and oleic acid was only evident in those rats fed the HFD for the third week of gestation or throughout gestation. This resonates as the rats were studied at a time when they were maintained on the diet containing high proportions of saturated FAs and oleic acid.

As reported in mice, HF feeding is likely to induce hepatic FA synthesis by chain elongation and subsequent desaturation rather than *de novo* synthesis [22] which may justify the unaltered palmitic acid but enhanced stearic and oleic acid in the livers of the mothers maintained on a HFD during the third week of gestation or throughout gestation, and studied near-term. A different scenario presents with the proportion of LA in the liver which was decreased near-term virtually in all the rats (apart from HF1 mothers) maintained on the HFD for any of the three weeks of gestation. However, the main PUFA derived from LA, AA, did not differ amongst the groups in either plasma or liver. Since the proportion of AA in the diets was very low, this suggested that the conversion of LA to AA was enhanced in those rats fed the HFD. An increase in the proportion of AA was previously reported in the liver of rat mothers, newborn pups and suckling pups that were fed a HFD 10 days prior to mating, throughout pregnancy, and during lactation [23]. These changes could be attributed to the known effects that HFDs have on the expression of genes involved in lipid metabolism that would facilitate LA elongation and desaturation in the synthesis of AA [24]. However, this situation cannot be sustained for DHA since levels of its EFA precursor, αLA, were very low in the diet and therefore the DHA levels mainly depend on its dietary availability which was greatly reduced in the HFD (~10-fold lower) compared to the control diet. The consequence was the consistent decline of DHA availability as demonstrated in the plasma, liver, and adipose tissue of rats fed the HFD for the last week of gestation or throughout gestation.

A similar rationale could be applied to understand the FA profile of placental neutral lipids (involved in lipid storage) and phospholipids (form cell membranes), where the most consistent changes were the decline in the proportions of DHA. The placenta plays a key role in the mother-fetus relationship, maintaining fetal homeostasis through the regulation of nutrient transfer [25] and is involved in materno-fetal exchanges, metabolism, endocrinology, and immune pathways, and is an active component for fetal growth [26]. Although lipogenesis occurs in the rat placenta [27], its rate seems to be slow [28,29] and, therefore, most placental FAs are a result of the balance between those taken up from maternal plasma and those released to the fetus. In the present study, DHA was the only FA that was consistently reduced in both placental neutral lipids and phospholipids in rats fed the HFD for the third week of gestation and throughout gestation. This change reflected the decrease of this PUFA in plasma and therefore may be a consequence of its limited uptake by the placenta from maternal circulation. The placenta is known to preferentially transfer PUFA, such as DHA, due to their absolute requirement for brain and retina development [30]. Further, the reduced placental phospholipid DHA profiles in rats maintained on the HFD for the third week of gestation or throughout gestation may also result in reduced transfer of this PUFA to their fetuses which may potentially stunt fetal brain and retina development. Interestingly, the fetal:maternal DHA ratio increased ~two-fold in rats maintained on the HFD for the third week of gestation or throughout gestation although the change *versus* the one value was not statistically significant. This finding resonates with the known magnification of this specific FA in the fetus in relation to the mother indicating a higher proportional placental transfer of DHA relative to other FAs [31], although absolute concentrations are lower in the fetus than in the mother under different dietary regimens [32] as also shown in humans [3].

The metabolic state and nutrition of mothers during pregnancy has developmental programming consequences for their progeny. PUFA dietary content, particularly a more balanced ω-6 to ω-3 ratio, may be a key dietary variable in the developmental programming of cardiometabolic function in adult offspring [33]. In rodent studies, the ω-6 to ω-3 FA ratio in the maternal diet may impact bone parameters and therefore indirectly also the body weight [34]. Modulation of dietary ω-6 to ω-3 ratio and/or early leptin levels may also have long-term effects on later metabolic parameters [35]. Increased maternal intake of ω-3 FAs led to a decreased growth rate, reduced adipose tissue mass, lower serum leptin concentrations [36], reduced fat accretion, and reduced the age-related decline in insulin sensitivity in progeny [37]. The reduced DHA in mothers maintained on a HFD for the third week of gestation or throughout gestation in the plasma, liver, adipose tissue, and placenta may predispose their offspring to metabolic disease.

In humans, DHA supplementation during normal pregnancy was associated with lower infant ponderal index at birth and decreased umbilical cord insulin concentrations compared to infants from mothers consuming placebos [38]. Higher cord plasma DHA concentrations and ω-3 to ω-6 PUFA ratios were associated with improved fetal insulin sensitivity, whereas cord plasma saturated FAs (namely stearic acid and arachidic acid (C20:0)) were negatively correlated with fetal insulin sensitivity, suggesting a positive impact of certain ω-3 FAs and a negative impact of saturated FAs on fetal insulin sensitivity [39]. This may be explained by PUFAs constituting important structural elements of cell membranes and, concomitant with their eicosanoid products, they also modulate gene expression [35]. In our study, in rats maintained on a HFD for the third week of gestation, plasma myristic and stearic acid proportions were elevated, whereas DHA proportions were reduced in both mothers maintained on a HFD during the third week of gestation or throughout gestation, which likely contributes to insulin insensitivity in their fetal offspring. Indeed, fetuses exposed to a HFD for the third week of fetal life were heaviest concomitant with elevated glycemia and insulin resistance [16] reflecting ,insulin insensitivity.

Unfortunately, the mechanisms involved cannot be derived from our data, although other studies provide some insight. Studies in pregnant mice reported that a HFD causes marked up-regulation of placental transport of specific nutrients, such as glucose and neutral amino acid transport [13]. Thus, since DHA is essential for normal fetal and neonatal growth and development [5,40], its deficiency in the HFD may enhance its placental transfer. The impact of dietary ω-3 on placental function is well recognized [41]. Another consideration is that an ω-3 deficient condition, as induced by the HF administration during gestation, could up-regulate the fetal synthesis of DHA from its EFA precursor, αLA. The near-term rat fetus has the capacity to synthesize DHA from αLA [42,43] via different desaturases and elongases [44–47]. Moreover in the adult rat, it was shown that an ω-3 deficient diet up-regulates the hepatic expression and activity of delta-6-desaturase [48] and the synthesis of DHA from αLA is enhanced by diets low in PUFA [49]. Additional studies are required to determine which of these mechanisms are in effect to justify the trend of the increase in the proportion of DHA in fetal plasma relative to their mothers under conditions of HF feeding during late pregnancy.

5. Conclusions

Mothers maintained on a HFD for the final week of gestation or throughout gestation had reduced DHA in plasma, liver, adipose tissue, and placenta. Altered circulating and hepatic FA profiles, particularly saturated FA elevation, and reduced key ω-3 and ω-6 PUFA, coinciding with the compromised maternal metabolic state of pregnancy, reflects altered lipid metabolism that may have adverse health outcomes. Low DHA maternal availability in rats fed the HFD may up-regulate its placental transfer or stimulate its fetal synthesis from its EFA precursor thereby allowing the maintenance of a higher proportion in fetal plasma relative to maternal plasma. Therefore, maternal intake of a HFD during the critical stage of peak fetal development should be avoided for stabilizing lipid profiles to promote healthy outcomes in mothers and their fetuses.

Supplementary Materials: Supplementary materials can be accessed at: http://www.mdpi.com/2072-6643/8/1/25/s1.

Acknowledgments: The authors extend their gratitude to Milagros Morante and Christo Muller for their expert technical assistance and the National Research Foundation of South Africa for funding. The study was also supported by a grant from Fundación Ramón Areces of Spain (grant CIVP16A1835).

Author Contributions: MEC's contributions were the conception and design; and analysis and interpretation of data; drafting of the article and critical revision for important intellectual content; and final approval of the version to be published. EH contributions were analysis and interpretation of data; critical revision for important intellectual content; and final approval of the version to be published.

Conflicts of Interest: The authors declare no conflict of interest.

References

1. Lorente-Cebrian, S.; Costa, A.G.; Navas-Carretero, S.; Zabala, M.; Alfredo Martinez, J.; Moreno-Aliaga, J. Role of omega-3 fatty acids in obesity, metabolic syndrome, and cardiovascular diseases: A review of the evidence. *J. Physiol. Biochem.* **2013**, *69*, 633–651. [CrossRef] [PubMed]
2. Russo, G.L. Dietary *n*-6 and *n*-3 polyunsaturated fatty acids: From biochemistry to clinical implications in cardiovascular prevention. *Biochem. Pharmacol.* **2009**, *77*, 937–946. [CrossRef] [PubMed]
3. Sakamoto, M.; Kubota, M. Plasma fatty acid profiles in 37 pairs of maternal and umbilical cord blood samples. *Environ. Health Prev. Med.* **2004**, *9*, 67–69. [CrossRef] [PubMed]
4. Le, H.D.; Meisel, J.A.; de Meijer, V.E.; Gura, K.M.; Puder, M. The essentiality of arachidonic acid and docosahexaenoic acid. *Prostaglandins Leukot. Essent. Fatty Acids* **2009**, *81*, 165–170. [CrossRef] [PubMed]
5. Innis, S.M. Essential fatty acids in growth and development. *Prog. Lipid Res.* **1991**, *30*, 39–103. [CrossRef]
6. Uauy, R.; Treen, M.; Hoffman, D.R. Essential fatty acid metabolism and requirements during development. *Semin. Perinatol.* **1989**, *13*, 118–130. [PubMed]
7. Burdge, G.C.; Lillycrop, K.A. Fatty acids and epigenetics. *Curr. Opin. Clin. Nutr. Metab. Care* **2014**, *17*, 156–161. [CrossRef] [PubMed]
8. Casas-Agustench, P.; Fernandes, F.S.; Tavares do Carmo, M.G.; Visioli, F.; Herrera, E.; Davalos, A. Consumption of distinct dietary lipids during early pregnancy differentially modulates the expression of microRNAs in mothers and offspring. *PLoS ONE* **2015**, *10*, e0117858. [CrossRef] [PubMed]
9. Herrera, E.; Ortega-Senovilla, H. Maternal lipid metabolism during normal pregnancy and its implications to fetal development. *Clin. Lipidol.* **2010**, *5*, 899–911. [CrossRef]
10. Hytten, F.E.; Leitch, I. The gross composition of the components of weight gain. In *The Physiology of Human Pregnancy*; Hytten, F.E., Leitch, I., Eds.; Blackwell: Oxford, UK, 1971; pp. 370–387.

11. Herrera, E.; Lasunción, M.A.; Gomez Coronado, D.; Aranda, P.; López-Luna, P.; Maier, I. Role of lipoprotein lipase activity on lipoprotein metabolism and the fate of circulating triglycerides in pregnancy. *Am. J. Obstet. Gynecol.* **1988**, *158*, 1575–1583. [CrossRef]

12. Herrera, E.; Ortega-Senovilla, H. Lipid metabolism during pregnancy and its implications for fetal growth. *Curr. Pharm. Biotechnol.* **2014**, *15*, 24–31. [CrossRef] [PubMed]

13. Jones, H.N.; Woollett, L.A.; Barbour, N.; Prasad, P.D.; Powell, T.L.; Jansson, T. High-fat diet before and during pregnancy causes marked up-regulation of placental nutrient transport and fetal overgrowth in C57/BL6 mice. *FASEB J.* **2009**, *23*, 271–278. [CrossRef] [PubMed]

14. Amusquivar, E.; Schiffner, S.; Herrera, E. Evaluation of two methods for plasma fatty acid analysis by GC. *Eur. J. Lipid Sci. Technol.* **2011**, *113*, 711–716. [CrossRef]

15. Folch, J.; Lees, M.; Sloane Stanley, G.H. A simple method for the isolation and purification of total lipids from animal tissues. *J. Biol. Chem.* **1957**, *226*, 497–509. [PubMed]

16. Cerf, M.E.; Louw, J.; Herrera, E. High fat diet exposure during late fetal life enhances hepatic omega 6 fatty acid profiles in fetal Wistar rats. *Nutrients* **2015**, *7*, 7231–7241. [CrossRef] [PubMed]

17. Mampel, T.; Villarroya, F.; Herrera, E. Hepatectomy-nephrectomy effects in the pregnant rat and fetus. *Biochem. Biophys. Res. Commun.* **1985**, *131*, 1219–1225. [CrossRef]

18. Mampel, T.; Camprodon, R.; Solsona, J.; Juncá, V.; Herrera, E. Changes in circulating glycerol, free fatty acids and glucose levels following liver transplant in the pig. *Arch. Int. Physiol. Biochim.* **1981**, *89*, 195–199. [CrossRef] [PubMed]

19. Wasfi, I.; Weinstein, I.; Heimberg, M. Increased formation of triglyceride from oleate in perfused livers from pregnant rats. *Endocrinology* **1980**, *107*, 584–590. [CrossRef] [PubMed]

20. Wasfi, I.; Weinstein, I.; Heimberg, M. Hepatic metabolism of [1-^{14}C] oleate in pregnancy. *Biochim. Biophys. Acta* **1980**, *619*, 471–481. [CrossRef]

21. Amusquivar, E.; Herrera, E. Influence of changes in dietary fatty acids during pregnancy on placental and fetal fatty acid profile in the rat. *Biol. Neonate* **2003**, *83*, 136–145. [CrossRef] [PubMed]

22. Oosterveer, M.H.; van Dijk, T.H.; Tietge, U.J.; Boer, T.; Havinga, R.; Stellaard, F.; Groen, A.K.; Kuipers, F.; Renjngound, D.J. High fat feeding induces hepatic fatty acid elongation in mice. *PLoS ONE* **2009**, *4*, e6066. [CrossRef] [PubMed]

23. Ghebremeskel, K.; Bitsanis, D.; Koukkou, E.; Lowy, C.; Poston, L.; Crawford, M.A. Maternal diet high in fat reduces docosahexaenoic acid in liver lipids of newborn and sucking rat pups. *Br. J. Nutr.* **1999**, *81*, 395–404. [PubMed]

24. Buettner, R.; Parhofer, K.G.; Woenckhaus, M.; Wrede, C.E.; Kunz-Schughart, L.A.; Schölmerich, J.; Bollheimer, L.C. Defining high-fat-diet rat models: Metabolic and molecular effects of different fat types. *J. Mol. Endocrinol.* **2006**, *36*, 485–501. [CrossRef] [PubMed]

25. Gabory, A.; Ferry, L.; Fajardy, I.; Vige, A.; Mayeur, S.; Attig, L.; Lesage, J.; Vieau, D.; Jais, J.P.; Junien, C. Maternal diets trigger sex-specific divergent trajectories of gene expression and epigenetic systems in mouse placenta. *PLoS ONE* **2012**, *7*, e47986. [CrossRef] [PubMed]

26. Tarrade, A.; Rousseau-Ralliard, D.; Aubriere, M.C.; Peynot, N.; Dahirel, M.; Bertrand-Michel, J.; Aguirre-Lavin, T.; Morel, O.; Beaujean, N.; Duranthon, V.; *et al.* Sexual dimorphism of the feto-placental phenotype in response to a high fat and control maternal diets in a rabbit model. *PLoS ONE* **2013**, *8*, e83458. [CrossRef] [PubMed]

27. Diamant, Y.Z.; Shafrir, E. Placental enzymes of glycolysis, gluconeogenesis and lipogenesis in the diabetic rat and in starvation. *Diabetologia* **1978**, *15*, 481–485. [CrossRef] [PubMed]

28. Hummel, L.; Zimmermann, T.; Schirrmeister, W.; Wagner, H. Synthesis, turnover and compartment analysis of the free fatty acids in the placenta of rats. *Acta Biol. Med. Ger.* **1976**, *35*, 1311–1316. [PubMed]

29. Vileisis, R.A.; Oh, W. Enhanced fatty acid synthesis in hyperinsulinemic rat fetuses. *J. Nutr.* **1983**, *113*, 246–252. [PubMed]

30. Dutta-Roy, A.K. Insulin mediated processes in platelets, erythrocytes and monocytes/macrophages: Effects of essential fatty acid metabolism. *Prostaglandins Leukot. Essent. Fatty Acids* **1994**, *51*, 385–399. [CrossRef]

31. Haggarty, P. Fatty acid supply to the human fetus. *Annu. Rev. Nutr.* **2010**, *30*, 237–255. [CrossRef] [PubMed]

32. Fernandes, F.S.; Tavares do Carmo, M.; Herrera, E. Influence of maternal diet during early pregnancy on the fatty acid profile in the fetus at late pregnancy in rats. *Lipids* **2012**, *47*, 505–517. [CrossRef] [PubMed]

33. Benyshek, D.C.; Kachinski, J.J.; Jin, H. F0 prenatal/lactation diets varying in saturated fat and long-chain polyunsaturated fatty acids alters the insulin sensitivity of F1 rats fed a high fat Western diet postweaning. *Open J. Endocr. Metab. Dis.* **2014**, *4*, 245–252. [CrossRef]

34. Korotkova, M.; Ohlsson, C.; Hanson, L.A.; Strandvik, B. Dietary *n*-6:*n*-3 fatty acid ratio in the perinatal period affects bone parameters in adult female rats. *Br. J. Nutr.* **2004**, *92*, 643–648. [CrossRef] [PubMed]

35. Korotkova, M.; Gabrielsson, B.G.; Holmang, A.; Larsson, B.-M.; Hanson, L.A.; Strandvik, B. Gender-related long-term effects in adult rats by perinatal dietary ratio of *n*-6/*n*-3 fatty acids. *Am. J. Physiol. Regul. Integr. Comp. Physiol.* **2005**, *288*, R575–R579. [CrossRef] [PubMed]

36. Korotkova, M.; Gabrielsson, B.; Lonn, M.; Hanson, L.-A.; Strandvik, B. Leptin levels in rat offspring are modified by the ratio of linoleic to alpha-linolenic acid in the maternal diet. *J. Lipid Res.* **2002**, *43*, 1743–1749. [CrossRef] [PubMed]

37. Sardinha, F.L.; Fernandes, F.S.; Tavares do Carmo, M.G.; Herrera, E. Sex-dependent nutritional programming: Fish oil intake during early pregnancy in rats reduces age-dependent insulin resistance in male, but not female, offspring. *Am. J. Physiol. Regul. Integr. Comp. Physiol.* **2013**, *304*, R313–R320. [CrossRef] [PubMed]

38. Courville, A.B.; Harel, O.; Lammi-Keefe, C.J. Consumption of a DHA-containing functional food during pregnancy is associated with lower infant ponderal index and cord plasma insulin concentration. *Br. J. Nutr.* **2011**, *106*, 208–212. [CrossRef] [PubMed]

39. Zhao, J.P.; Levy, E.; Fraser, W.D.; Julien, P.; Delvin, E.; Montouids, A.; Spahis, S.; Garofalo, C.; Nuyt, A.M.; Luo, Z.C. Circulating docosahexaenoic acid levels are associated with fetal insulin sensitivity. *PLoS ONE* **2014**, *9*, e85054. [PubMed]

40. Uauy, R.; Peirano, P.; Hoffman, D.; Mena, P.; Birch, D.; Birch, E. Role of essential fatty acids in the function of the developing nervous system. *Lipids* **1996**, *31*, S167–S176. [CrossRef] [PubMed]

41. Jones, M.L.; Mark, P.J.; Waddell, B.J. Maternal dietary omega-3 fatty acids and placental function. *Reproduction* **2014**, *147*, R143–R152. [CrossRef] [PubMed]

42. Sanders, T.A.; Naismith, D.J. The metabolism of alpha-linolenic acid by the foetal rat. *Br. J. Nutr.* **1980**, *44*, 205–208. [CrossRef] [PubMed]

43. Sanders, T.A.; Rana, S.K. Comparison of the metabolism of linoleic and linolenic acids in the fetal rat. *Ann. Nutr. Metab.* **1987**, *31*, 349–353. [CrossRef] [PubMed]

44. Cho, H.P.; Nakamura, M.; Clarke, S.D. Cloning, expression, and fatty acid regulation of the human delta-5 desaturase. *J. Biol. Chem.* **1999**, *274*, 37335–37339. [CrossRef] [PubMed]

45. Cho, H.P.; Nakamura, M.T.; Clarke, S.D. Cloning, expression, and nutritional regulation of the mammalian delta-6 desaturase. *J. Biol. Chem.* **1999**, *274*, 471–477. [CrossRef] [PubMed]

46. Wang, Y.; Botolin, D.; Christian, B.; Busik, J.; Xu, J.; Jump, D.B. Tissue-specific, nutritional, and developmental regulation of rat fatty acid elongases. *J. Lipid Res.* **2005**, *46*, 706–715. [CrossRef] [PubMed]

47. Zheng, X.; Tocher, D.R.; Dickson, C.A.; Bell, J.G.; Teale, A.J. Highly unsaturated fatty acid synthesis in vertebrates: New insights with the cloning and characterization of a delta-6-desaturase of Atlantic salmon. *Lipids* **2005**, *40*, 13–24. [CrossRef] [PubMed]

48. Hofacer, R.; Jandacek, R.; Rider, T.; Tso, P.; Magrisso, J.; Benoit, S.C.; McNamara, R.K. Omega-3 fatty acid deficiency selectively up-regulates delta6-desaturase expression and activity indices in rat liver: Prevention by normalization of omega-3 fatty acid status. *Nutr. Res.* **2011**, *31*, 715–722. [CrossRef] [PubMed]

49. Gibson, R.A.; Neumann, M.A.; Lien, E.L.; Boyd, K.A.; Tu, W.C. Docosahexaenoic acid synthesis from alpha-linolenic acid is inhibited by diets high in polyunsaturated fatty acids. *Prostaglandins Leukot. Essent. Fatty Acids* **2013**, *88*, 139–146. [CrossRef] [PubMed]

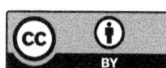

nutrients

MDPI

Article

Protective Effect of Vanillic Acid against Hyperinsulinemia, Hyperglycemia and Hyperlipidemia via Alleviating Hepatic Insulin Resistance and Inflammation in High-Fat Diet (HFD)-Fed Rats

Wen-Chang Chang [1], James Swi-Bea Wu [1], Chen-Wen Chen [1], Po-Ling Kuo [2], Hsu-Min Chien [3], Yuh-Tai Wang [4] and Szu-Chuan Shen [2,*]

[1] Graduate Institute of Food Science and Technology, National Taiwan University, P.O. Box 23-14, Taipei 10672, Taiwan; d99641001@ntu.edu.tw (W.-C.C.); jsbwu@ntu.edu.tw (J.S.-B.W.); jenwen0813@hotmail.com (C.-W.C.)
[2] Department of Human Development and Family Studies, National Taiwan Normal University, No. 162, Sec. 1, Heping East Road, Taipei 10610, Taiwan; maplebling@gmail.com
[3] Department of Nursing, Taipei City Hospital, Renai Branch, No. 10, Sec. 4, Renai Road, Taipei 10629, Taiwan; B1465@tpech.gov.tw
[4] Life Science Center, Hsing Wu Institute of Technology, No. 101, Sec. 1, Fen-Liao Road, Lin-Kou District, New Taipei City 244, Taiwan; yuhtai@yahoo.com
*   Correspondence: scs@ntnu.edu.tw; Tel.: +886-2-77341437; Fax: +886-2-23639635

Received: 24 September 2015; Accepted: 24 November 2015; Published: 2 December 2015

Abstract: Excess free fatty acid accumulation from abnormal lipid metabolism results in the insulin resistance in peripheral cells, subsequently causing hyperinsulinemia, hyperglycemia and/or hyperlipidemia in diabetes mellitus (DM) patients. Herein, we investigated the effect of phenolic acids on glucose uptake in an insulin-resistant cell-culture model and on hepatic insulin resistance and inflammation in rats fed a high-fat diet (HFD). The results show that vanillic acid (VA) demonstrated the highest glucose uptake ability among all tested phenolic acids in insulin-resistant FL83B mouse hepatocytes. Furthermore, rats fed HFD for 16 weeks were orally administered with VA daily (30 mg/kg body weight) at weeks 13–16. The results show that levels of serum insulin, glucose, triglyceride, and free fatty acid were significantly decreased in VA-treated HFD rats ($p < 0.05$), indicating the protective effects of VA against hyperinsulinemia, hyperglycemia and hyperlipidemia in HFD rats. Moreover, VA significantly reduced values of area under the curve for glucose ($AUC_{glucose}$) in oral glucose tolerance test and homeostasis model assessment-insulin resistance (HOMA-IR) index, suggesting the improving effect on glucose tolerance and insulin resistance in HFD rats. The Western blot analysis revealed that VA significantly up-regulated expression of hepatic insulin-signaling and lipid metabolism-related protein, including insulin receptor, phosphatidylinositol-3 kinase, glucose transporter 2, and phosphorylated acetyl CoA carboxylase in HFD rats. VA also significantly down-regulated hepatic inflammation-related proteins, including cyclooxygenase-2 and monocyte chemoattractant protein-1 expressions in HFD rats. These results indicate that VA might ameliorate insulin resistance via improving hepatic insulin signaling and alleviating inflammation pathways in HFD rats. These findings also suggest the potential of VA in preventing the progression of DM.

Keywords: vanillic acid; insulin resistance; hyperinsulinemia; hyperglycemia; hyperlipidemia

1. Introduction

As advanced medical technology and improved living standards extend the expectancy of human life, chronic diseases have become a major threat to the health of people. Diabetes mellitus (DM) is one of the fastest-growing chronic diseases. The World Health Organization (WHO) reported that there were more than 347 million people suffering from DM worldwide, and predicted the patient number would double (694 million) by 2030 [1]. The process of DM development involves an initial prediabetes state, and develops into DM if the condition is not appropriately controlled. Therefore, effectively maintaining blood glucose homeostasis has become a crucial issue in DM prevention.

After consuming high-calorie foods, the body is in a hyperglycemic state with an increased insulin secretion, reducing serum glucose to maintain a steady level of serum glucose. Long-term excess intake of high-calorie or high-fat diet (HFD) resulted in increasing blood glucose level and free fatty acid content and induced metabolic related diseases, such as obesity, dyslipidemia, type 2 diabetes mellitus (T2DM), and fatty liver disease [2–4]. The increased blood glucose level caused islet cells to continuously secrete insulin, while the increased free fatty acid content caused an increased lipid synthesis, leading to the accumulation of diacylglycerol in the liver and activation of protein kinase Cε (PKCε). Activated PKCε inhibits the insulin signaling, consequently resulting in hepatic insulin resistance [4]. HFD also tends to be obesity associated. Previous studies indicated that insulin resistance that occurred via obesity is correlated with internal chronic inflammation, which is among the major causes of insulin resistance [5–7]. Increased release of free fatty acids from adipocytes into blood was reported to activate protein kinases, e.g., protein kinase C, which subsequently affected the expression of inhibitor of kappa β kinase, c-Jun N-terminal kinases (JNK), and p38 mitogen-activated protein kinases, stimulating the release of inflammatory factors such as tumor necrosis factor-alpha (TNF-α) and interleukin-6 (IL-6), and causing internal inflammatory responses [8].

Phenolic acids are phytochemicals abundant in various vegetables and fruits. Hydroxybenzoic acid derivatives and hydroxycinnamic acid derivatives are two major categories of phenolic acid [9]. Hydroxycinnamic acid derivative *p*-methoxycinnamic acid promoted glycolysis, reduced gluconeogenesis in the liver of diabetic rats, and increased the secretion of insulin to reduce hyperglycemia in streptozotocin (STZ)-induced diabetic rats [10]. Ferulic acid improved the serum glucose levels and counteracted lipid peroxidation in STZ-induced diabetic mice and KK-Ay spontaneous diabetic mice [11]. Caffeic acid was reported to increase the utilization of glucose by the liver and adipocytes to reduce serum glucose levels in type 2 diabetic mice [12]. Various phenolic acids were found to alleviate the DM and its associated syndromes [9–12]. However, the study of phenolic acids against HFD-induced hyperinsulinemia, hyperglycemia and hyperlipidemia is limited. The aim of the present study is to assess the glucose uptake-enhancing effect *in vitro* and investigate the hypoinsulinemic, hypoglycemic and hypolipidemic effect *in vivo* of phenolic acids. The mechanism of the selected phenolic acid on attenuating insulin resistance in HFD rats is also elucidated.

2. Materials and Methods

2.1. Chemicals

Bovine serum albumin (BSA), caffeic acid, chlorogenic acid, cinnamic acid, D-(+)-glucose, dimethyl sulfoxide (DMSO), disodium hydrogen phosphate (Na_2HPO_4), ferulic acid, 4-(2-hydroxyethyl)-1-piperazineethanesulfonic acid (HEPES), insulin, pioglitazone hydrochloride (Pio), potassium chloride (KCl), potassium dihydrogen phosphate (KH_2PO_4), protocatechuic acid, sinapic acid, sodium chloride (NaCl), sodium phosphate dibasic (Na_2HPO_4), syringic acid, vanillic acid (VA), recombinant mouse tumor necrosis factor (TNF)-α, sulfuric acid (H_2SO_4), Triton X-100, TEMED (*N*,*N*,*N*,*N'*-Tetramethyl-eyhylenediamine), 3-(4,5-dimethylthiazol-2-yl)-2,5-diphenyl-tetrazolium bromide (MTT reagent), and F12 Ham Kaighn's modification (F12K) medium were purchased from Sigma-Aldrich Co. (St. Louis, MO, USA). Fetal bovine serum (FBS) was obtained from Gemini Bio-Products (Woodland, CA, USA). The fluorescent dye 2-(N-(7-nitrobenz-2-oxa-1,3-diazol-4-yl)amino)-2-deoxyglucose (2-NBDG) was purchased from Invitrogen (Camarillo, CA, USA). Bio-Rad protein assay dye reagent was obtained from Bio-Rad Laoboratories (Richmond, VA, USA). All of the chemicals used in this study were of analytical grade.

2.2. Cell Culture

Experiments were performed on a hepatocyte cell line (FL83B) deriving from a fetal mouse (15–17 days). The FL83B cells were incubated in F12K medium containing 10% fetal bovine serum and 1% penicillin and streptomycin (Invitrogen Corporation, Camarillo, CA, USA) in 10 cm Petri dishes at 37 °C and 5% carbon dioxide. Experiments were performed when cells were 80%–90% confluent.

2.3. Tumor Necrosis Factor-Alpha (TNF-α) Induction of Insulin Resistance

The induction of insulin resistance in hepatocytes referred to the method reported by Chang and Shen with minor modifications [13]. FL83B cells were seeded in 10 cm dishes and incubated at 37 °C for 48 h to 80% confluence. Serum-free F12K medium containing 20 ng/mL recombinant mouse TNF-α was then added and incubated for 5 h to induce insulin resistance.

2.4. Uptake of Fluorescent 2-(N-(7-Nitrobenz-2-oxa-1,3-Diazol-4-yl)Amino)-2-Deoxyglucose in FL83B Mouse Hepatocytes

The FL83B cells were detached with trypsin and suspended in 1200 μL of Krebs-Ringer bicarbonate buffer containing 1 μM insulin. Aliquots of the cell suspension (172 μL) were transferred to Eppendorf tubes and co-incubated with 20 μL of 6.25 ng/mL VA and 8 μL of the fluorescent dye 2-NBDG (to a final concentration of 200 μM) in a water bath at 37 °C for 1 h in the dark. The reaction was stopped on ice. The cell suspension was centrifuged at 3000× g (4 °C) for 5 min to remove the supernatant. The pellet was washed with phosphate-buffered saline (PBS) and centrifuged 3 times before being suspended in 1 mL of PBS. The fluorescence intensity of the cell suspension was evaluated using flow cytometry (FACScan, Becton Dickinson, Bellport, NY, USA) at an excitation wavelength of 488 nm and an emission wavelength of 542 nm. Fluorescence intensity reflected the cellular uptake of 2-NBDG.

$$\text{Amelioration rate (\%)} = \frac{((\text{fluorescence intensity of phenolic acid} - \text{treated group}) - (\text{fluorescence intensity of TNF} - \alpha - \text{treated group}))}{(\text{fluorescence intensity of TNF} - \alpha - \text{treated group})} \times 100\ (\%). \tag{1}$$

2.5. Animals and Diets

Male Sprague-Dawley (SD) rats (5 weeks old) were obtained from the National Laboratory Animal Center, Taipei, Taiwan. The rats were maintained in standard laboratory conditions (22 ± 1 °C and a 12 h light/12 h dark cycle) with free access to food and water. Rats were fed a normal diet for 1 week and had a body weight of approximately 250 g. The rats were divided into 4 groups, with each group containing 6 rats. One group was fed a normal diet for 16 weeks (Control group). A second group was fed an HFD (60% calories from fat) throughout the experimental period (HFD group). A third group was provided an HFD for 16 weeks and daily administered Pio (30 mg/kg body weight) on a daily basis during weeks 13–16 (HFD + Pio group). A final group was provided an HFD for 16 weeks, and orally administered VA (30 mg/kg body weight) on a daily basis during weeks 13–16 (HFD + VA group). The rats were sacrificed at the end of the experiment before the blood samples were collected and the biochemical analysis conducted. The organs such as liver, kidney, perirenal and epididymal adipose tissues were isolated from animals and weighed. The liver was stored at −80 °C for the free fatty acid assay and Western blot analysis.

2.6. Blood Sample Preparation

Blood samples were collected and allowed to clot for 30 min at room temperature and then centrifuged at 3000× g for 20 min to obtain the serum, which was stored at −80 °C before use.

2.7. Biochemical Measurements

Enzyme-linked immunosorbent assay kits for rat insulin, total bilirubin, blood urea nitrogen, creatinine, total cholesterol, triglyceride, free fatty acid, and leptin were purchased from Randox Laboratories (Crumlin Co., Antrim, UK). Biochemical analyses were performed according to the manufacturer's protocols.

2.8. Oral Glucose Tolerance Test (OGTT)

The OGTT was performed on rats in all groups after an overnight fast at week 16. All animals were orally administered 1.5 g of glucose/kg body weight. Blood was sampled from the tail vessels of conscious animals before (t = 0) and 30, 60, 90, and 120 min after glucose administration. The samples were allowed to clot for 30 min and then centrifuged (4 °C, 3000× g, 20 min) to obtain the serum. Glucose concentration was determined using a glucose enzymatic kit (Crumlin Co.). The obtained glucose concentration values were plotted against time to provide a curve showing the changes in glucose levels with time, expressed as an integrated area under the curve for glucose ($AUC_{glucose}$).

2.9. Homeostasis Model Assessment of Insulin Resistance (HOMA-IR) Index [14]

The HOMA-IR index was calculated using the following equation:

$$HOMA - IR\,index\ =\ fasting\,serum\,insulin\,(mU/L) \times fasting\,glucose\,(mmol/L)/22.5 \qquad (2)$$

2.10. Western Blot Analysis

Aliquots of supernatants, each containing 50 μg protein, were used to evaluate the expression of insulin receptor (IR), phosphatidylinositol-3 kinase (PI3K), glucose transporter 2 (GLUT-2), cyclooxygenase-2 (COX-2), monocyte chemoattractant protein-1 (MCP-1), and acetyl CoA carboxylase (ACC), phospho-acetyl CoA carboxylase (pACC). The samples were subjected to 10% sodium dodecyl sulfate polyacrylamide gel electrophoresis, and the proteins were electrotransferred to a polyvinylidene difluoride membrane. The membrane was incubated with block buffer (PBS containing 0.05% Tween-20 and 5% *w/v* nonfat dry milk) for 1 h, washed with PBS containing 0.05% Tween-20 (PBST) 3 times, and then probed with 1:2000 diluted solutions of anti-IR, anti-PI3K, anti-GLUT-2, anti-COX-2, anti-MCP-1, and anti-ACC, anti-pACC, antibodies (Gene Tex, Irvine, CA, USA) overnight at 4 °C. The intensity of the blot probed with a 1:4000 diluted solution of mouse monoclonal antibody to bind actin (Gene Tex) was used as a control to ensure that a constant amount of protein was loaded into each lane of the gel. The membrane was washed 3 times (5 min each time) in PBST, shaken in a solution of horseradish peroxidase-linked anti-mouse IgG or anti-rabbit IgG secondary antibody, washed 3 more times (5 min each time) in PBST, and then exposed to enhanced chemiluminescence reagent (Millipore) according to the manufacturer's instructions. The films were scanned and analyzed using a UVP Biospectrum image system (Level, Cambridge, UK).

2.11. Statistical Analysis

Results presented as mean ± standard deviation (SD) were analyzed using one-way ANOVA and Duncan's new multiple range tests. All comparisons were made relative to controls, and $p < 0.05$ was considered significant.

3. Results and Discussion

3.1. Effect of Phenolic Acids on Cell Viability and Glucose Uptake Ability in Insulin-Resistant FL83B Mouse Hepatocytes

The *in vitro* MTT assay is typically used to evaluate the cellular growth inhibition and assess toxicity of drugs or chemicals [15]. Phenolic acids are known to possess antiviral, antioxidative, anticancer, and antihyperglycemic bioactivities [16–18]. However, the effect of phenolic acid on bioactivity and the cytotoxicity in FL83B mouse hepatocytes have not been systematically investigated. Table 1 shows the growth inhibitory of concentration effect of eight naturally occurred phenolic acids on FL83B cells. The results from the cell viability test reveal that the all tested phenolic acids at the concentration of 12.5 μM show above 80%, indicating non-toxicity to FL83B mouse hepatocytes. Therefore, this concentration (12.5 μM) was used to evaluate the glucose uptake-enhancing effect of phenolic acids in insulin resistance cell model.

Table 1. Effects of various concentrations of phenolic acids on cell viability and amelioration rate of glucose uptake in insulin-resistant FL83B cells.

Phenolic Acids \ Concentrations	Cell Viability (%) [a]				Amelioration Rate (%) [b] (12.5 μM Phenolic Acid)
	12.5 μM	25 μM	50 μM	100 μM	
Caffeic acid	102.8 ± 15.8	99.4 ± 16.8	82.0 ± 14.3	74.3 ± 8.6	−6.60
Cinnamic acid	86.2 ± 2.1	88.7 ± 2.5	88.6 ± 6.7	89.6 ± 0.1	−11.30
Ferulic acid	92.7 ± 7.3	88.9 ± 9.1	86.7 ± 6.7	77.4 ± 28.2	−22.01
Protocatechuic acid	91.7 ± 10.4	91.8 ± 9.0	75.4 ± 8.1	71.8 ± 9.0	−12.90
Rosmarinic acid	104.3 ± 17.6	97.2 ± 13.1	102.5 ± 16.5	90.7 ± 22.4	−10.28
Sinapic acid	97.2 ± 2.9	102.1 ± 10.1	102.0 ± 10.5	80.0 ± 9.2	−15.37
Syringic acid	90.9 ± 2.2	79.8 ± 17.4	70.2 ± 13.1	64.6 ± 14.5	8.36
Vanillic acid	114.2 ± 26.3	114.8 ± 18.5	109.8 ± 25.5	116.7 ± 17.6	13.66

[a] Cell viability (%) = (A_{570} of sample group)/(A_{570} of control group) × 100 (%); [b] Amelioration rate (%) = ((fluorescence intensity of phenolic acid-treated group) − (fluorescence intensity of TNF-α-treated group))/(fluorescence intensity of TNF-α-treated group) × 100 (%). Data are expressed as percentage relative to control value (100%) or mean ± SD ($n = 3$).

TNF-α is a cytokine found to interfere with the transmission of insulin signaling and the abilities of liver cells, myofibroblasts, and adipocytes to absorb and metabolize glucose [19–21]. Previously, the 2-NBDG, a modified D-glucose fluorescent derivative, was used to assess the viability of yeast and *Escherichia coli*, and the ability of glucose uptake in FL83B cells treated with TNF-α to induce insulin resistance [13,22,23]. In the present study, fluorescent 2-NBDG was used to evaluate the effect of phenolic acids on glucose uptake ability in insulin-resistant FL83B mouse hepatocytes. As shown in Table 1, VA at concentration of 12.5 μM showed the highest potential for reducing insulin resistance (amelioration rate, 13.66%) among tested phenolic acids. VA was thus used in the subsequent animal experiments.

3.2. Effect of Vanillic Acid on Glucose Tolerance, Serum Insulin and Insulin Resistance Index in High-Fat Diet (HFD)-Fed Rats

HFD is associated with insulin resistance and reduced insulin secretion by β-cells in the pancreas, leading to abnormal glucose tolerance in animal [24–27]. Figure 1a shows the results of OGTT in rats fed HFD for 16 weeks and orally administered with VA daily during the last 4 weeks. The serum glucose levels of rats in the HFD group increased significantly after 30 min, and then decreased slowly. HFD rats treated with Pio or VA exhibited similar changes in serum glucose levels. The $AUC_{glucose}$ for the OGTT, indicating the degree of glucose tolerance in the rats, remained at high levels, thereby indicating low glucose tolerance in the present study. The HFD rats exhibited significantly ($p < 0.05$) lower glucose tolerance than the control rats and VA-treated HFD rats (Figure 1b). In other words, VA can ameliorate the HFD-induced glucose intolerance.

Hyperinsulinemia is likely a marker of insulin resistance, rather than a major, direct contributor to the process [28]. Under hyperglycemic conditions, the pancreas compensates for the decreased insulin response by increasing the insulin secretion; however, the result is hyperinsulinemia to maintain the stable plasma glucose. This process will continue until the reserve capacity is surpassed by metabolic demands and insulin secretion is no longer sufficient; then, blood glucose concentration rises and glucose intolerance and T2DM develop [29–31]. HFD is also reported to be associated with the hyperinsulinemia of rats [32]. In this study, the fasting serum insulin concentration of rats in the HFD group (4.30 ± 1.14 μg/L) was 347.9% higher than that in the control (normal diet) group (0.96 ± 0.33 μg/L) (Figure 1c), indicating the hyperinsulinemia in the HFD rats. However, the serum insulin level of VA-treated HFD rats (2.13 ± 0.64 μg/L) was significantly lower than that in HFD-fed rats, indicating the hypoinsulinemic ability of VA. The rats fed HFD over the long term will develop diabetic symptoms such as insulin resistance [33]. Matthews *et al.* proposed methods using the fasting serum insulin and glucose levels during leisure time to calculate the HOMA-IR index, which is considered a sensitive indicator to assess the degree of insulin resistance [14]. A high HOMA-IR value represents high insulin resistance [14,34]. The advantages of the HOMA-IR are ease of calculation of fasting serum insulin and glucose levels, and potential for extensive use in epidemiological research. As shown in Figure 1d, the HOMA-IR index of VA-treated HFD rats was significantly lower than that of HFD rats, indicating VA may ameliorate the insulin resistance in HFD rats. VA derivative was previously reported to inhibit protein-tyrosine phosphatase 1B (PTP1B) activity, reduce the interference on insulin-signaling proteins, and lead to the alleviation of insulin resistance in T2DM patients [35].

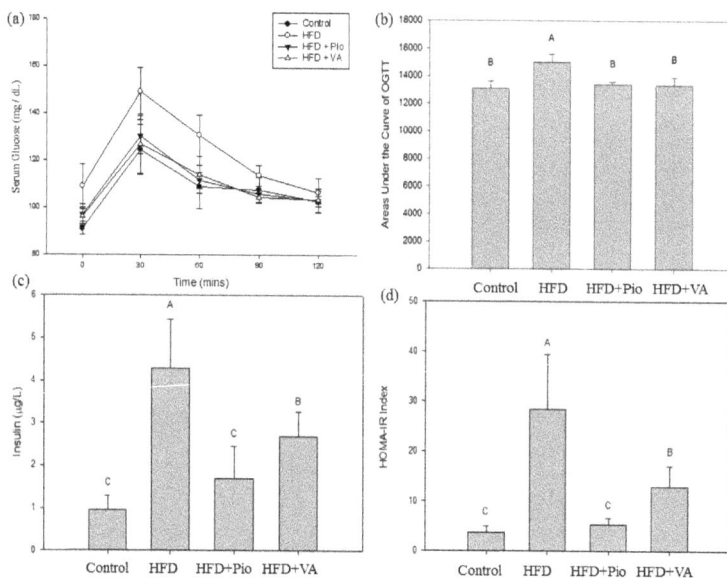

Figure 1. (a) Oral glucose tolerance test (OGTT); (b) area under the curve for glucose ($AUC_{glucose}$) of OGTT; (c) fasting serum insulin, and (d) homeostasis model assessment of insulin resistance (HOMA-IR) in rats fed high-fat diet for 16 weeks and orally administered with vanillic acid during the last 4 weeks. Control: normal diet; HFD: high-fat diet (60 kcal % fat); HFD + Pio: HFD (60 kcal % fat) + pioglitazone (30 mg/kg body weight); HFD + VA: HFD (60 kcal % fat) + vanillic acid (30 mg/kg body weight); (A–C) indicate statistically significant differences $p < 0.05$. Data are presented as mean ± SD (6 rats in each group).

3.3. Effect of Vanillic Acid on Energy Intake, Body Weight, and Selected Organ Weight in HFD-Fed Rats

No significant difference ($p > 0.05$) in the energy intakes among tested groups was observed, indicating that orally administered VA exerts no significant effect on energy intake in HFD rats (Table 2). There was no significant difference in the kidney weights of each group (Table 2). However, after 4 weeks of treatment, the average body, liver and adipose tissue weights of HFD rats were significantly higher than those of Pio and VA-treated HFD rats ($p < 0.05$). HFD was reported to increase serum triglyceride and non-esterified free fatty acid (NEFA) content, thereby resulting in increased lipogenesis in rats [36]. Pio was reported to restrict the increase of adipose tissue and body weight in obese women [37]. Thus, VA was postulated to possess the similar effect as Pio on suppressing accumulation of body fat in HFD-fed rats via the inhibition of lipid synthesis or lipogenesis.

Table 2. The body weight, selected tissue weight, and energy intake in rats fed a high-fat diet for 16 weeks and orally administered with vanillic acid during the last 4 weeks.

Items/Groups	Control	HFD	HFD + Pio	HFD + VA
Body weight (g)	627.1 ± 28.7 [C]	760.7 ± 63.1 [A]	686.0 ± 30.4 [B]	676.9 ± 70.2 [B]
Diet intake (kcal/rat/day)	104.45 ± 4.43 [A]	110.04 ± 11.33 [A]	101.63 ± 5.77 [A]	104.97 ± 9.91 [A]
Liver weight (g)	14.6 ± 0.7 [B]	18.5 ± 2.2 [A]	13.9 ± 1.4 [B]	13.9 ± 1.6 [B]
Kidney weight (g)	1.1 ± 0.4 [A]	1.4 ± 0.5 [A]	1.7 ± 0.2 [A]	0.9 ± 0.6 [A]
Adipose weight (g)	17.7 ± 4.6 [C]	56.1 ± 12.7 [A]	36.7 ± 6.4 [B]	35.3 ± 12.7 [B]

Control: normal diet; HFD: high-fat diet (60 kcal % fat); HFD+Pio: HFD (60 kcal % fat) + pioglitazone (30 mg/kg body weight); HFD + VA: HFD (60 kcal % fat) + vanillic acid (30 mg/kg body weight). Adipose weight: total weight of perirenal and epididymal adipose tissues. ([A–C]) indicate statistically significant differences $p < 0.05$. Data are presented as mean $\pm$ SD ($n = 6$/group). Adipose weight includes epididymal fat pad and abdominal adipose tissue weight.

3.4. Effect of Vanillic Acid on Serum Biochemical Parameters in HFD-Fed Rats

Long term consumption HFD resulting in the increment of adipose tissues. The fatty acids from adipocytes are subsequently released into the blood then transported to periphery tissues such as liver and muscle. The process inhibits the utilization of glycogen and glucose and induces insulin resistance in peripheral tissues. HFD was reported to induce dyslipidemia, resulting in elevated serum glucose, triglyceride, NEFA levels and reduced high-density lipoprotein levels in rats [33,38]. After feeding rats for 16 weeks, the fasting serum glucose of the HFD group was 18.1% higher than that of control group (Table 3). The significant difference ($p < 0.05$) between these two groups was consistent to the previous study and revealed that hyperglycemia was induced in HFD-fed rats in the present study [38]. Furthermore, the fasting serum glucose level in VA-treated rats (94.5 ± 1.9 mg/L) was significantly lower than that in the HFD rats ($p < 0.05$) (Table 3), indicating the hypoglycemic ability of VA.

Moreover, the fasting serum triglyceride and free fatty acid concentration of rats in the HFD group are higher than those in the control group by 20.8% and 27.2%, respectively (Table 3), indicating the hyperlipidemia in the HFD rats. However, the fasting serum triglyceride and free fatty acid were significantly reduced in HFD rats supplemented with VA (71.63 ± 13.42 µg/L, 0.76 ± 0.14 mmol/L) compared to the HFD rats ($p < 0.05$), suggesting the hypolipidemic ability of VA.

Leptin is a hormone secreted by adipose tissues and regulates utilization of lipid in human body. The serum leptin concentration of in the HFD rats was significantly ($p < 0.05$) higher than that in control group (Table 3). Comparatively, the serum leptin level was significantly reduced ($p < 0.05$) in HFD rats after 4-weeks VA treatment (Table 3). Previous studies reported a positive correlation between serum leptin concentration and body fat content, and suggested that people with obesity or T2DM have higher serum leptin levels than healthy people do [39,40]. Studies have also indicated that leptin reduces body weight, body fat, energy intake, serum glucose levels, and insulin concentration in mice [41,42]. However, the mechanism underlying such effects was still unidentified. We speculate that HFD promotes leptin production and is involved in the accumulation of hepatic NEFA and the induction of hepatic insulin resistance in rats subsequently.

Table 3. The fasting serum parameters in rats fed high-fat diet for 16 weeks and orally administered with vanillic acid during the last 4 weeks.

Items/Groups	Control	HFD	HFD + Pio	HFD + VA
Glucose (mg/dL)	90.8 ± 1.7 [B]	107.2 ± 5.5 [A]	97.0 ± 3.7 [B]	94.5 ± 1.9 [B]
Triglyceride (mg/dL)	74.13 ± 18.20 [B]	89.50 ± 11.70 [A]	61.50 ± 9.80 [B]	71.63 ± 13.42 [B]
Free fatty acid (mmol/L)	0.92 ± 0.09 [B]	1.17 ± 0.26 [A]	0.69 ± 0.16 [C]	0.76 ± 0.14 [B,C]
Total cholesterol (mg/dL)	62.38 ± 9.71 [A]	51.63 ± 14.35 [A]	58.13 ± 9.95 [A]	40.00 ± 6.41 [B]
Leptin (ng/mL)	162.3 ± 32.6 [B]	986.3 ± 413.8 [A]	429 ± 69.7 [B]	303.2 ± 84.2 [B]
Bili-total (mg/dL)	0.08 ± 0.01 [A]	0.07 ± 0.01 [A]	0.05 ± 0.01 [B]	0.07 ± 0.02 [A]
BUN (mg/dL)	15.33 ± 1.25 [A]	9.55 ± 0.91 [C]	12.80 ± 1.05 [B]	10.96 ± 2.11 [C]
Creatinine (mg/dL)	0.35 ± 0.05 [AB]	0.38 ± 0.05 [A]	0.31 ± 0.04 [B]	0.38 ± 0.05 [A]

Bili-total: total bilirubin; BUN: blood urea nitrogen. Control: normal diet; HFD: high-fat diet (60 kcal % fat); HFD + Pio: HFD (60 kcal % fat) + pioglitazone (30 mg/kg body weight); HFD + VA: HFD (60 kcal % fat) + vanillic acid (30 mg/kg body weight); $(^{A-C})$ indicate statistically significant differences $p < 0.05$. Data are presented as mean ± SD (6 rats in each group).

3.5. Effect of Vanillic Acid on Hepatic Insulin Signaling, Inflammation and NEFA Formation in HFD-Fed Rats

Insulin is a hormone with multiple effects. Binding of insulin to the α-subunit of the insulin receptor molecule induces rapid auto-phosphorylation of the β-subunit, which leads to an increase of its tyrosine kinase activity [43]. Tyrosine phosphorylation of insulin receptor proteins induces the cytoplasmic binding activity of insulin receptor substrate-1 (IRS-1) to insulin receptor. IRS-1 plays a pivotal role in transmitting signals from insulin receptors to intracellular PI3K/Akt pathway, which eventually results in the second intracellular step of insulin action, targeting tyrosine-phosphorylated insulin receptor β and IRS-1 [29,43–45]. IR is a condition in which defects in the action of insulin are such that normal levels of insulin do not operate as the signal for glucose uptake [43]. After a 4-week administration of VA, a down-regulation of hepatic insulin signaling-related proteins, such as IR, PI3K, and GLUT-2, was found in HFD group rats as compared with the control group (Figure 2). These results suggested that VA normalizes hepatic insulin signaling and alleviates hepatic insulin resistance in the liver of HFD-fed rats.

The chronic inflammation increases the development of obesity-related insulin resistance [5]. COX-2, an enzyme involved in inflammatory responses, is barely detectable in normal conditions and rapidly up-regulated in the inflammation conditions [28]. MCP-1, an inflammatory cytokine, is up-regulated in the conditions of hyperlipidemia and inflammation [46]. As shown in Figure 3, HFD up-regulated the hepatic COX-2 and MCP-1 protein expressions as compared with the control group. In contrast, the expressions of COX-2 and MCP-1 protein were down-regulated ($p < 0.05$) after a 4-week VA treatment in HFD-fed rats. Diet-induced obesity is a type of inflammatory response, with up-regulated COX-2 and MCP-1 protein expressions observed in the internal tissues of obese rats [47,48].

HFD increases the lipid synthesis in liver and adipose tissues, induces chronic inflammatory responses thus leading to insulin resistance in mice [28,37]. Acetyl CoA carboxylase (ACC), an essential enzyme in fatty acid synthesis, is activated by dephosphorylation and transforms acetyl CoA into malonyl CoA through carboxylation. Enhancing phosphorylation of ACC protein may thus reduce adipose tissue formation and NEFA accumulation in peripheral tissue, including liver [49]. Excess NEFA from adiposity was reported to cause insulin resistance by inhibiting insulin signaling in T2DM [49]. In the present study, the phosphorylated ACC/ACC protein expression of liver significantly decreased, indicating the increment of hepatic lipogenesis in the HFD rats (Figure 4a). The expression of hepatic phosphorylated ACC/ACC protein expression was increased, and the hepatic NEFA level reduced in HFD rats treated with VA for 4 weeks (Figure 4b). The current study suggests that VA may reduce hepatic NEFA accumulation via promoting the phosphorylation of ACC protein expression in liver of HFD rats.

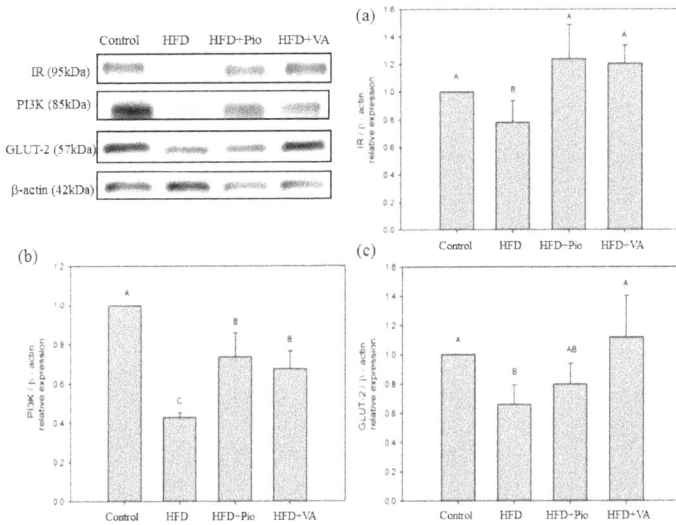

Figure 2. Hepatic (**a**) insulin receptor (IR); (**b**) phosphoinositide 3-kinase (PI3K); and (**c**) glucose transporter 2 (GLUT-2) proteins expression in rat fed high-fat diet for 16 weeks and orally administered vanillic acid during the last 4 weeks. Control: normal diet; HFD: high-fat diet (60 kcal % fat); HFD + Pio: HFD (60 kcal % fat) + pioglitazone (30 mg/kg body weight); HFD + VA: HFD (60 kcal % fat) + vanillic acid (30 mg/kg body weight); (A–C) indicate statistically significant differences $p < 0.05$. Data are presented as mean ± SD (3 rats in each group).

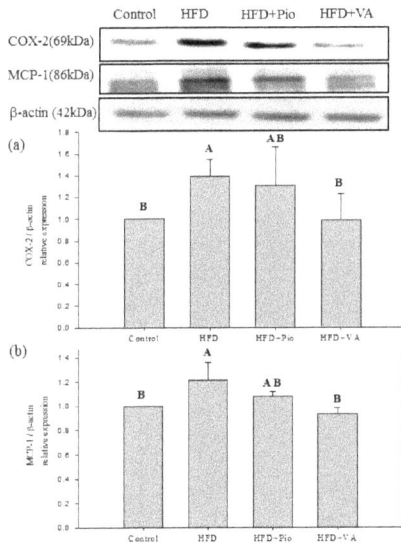

Figure 3. Hepatic (**a**) cyclooxygenase 2 (COX-2) and (**b**) monocyte chemoattractant protein-1 (MCP-1) protein expression in rats fed high-fat diet for 16 weeks and orally administered with vanillic acid during the last 4 weeks. Control: normal diet; HFD: high-fat diet (60 kcal % fat); HFD + Pio: HFD (60 kcal % fat) + pioglitazone (30 mg/kg body weight); HFD + VA: HFD (60 kcal % fat) + vanillic acid (30 mg/kg body weight); (A–C) indicate statistically significant differences $p < 0.05$. Data are presented as mean ± SD (3 rats in each group).

45

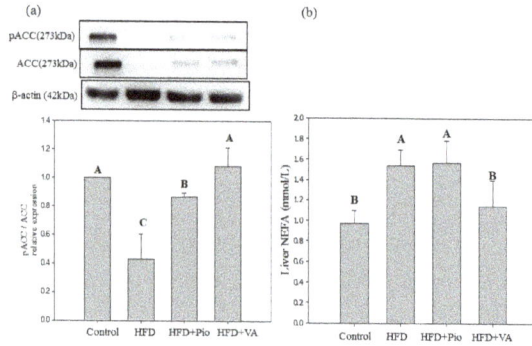

Figure 4. (**a**) Hepatic phosphorylated acetyl-CoA carboxylase/acetyl-CoA carboxylase (pACC/ACC) protein expression; and (**b**) non-esterified free fatty acid (NEFA) in rats fed high-fat diet for 16 weeks and orally administered with vanillic acid during the last 4 weeks. Control: normal diet; HFD: high-fat diet (60 kcal % fat); HFD + Pio: HFD (60 kcal % fat) + pioglitazone (30 mg/kg body weight); HFD + VA: HFD (60 kcal % fat) + vanillic acid (30 mg/kg body weight); NEFA: non-esterified free fatty acid in supernatant of liver homogenate. The liver tissue was homogenized with PBS (1/4; *w/v* and centrifuged at 4 °C for 60 min to obtain the supernatant; (A–C) indicate statistically significant differences $p < 0.05$. Data are presented as mean ± SD (6 rats in each group).

Previous studies indicated that high concentration of NEFA was associated with increased expression of MCP-1 or COX-2 [50,51]. Recent reports also suggest that chronic MCP-1 or COX-2-mediated inflammation in fat is crucial for obesity-linked insulin resistance [52,53]. Phenolic acids were previously reported to exert counteractive effect on inflammation, and prevent the processing of chronic diseases [18]. The results from this study elucidate that VA may reduce hepatic NEFA level, decrease hepatic inflammatory responses and subsequently alleviate insulin resistance in HFD rats.

4. Conclusions

VA is a naturally occurring phenolic acid widely existing in various plant foods. The present study demonstrates that the protective effect of VA against hyperinsulinemia, hyperglycemia and hyperlipidemia is through decreasing hepatic NEFA accumulation, alleviating hepatic inflammation as well as hepatic insulin resistance in HFD-fed rats (Figure 5). Our findings support that VA exerts therapeutic effects and has the potential to be used in clinical medicine or as a dietary supplement for preventing the progression of DM.

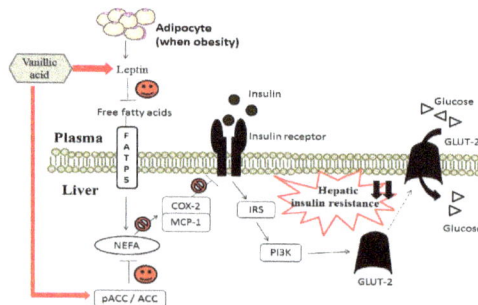

Figure 5. The postulated mechanisms underlying the effect of vanillic acid on hepatic insulin resistance by regulating insulin signaling and inflammation pathways in rats fed an HFD.

Acknowledgments: The authors would like to thank the Ministry of Science and Technology of the Republic of China (ROC), Taiwan, for financially supporting this research under contract No. NSC 100-2313-B-003-001. Our gratitude also goes to the Academic Paper Editing Clinic, National Taiwan Normal University.

Author Contributions: Wen-Chang Chang, James Swi-Bea Wu, Hsu-Min Chien and Szu-Chuan Shen designed the research; Chen-Wen Chen, Po-Ling Kuo and Wen-Chang Chang performed the experimental work; Szu-Chuan Shen, Wen-Chang Chang and Yuh-Tai Wang wrote the manuscript. All authors discussed, edited and approved the final version.

Conflicts of Interest: The authors declare no conflict of interest.

References

1. World Health Organization. Preventing Diabetes is Essential for Keeping Health and Well-Being in Tajikistan. 2011. Available online: http://www.euro.who.int/en/health-topics/noncommunicable-diseases/diabetes/news/news/2011/11/preventing-diabetes-is-essential-for-keeping-health-and-well-being-in-tajikistan (accessed on 21 November 2011).

2. Buettner, R.; Parhofer, K.G.; Woenckhaus, M.; Wrede, C.E.; Kunz-Schughart, L.A.; Scholmerich, J.; Bollheimer, L.C. Defining high-fat-diet rat models: Metabolic and molecular effect of different fat types. *Mol. Endocrinol.* **2006**, *36*, 485–501. [CrossRef] [PubMed]

3. Okabayashi, Y.; Maddux, B.A.; Mcdonald, A.R.; Logsdon, C.D.; Williams, J.A.; Goldfine, I.D. Mechanisms of insulin-induced insulin-receptor downregulation: Decrease of receptor biosynthesis and mRNA levels. *Diabetes* **1989**, *38*, 182–187. [CrossRef] [PubMed]

4. Samuel, V.T. Fructose induced lipogenesis: From sugar to fat to insulin resistance. *Trends Endocrinol. Metab.* **2011**, *22*, 60–65. [CrossRef] [PubMed]

5. Xu, H.; Barnes, G.T.; Yang, Q.; Tan, G.; Yang, D.; Chou, C.J.; Sole, J.; Nichols, A.; Ross, J.S.; Tartaglia, L.A.; *et al.* Chronic inflammation in fat plays a crucial role in the development of obesity-related insulin resistance. *J. Clin. Investig.* **2003**, *112*, 1821–1830. [CrossRef] [PubMed]

6. Arkan, M.C.; Hevener, A.L.; Greten, F.R.; Maeda, S.; Li, Z.W.; Long, J.M.; Wynshaw-Boris, A.; Poli, G.; Olefsky, J.; Karin, M. IKK-β links inflammation to obesity-induced insulin resistance. *Nat. Med.* **2005**, *11*, 191–198. [CrossRef] [PubMed]

7. Cai, D.; Yuan, M.; Frantz, D.F.; Melendez, P.A.; Hansen, L.; Lee, J.; Shoelson, S.E. Local and systemic insulin resistance resulting from hepatic activation of IKKβ and NF-κB. *Nat. Med.* **2005**, *11*, 183–190. [CrossRef] [PubMed]

8. Qatanani, M.; Lazar, M.A. Mechanisms of obesity-associated insulin resistance: Many choices on the menu. *Gene. Dev.* **2007**, *21*, 1443–1455. [CrossRef] [PubMed]

9. Kilmartin, P.A.; Zou, H.; Waterhouse, A.L. A cyclic voltammetry method suitable for characterizing antioxidant properties of wine and wine phenolics. *J. Agric. Food Chem.* **2001**, *49*, 1957–1965. [CrossRef]

10. Adisakwattana, S.; Roengsamran, S.; Hsu, W.H.; Yibchok-Anun, S. Mechanisms of antihyperglycemic effect of *p*-methoxycinnamic acid in normal and streptozotocin-induced diabetic rats. *Life Sci.* **2005**, *78*, 406–412. [CrossRef] [PubMed]

11. Ohnishi, M.; Matuo, T.; Tsuno, T.; Hosoda, A.; Normura, E.; Taniguchi, H.; Sasaki, H.; Morishita, H. Antioxidation activity and hypoglycemic effect of ferulic acid in STZ-induced diabetic mice and KK-Ay mice. *Biofactors* **2004**, *21*, 315–319. [CrossRef] [PubMed]

12. Jung, U.J.; Lee, M.K.; Park, Y.B.; Jeon, S.M.; Choi, M.S. Antihyperglycemic and antioxidant properties of caffeic acid I *db/db* mice. *J. Pharmacol. Exp. Ther.* **2006**, *318*, 476–483. [CrossRef] [PubMed]

13. Chang, W.C.; Shen, S.C. Effect of water extracts from edible Myrtaceae plants on uptake of 2-(*N*-(7-nitrobenz-2-oxa-1,3-diazol-4-yl)amino)-2-deoxyglucose (2-NBDG) in tumor necrosis factor-α-treated FL83B mouse hepatocytes. *Phytother. Res.* **2013**, *27*, 236–243. [CrossRef] [PubMed]

14. Matthews, D.R.; Hosker, J.P.; Rudenski, A.S.; Naylor, B.A.; Treacher, D.F.; Turner, R.C. Homeostasis model assessment: Insulin resistance and beta-cell function from fasting plasma glucose and insulin concentrations in man. *Diavetologia* **1985**, *28*, 412–419. [CrossRef]

15. Sargent, J.M. The use of the MTT assay to study drug resistance in fresh tumor samples. *Recent Results Cancer Res.* **2003**, *161*, 13–25.
16. Bahorun, T.; Luximon-Ramma, A.; Crozier, A.; Aruoma, O.I. Total phenol, flavonoid, proanthocyanidin and vitamin C levels and antioxidant activities of Mauritian vegetables. *J. Sci. Food Agric.* **2004**, *84*, 1553–1561. [CrossRef]
17. Inoue, M.; Suzuki, R.; Sakaguchi, N.; Li, Z.; Takeda, T.; Ogihara, Y.; Jiang, B.Y.; Chen, Y. Selective induction of cell death in cancer cells by gallic acid. *Biol. Pharm. Bull.* **1995**, *18*, 1526–1530. [CrossRef]
18. Scalbert, A.R.; Johnson, I.T.; Saltmarsh, M. Polyphenols: Antioxidants and beyond. *Am. J. Clin. Nutr.* **2005**, *81*, 215S–217S. [PubMed]
19. Feinstein, R.; Kanety, H.; Papa, M.Z.; Lunenfeld, B.; Karasik, A. Tumor necrosis factor-alpha suppresses insulin-induced tyrosine phosphorylation of insulin receptor and its substrates. *J. Biol. Chem.* **1993**, *268*, 26055–26058.
20. Peraldi, P.; Hotamisligil, G.S.; Buurman, W.A.; White, M.F.; Spiegelman, B.M. Tumor necrosis factor (TNF-α) inhibits insulin signaling through stimulation of the p55 TNF receptor and activation of sphingomyelinase. *J. Biol. Chem.* **1996**, *271*, 13018–13022.
21. Kroder, G.; Bossenmayer, B.; Kellerer, M.; Capp, E.; Stoyanov, B.; Muhlhofer, A.; Berti, L.; Horikoshi, H.; Ullrich, A.; Haring, H. Tumor necrosis factor-alpha and hyperglycemia-induced insulin resistance. *J. Clin. Investig.* **1996**, *97*, 1471–1477. [CrossRef] [PubMed]
22. Yoshioka, K.; Oh, K.B.; Saito, M.; Nemoto, Y.; Matsuoka, H. Evaluation of 2-[*N*-(7-nitrobenz-2-oxa-1,3-diazol-4-yl)amino]-2-deoxy-D-glucose, a new fluorescent derivative of glucose, for viability assessment of yeast *Candida albicans*. *Appl. Microbiol. Biotechnol.* **1996**, *46*, 400–404.
23. Louzao, M.C.; Espiña, B.; Vieytes, M.R.; Vega, F.V.; Rubiolo, J.A.; Baba, O.; Terashima, T.; Botana, L.M. "Fluorescent glycogen" formation with sensibility for *in vivo* and *in vitro* detection. *Glycoconj. J.* **2008**, *25*, 503–510. [CrossRef] [PubMed]
24. Kraegen, E.W.; James, D.E.; Storlien, L.H.; Burleigh, K.M.; Chisholm, D.J. *In vivo* insulin resistance in individual peripheral tissues of the high fat fed rat: Assessment by euglycaemic clamp plus deoxyglucose administration. *Diabetologia* **1986**, *29*, 192–198. [CrossRef]
25. Pedersen, O.; Kahn, C.R.; Flier, J.S.; Kahn, B.B. High fat feeding causes insulin resistance and a marked decrease in the expression of glucose transporters (Glut 4) in fat cells of rats. *Endocrinology* **1991**, *129*, 771–777. [CrossRef] [PubMed]
26. Ahren, B.; Gudbjartsson, T.; Al-Amin, A.N. Islet perturbations in rats fed a high-fat diet. *Pancreas* **1999**, *18*, 75–83. [CrossRef] [PubMed]
27. Kaiyala, K.J.; Prigeon, R.L.; Kahn, S.E.; Woods, S.C.; Porte, D.; Schwartz, M.W. Reduced β-cell function contributes to impaired glucose tolerance in dogs made obese by high-fat feeding. *Am. J. Physiol.* **1999**, *277*, E659–E667. [PubMed]
28. Ginsberg, H.N. Insulin resistance and cardiovascular disease. *J. Clin. Investig.* **2000**, *106*, 453–458. [CrossRef] [PubMed]
29. Jellinger, P.S. Metabolic consequences of hyperglycemia and insulin resistance. *Clin. Cornerstone* **2007**, *8*, S30–S42. [CrossRef]
30. Bahadoran, Z.; Mirmiran, P.; Azizi, F. Potential efficacy of broccoli sprouts as a unique supplement for management of type 2 diabetes and its complications. *J. Med. Food* **2013**, *16*, 375–382. [CrossRef] [PubMed]
31. Hekmatdoost, A.; Mirmiran, P.; Hosseini-Esfahani, F.; Azizi, F. Dietary fatty acid composition and metabolic syndrome in Tehranian adults. *Nutrition* **2011**, *27*, 1002–1007. [CrossRef] [PubMed]
32. Prada, P.O.; Zecchin, H.G.; Gasparetti, A.L.; Torsoni, M.A.; Ueno, M.; Hirata, A.E.; do Amaral, M.E.; Höer, N.F.; Boschero, A.C.; Saad, M.J. Western diet modulates insulin signaling, c-Jun N-terminal kinase activity, and insulin receptor substrate-1ser307 phosphorylation in a tissue-specific fashion. *Endocrinology* **2005**, *146*, 1576–1587. [CrossRef] [PubMed]
33. Huang, B.W.; Chiang, M.T.; Yao, H.T.; Chiang, W. The effect of high-fat and high-fructose diets on glucose tolerance and plasma lipid and leptin levels in rats. *Diabetes Obes. Metab.* **2004**, *6*, 120–126. [CrossRef]

34. Bonora, E.; Targher, G.; Alberiche, M.; Bonadonna, R.C.; Saggiani, F.; Zenere, M.B.; Monauni, T.; Muggeo, M. Homeostasis model assessment closely mirrors the glucose clamp technique in the assessment of insulin sensitivity: Studies in subjects with various degrees of glucose tolerance and insulin sensitivity. *Diabetes Care* **2000**, *23*, 57–63. [CrossRef] [PubMed]

35. Feng, Y.; Carroll, A.R.; Addepalli, R.; Fechner, G.A.; Avery, V.M.; Quinn, R.J. Vanillic acid derivatives from the green algae *Cladophora socialis* as potent protein tyrosine phosphatase 1B inhibitors. *J. Nat. Prod.* **2007**, *70*, 1790–1792. [CrossRef] [PubMed]

36. Fraze, E.; Chiou, M.; Chen, Y.; Reaven, G.M. Age-related changes in postprandial plasma glucose, insulin, and free fatty acid concentrations in nondiabetic individuals. *J. Am. Geriatr. Soc.* **1987**, *35*, 224–228. [CrossRef] [PubMed]

37. Jensen, M.D.; Haymond, M.W.; Rizza, R.A.; Cryer, P.E.; Miles, J.M. Influence of body fat distribution on free fatty acid metabolism in obesity. *J. Clin. Investig.* **1989**, *83*, 1168–1173. [CrossRef] [PubMed]

38. Wang, Y.; Wang, P.Y.; Qin, L.Q.; Davaasambuu, G.; Kaneko, T.; Xu, J.; Murata, S.I.; Katoh, R.; Sato, A. The development of diabetes mellitus in wistar rats kept on a high-fat low-carbohydrate diet for long periods. *Endocrine* **2003**, *22*, 85–92. [CrossRef]

39. Considine, R.V.; Sinha, M.K.; Heiman, M.L.; Kriauciunas, A.; Stephens, T.W.; Nyce, M.R.; Ohannesian, J.P.; Marco, C.C.; Mckee, L.J.; Baur, T.L.; *et al.* Serum immunoreative-leptin concentrations in normal weight and obese human. *N. Engl. J. Med.* **1996**, *334*, 292–295. [CrossRef] [PubMed]

40. Maffei, M.; Halaas, J.; Ravussin, E.; Pratley, R.E.; Lee, G.H.; Zhang, Y.; Fei, H.; Kim, S.; Lallone, R.; Ranganathan, S.; *et al.* Leptin levels in human and rodent: Measurement of plasma leptin and *ob* RNA in obese and weight-reduced subjects. *Nat. Med.* **1995**, *1*, 1155–1161. [CrossRef]

41. Pelleymounter, M.A.; Cullen, M.J.; Baker, M.B.; Hecht, R.; Winters, D.; Boone, T.; Collins, F. Effects of the obese gene product on body weight regulation in ob/ob mice. *Science* **1995**, *269*, 540–543. [CrossRef] [PubMed]

42. Halaas, J.L.; Gajiwala, K.S.; Maffei, M.; Cohen, S.L.; Chait, B.T.; Rabinowitz, D.; Lallone, R.L.; Burley, S.K.; Friedman, J.M. Weight-reducing effects of the plasma protein encoded by the obese gene. *Science* **1995**, *269*, 543–546. [CrossRef]

43. Ghorbani, Z.; Hekmatdoost, A.; Mirmiran, P. Anti-hyperglycemic and insulin sensitizer effects of turmeric and its principle constituent curcumin. *Int. J. Endocrinol. Metab.* **2014**, *12*. [CrossRef] [PubMed]

44. Panzhinskiy, E.; Hua, Y.; Lapchak, P.A.; Topchiy, E.; Lehmann, T.E.; Ren, J.; Nair, S. Novel curcumin derivative CNB-001 mitigates obesity-associated insulin resistance. *J. Pharmacol. Exp. Ther.* **2014**, *349*, 248–257. [CrossRef] [PubMed]

45. Martyn, J.A.; Kaneki, M.; Yasuhara, S. Obesity-induced insulin resistance and hyperglycemia: Etiologic factors and molecular mechanisms. *Anesthesiology* **2008**, *109*, 137–148. [CrossRef] [PubMed]

46. Bose, T.; Alvarenga, J.C.; Tejero, M.E.; Voruganti, V.S.; Proffitt, J.M.; Freeland-Graves, J.H. Association of monocyte chemoattractant protein-1 with adipocyte number, insulin resistance and liver function markers. *J. Med. Primatol.* **2009**, *38*, 418–424. [CrossRef] [PubMed]

47. Weisberg, S.P.; Hunter, D.; Huber, R.; Lemieux, J.; Slaymaker, S.; Vaddi, K.; Charo, I.; Leibel, R.L.; Ferrante, A.W. CCR2 modulates inflammatory and metabolic effects of high-fat feeding. *J. Clin. Investig.* **2006**, *116*, 115–124. [CrossRef] [PubMed]

48. Esposito, E.; Iacono, A.; Bianco, G.; Autore, G.; Cuzzocrea, S.; Vajro, P.; Canani, R.B.; Calignano, A.; Raso, G.M.; Meli, R. Probiotics reduce the inflammatory response induced by a high-fat diet in the liver of young rats. *J. Nutr.* **2009**, *139*, 905–911. [CrossRef] [PubMed]

49. Capurso, C.; Capurso, A. From excess adiposity to insulin resistance: The role of free fatty acids. *Vascul. Pharmacol.* **2012**, *57*, 91–97. [CrossRef] [PubMed]

50. Jiang, C.H.; Yao, N.; Wang, Q.Q.; Zhang, J.H.; Sun, Y.; Xiao, N.; Liu, K.; Huang, F.; Fang, S.Z.; Shang, X.L.; *et al.* Cyclocarya paliurus extract modulates adipokine expression and improves insulin sensitivity by inhibition of inflammation in mice. *J. Ethnopharmacol.* **2014**, *153*, 344–351. [CrossRef] [PubMed]

51. Hsieh, P.S.; Jin, J.S.; Chiang, C.F.; Chan, P.C.; Chen, C.H.; Shih, K.C. COX-2-mediated inflammation in fat is crucial for obesity-linked insulin resistance and fatty liver. *Obesity* **2009**, *17*, 1150–1157. [CrossRef] [PubMed]

52. Lloyd, E.E.; Gaubatz, J.W.; Burns, A.R.; Pownall, H.J. Sustained elevations in NEFA induce cyclooxygenase-2 activity and potentiate THP-1 macrophage foam cell formation. *Atherosclerosis* **2007**, *192*, 49–55. [CrossRef] [PubMed]

53. Mas, S.; Martínez-Pinna, R.; Martín-Ventura, J.L.; Pérez, R.; Gomez-Garre, D.; Ortiz, A.; Fernandez-Cruz, A.; Vivanco, F.; Egido, J. Local non-esterified fatty acids correlate with inflammation in atheroma plaques of patients with type 2 diabetes. *Diabetes* **2010**, *59*, 1292–301. [CrossRef] [PubMed]

nutrients

MDPI

Article

Involvement of the Niacin Receptor GPR109a in the Local Control of Glucose Uptake in Small Intestine of Type 2 Diabetic Mice

Tung Po Wong, Leo Ka Yu Chan and Po Sing Leung *

School of Biomedical Sciences, Faculty of Medicine, The Chinese University of Hong Kong, Shatin, Hong Kong, China; wongtp@cuhk.edu.hk (T.P.W.); leokychan@link.cuhk.edu.hk (L.K.Y.C.)

* Correspondence: psleung@cuhk.edu.hk; Tel.: +852-3943-6879 (ext. 36879); Fax: +852-2603-5139.

Received: 3 August 2015; Accepted: 26 August 2015; Published: 8 September 2015

Abstract: Niacin is a popular nutritional supplement known to reduce the risk of cardiovascular diseases by enhancing high-density lipoprotein levels. Despite such health benefits, niacin impairs fasting blood glucose. In type 2 diabetes (T2DM), an increase in jejunal glucose transport has been well documented; however, this is intriguingly decreased during niacin deficient state. In this regard, the role of the niacin receptor GPR109a in T2DM jejunal glucose transport remains unknown. Therefore, the effects of diabetes and high-glucose conditions on GPR109a expression were studied using jejunal enterocytes of 10-week-old *m+/db* and *db/db* mice, as well as Caco-2 cells cultured in 5.6 or 25.2 mM glucose concentrations. Expression of the target genes and proteins were quantified using real-time polymerase chain reaction (RT-PCR) and Western blotting. Glucose uptake in Caco-2 cells and everted mouse jejunum was measured using liquid scintillation counting. 10-week T2DM increased mRNA and protein expression levels of GPR109a in jejunum by 195.0% and 75.9%, respectively, as compared with the respective *m+/db* control; high-glucose concentrations increased mRNA and protein expression of GPR109a in Caco-2 cells by 130.2% and 69.0%, respectively, which was also confirmed by immunohistochemistry. In conclusion, the enhanced GPR109a expression in jejunal enterocytes of T2DM mice and high-glucose treated Caco-2 cells suggests that GPR109a is involved in elevating intestinal glucose transport observed in diabetes.

Keywords: enterocytes; jejunum; glucose transport; SGLT1; GLUT2; Caco-2; hyperglycemia; hyperlipidemia

1. Introduction

Diabetes mellitus is classically one of the most common chronic metabolic disorders, which is characterized by a plethora of clinical complications; they include, but are not limited to, cardiovascular disease, end-stage renal diseases, diabetic foot disorders, and blindness. One of the most notable clinical manifestations of diabetic patients is dyslipidemia, which is the major risk factor for cardiovascular disease in type 2 diabetes mellitus (T2DM). It has been reported that diabetics have significantly higher coronary-event-associated deaths than the non-diabetics [1]. Furthermore, diabetic individuals without known clinical coronary heart disease (CHD) are exposed to comparable risk of mortality compared to those non-diabetics who have experienced a myocardial infarction [2], thus leading to the recognition of diabetes as a CHD-risk-equivalent condition [3].

In order to address this issue, scientists have taken strides to develop novel therapeutic agents that ameliorate cardiovascular disease by specifically targeting dyslipidemia in diabetic patients. In recent years, niacin, also known as nicotinic acid or Vitamin B3, has been a popular nutritional supplement; in fact, it is widely used to treat cardiovascular disease which is associated with dyslipidemia by lowering the level of low-density lipoprotein and triglycerides, while raising the level of high-density lipoprotein simultaneously [4]. Notwithstanding the existence of these health benefits, niacin has been shown to induce glucose intolerance in patients, as evidenced by significant increases in blood glucose levels (5.83 mg/dL) after three years of niacin treatment in euglycemic patients (9.88 mg/dL for niacin *vs.* 4.05 mg/dL for without niacin) [5]. Meanwhile, the incidence rate of impaired fasting blood glucose was increased by 29%. In patients suffering from hyperglycemia, high doses of niacin also increased their level of Hemoglobin A1c by about 0.3% [6]. It is recognized that oral niacin elevated blood glucose levels and thereby deteriorated diabetes in some patients; however, the precise mechanism still remains unknown [7]. In contrast, a lower V_{max} for jejunal glucose uptake *vs.* control group was observed in rats fed with niacin deficient diet [8]. Niacin deficiency also significantly lowers the active electrogenic absorption of glucose across jejunal mucosa [9]. Collectively, these findings have shown that niacin, to a certain extent, might not be beneficial in terms of its adverse effects on glucose homeostasis observed in diabetic patients.

Of interest in this context is our recent data showing that such a niacin-induced hyperglycemia is probably mediated via the activation of niacin receptor GPR109A-mediated ROS-PPARγ-UCP2 (reactive oxygen species-peroxisome proliferator-activated receptor-γ-uncoupling protein 2) signaling pathway in the pancreatic islet β-cells [10]. In addition, previous studies have shown that niacin exerts its effects by binding to its specific G protein-coupled receptors HM74 (GPR109B) and its homologues HM74A (GPR109A) [11–13]. In terms of its potency, niacin activates GPR109A and GPR109B with half maximal effective concentration (EC_{50}) values of 0.1 mM and 100 mM, respectively [14]. Both GPR109A and GPR109B have been expressed in the human colon and localized to the apical membrane of colonocytes [15]. In mice, GPR109A is expressed in both small and large intestines [12,16]. Despite these findings, the role of GPR109A in jejunal glucose uptake is still elusive. Interestingly, jejunal glucose transport via both sodium-dependent glucose transporter (SGLT1) and glucose transporter 2 (GLUT2) is greatly increased in early diabetes [17]. In this respect, SGLT1 is a high-affinity, low-capacity transporter localized at the brush border membrane (BBM) of jejunal enterocytes, which is responsible for active uptake of glucose from the intestinal lumen; however, GLUT2 is a glucose transporter normally situated on the basolateral membrane of the jejunal enterocytes but it is translocated and inserted into the BBM during enhanced SGLT1-mediated glucose uptake [18–20]. In this way, glucose transport capability of GLUT2 can be up to three times greater than that of SGLT1 [21].

Given the fact that dietary glucose is a critical component in determining our blood glucose homeostasis and in light of the above-mentioned findings, the present study was designed to unravel the undiscovered role of niacin in the regulation of intestinal glucose uptake, with particular emphasis on T2DM, and its potential interaction with the intestinal glucose transporters, SGLT1 and GLUT2, thus its consequence on glucose homeostasis.

2. Experimental Section

2.1. Animals

4- to 12-week-old male *m+/db* and *db/db* mice in this study were used and supplied by the Laboratory Animal Services Centre at The Chinese University of Hong Kong. Animals were maintained on a standard chow (Prolab RMH 2500, 5P14; Lab Diet, St. Louis, MO, United States) and water *ad libitum* up to the time of experiment. Only those diabetic mice with blood glucose levels above 10 mM were included in the diabetic group. Anesthesia before experimentation was achieved with pentobarbitone sodium (50 mg/kg) intraperitoneally. All procedures have been approved by the Animal Experimentation Ethics Committee of the Chinese University of Hong Kong (No. 10/064/MIS).

2.2. Isolation of Enterocytes

Enterocytes were prepared from 4 cm long jejunal segments, beginning 4 cm distal to the ligament of Treitz. Intestinal epithelia cells were isolated and harvested by a Ca^{2+}-chelation technique [22]. Briefly, isolated intestinal segments were flushed through with ice-cold saline followed by air. The segment was tied off at one end and filled with Ca^{2+}-free hypertonic isolation buffer (7 mM K_2SO_4,

44 mM K_2HPO_4, 9 mM $NaHCO_3$, 10 mM HEPES, 2 mM L-glutamine, 0.5 mM dithiothreitol, 1 mM Na_2EDTA, and 180 mM glucose, pH 7.4), equilibrated with 95% O_2 and 5% CO_2, where over-distention was avoided. The segment was then tied off to form a closed sac and incubated in 0.9% saline at 37 °C with gentle shaking for 16 min. Cells were dislodged manually, and the resulting suspension was collected and centrifuged for 30 s at 500 g; the pellet was re-suspended in freshly prepared cold buffer and this procedure was repeated twice, as we reported previously [23,24].

2.3. Western Blot Analysis

The procedures of Western blot have been described previously [25]. Proteins from the enterocyte and Caco-2 cells were extracted using the CytoBuster protein extraction reagent (Novagen, Darmstadt, Germany) and quantified using Bio-Rad Bradford assay kit (Bio-Rad, Munich, Germany). Proteins (10 µg/lane) were subjected to electrophoresis on a 10% (weight (wt)/volume (vol)) polyacrylamide gel. Proteins from the polyacrylamide gel were transferred to the polyvinylidene difluoride membrane using a semi-dry transblot unit (Bio-Rad, Munich, Germany). The protein-blotted membrane was saturated by submersion in 5% (wt/vol) nonfat skimmed milk in phosphate buffered saline (PBS) (pH 7.4) with 0.1% (vol/vol) Tween-20 for one hour at room temperature. The membranes were incubated with anti-HM74(M-65) receptor rabbit polyclonal antibodies (SC-134583; Santa Cruz Biotechnology, Dallas, TX, United States)(1:100), anti-NIACR1 (Niacin receptor 1) rabbit polyclonal antibodies (NBP1-92180, Novus Biologicals, Littleton, CO, United States) (1:100), and anti-β-actin mouse polyclonal antibodies (EMD Millipore, Danvers, Massachusetts, United States) (1:5000) overnight at 4 °C. After washing with 0.1% Tween-20 in Phosphate-buffered saline (PBS), membranes were incubated with the following corresponding peroxidase-labeled secondary antibodies for one hour at room temperature: anti-rabbit Immunoglobulin G (IgG) antibody (GE Healthcare Bio-Sciences, Pittsburgh, PA, United States) (1:1300) and anti-mouse IgG antibody (GE Healthcare Bio-Sciences, Pittsburgh, PA, United States) (1:2500). The positive signal was revealed using Enhanced Chemiluminescence-plus (ECL-plus); GE Healthcare Bio-Sciences, Pittsburgh, PA, United States) western blotting detection reagent and Fuji Medical Super RX-N autoradiography film (FUJIFILM, Valhalla, NY, United States). The intensity of the bands was quantified using FluorChem software (ProteinSimple, San Jose, CA, United States). The corresponding expression of β-actin of each sample was used to normalize its expression of the target protein.

2.4. Real-Time PCR Analysis

Quantitative RT-PCR was performed using StepOne™ Real-Time PCR Systems (ThermoFisher Scientific, Grand Island, NY, United States). The procedure has been described previously [26]. Briefly, total RNA was extracted from freshly prepared enterocytes or Caco-2 cells grown in 5.6, 11.2, or 25.2 mM glucose using Trizol reagent (ThermoFisher Scientific, Grand Island, NY, United States) according to the manufacturer's instructions. RNase Out (ThermoFisher Scientific, Grand Island, NY, United States) was added to the RNA solutions to prevent degradation by RNase. Total RNA served as the template for cDNA preparation using iScript™ Select cDNA Synthesis Kit (Bio-Rad Laboratories, Munich, Germany). Primers were designed from mice and human cDNA sequences using Primer Express Software provided by ThermoFisher Scientific. Mice β-actin and Human β-actin were used as reference genes to normalize the relative expression of each target gene. The sequences of primers used are shown in Table 1. Sybergreen reactions were set up in a volume of 25 µL with ABI two-step sybergreen PCR reagents (ThermoFisher Scientific, Grand Island, NY, United States). Each reaction consisted of 12.5 µL PCR master mix, 0.05 to 0.30 µM of each amplification primer, and 1 µL cDNA. Each sample was run in duplicate with an initial 10-min period at 95 °C to enable the reaction, followed by 40 cycles at 95 °C for 15 s and 60 °C for 1 min. The samples were heated to 60 °C for 1 min, then to 95 °C over the next minute, and finally cooled slowly from 95 °C to 60 °C over 20 min to collect data for the analysis of dissociation curve. Amplification data were collected by the detector of the StepOne™ Real-Time PCR Systems and analyzed with Sequence Detection System software

(ThermoFisher Scientific, Grand Island, NY, United States). The threshold cycle (C_T) of each sample was determined from the time point where fluorescence was first detected, with the cycle number being inversely related to cDNA concentration. The fold changes in mRNA expression were calculated using the $2^{-\Delta\Delta CT}$ method [27].

Table 1. Sequences of specific primers used for real-time quantitative RT-PCR.

Gene	Forward Primer	Reverse Primer
Mouse β-actin (NM_007393.4)	TCCTCCTGAGCGCAAGTACTC	GTGGACAGTAGTGAGGCCAGGT
Mouse GPR109a (NM_030701.3)	GGCGTGGTGCAGTGAGCAGT	GGCCCACGGACAGGCTAGGT
Human β-actin (NC_000007.14)	GGCACCCAGCACAATGAAGATC	ATGCTTCTAGGCGGACTATGACTT
Human GPR109a (NM_177551.3)	TGCCGCCCTTCCTGATGGACA	TGTTCAGGGCGTGGTGGGGA

2.5. Immunohistochemistry

Immunofluorescence was carried out as described previously with some modifications to determine the mucosal localization of niacin receptors [23]. Isolated jejunal segments were rinsed with cold saline and then quickly transferred to ice-cold 4% paraformaldehyde (PFA) in 0.1 M PBS (pH 7.4) and incubated at 4 °C overnight. Tissue segments were rinsed with PBS and incubated with 20% sucrose in PBS at 4 °C overnight and later embedded in optimum cutting temperature medium (Tissue-Tek, Sakura Finetek Europe B.V., Zoeterwoude, The Netherlands). Sections (6 μm) were collected on Superforst slides (Gerhard Menzel GmbH, Braunschweig, Germany), and these were boiled in 10 mM citrate buffer for 10 min to retrieve the antigens. Sections were incubated with 1% (wt/vol) bovine serum albumin (BSA) and 6% (wt/vol) normal donkey serum (NDS) (Jackson Immuno Research, West Grove, PA, United States) for one hour at room temperature to block nonspecific antibody binding. The slides were incubated overnight at 4 °C with primary antibody (SC-134583; Santa Cruz Biotechnology, Dallas, TX, United States) (1:100), diluted in PBS with 2% NDS and 0.1% Triton X-100. After three washes with PBS, bound primary antibodies were detected by incubation with their corresponding secondary antibodies labeled with Cyc-3 (Jackson Immuno Research, West Grove, PA, United States) (1:100, diluted with 0.1 M PBS containing 2% NDS) at room temperature for 1 h. Immunoreactivity was captured with a fluorescent microscope equipped with a DC480 digital camera (Leica Microsystems, Buffalo Grove, IL, United States). Human Caco-2 cells were grown on silane-coated cover slips, incubated with ice-cold 4% PFA in 0.1 M PBS (pH 7.4) for 8 min, and washed three times with 0.1 M PBS, followed by the same steps as the immunostaining procedures mentioned above starting from the incubation with 1% BSA and 6% NDS (wt/vol), except that anti-NIACR1 rabbit polyclonal antibodies (NBP1-92180) (1:100) was used as the primary antibody.

2.6. Glucose Uptake by Everted Jejunal Sleeves

Prior to measurements of glucose uptake, long jejunal segments (3 to 4 cm long) were taken 3 cm distal to the ligament of Treitz. Glucose uptake was measured using everted jejunal sleeves [28,29]. In brief, isolated jejunal segments were rinsed with cold saline and everted over a glass rod. The tissue was tied securely to the rod and pre-incubated in gassed carbogen (95% O_2, 5% CO_2) bicarbonate buffer (128 mM NaCl, 4.7 mM KCl, 2.5 mM $CaCl_2$, 1.2 mM KH_2PO_4, 1.2 mM $MgSO_4$, and 20 mM $NaHCO_3$) without glucose for 4 min at 37 °C followed by 15 min using the same buffer, with 0.1 μM to 2 mM of niacin (Sigma-Aldrich, St Louis, MO, United States). Then, concentrated D-glucose was added to the buffer to make up to a final glucose concentration of 50 mM with 0.2 μCi/mL D-[^{14}C]glucose (GE Healthcare Bio-Sciences, Pittsburgh, PA, United States) with trace amounts of 0.1 μCi/mL L-[^{3}H]glucose (Sigma-Aldrich, St Louis, MO, United States) to correct for non-specific uptake. After a 2 min incubation, the segments were washed rapidly with ice-cold saline containing 0.3 mM phlorizin with stirring for 1 min. The tissue was removed from the rod, oven-dried, and weighed. The dried residue was incubated with Soluene-350 (Perkin-Elmer, Waltham, MA, United States) at 60 °C for 4 h. Scintillation fluid (Ultima Gold; Perkin-Elmer, Waltham, MA, United States) was added, and counting of radioactivity was carried out. The rate of glucose uptake was calculated as picomole per milligram dry weight intestine per second.

2.7. Glucose Uptake by Caco-2 Cells

Caco-2 cells were purchased from ATCC (catalog no. HTB-37). Cells were grown at 37 °C in minimum essential medium (M2279; Sigma-Aldrich, St Louis, MO, United States) with 20% fetal bovine serum (FBS), 1% nonessential amino acids (#11140; ThermoFisher Scientific, Grand Island, NY, United States), and 1% penicillin-streptomycin and gassed with 95% air–5% CO_2. Cells were subcultured at ~80% confluence, at a cell density of between 8×10^4 and 1×10^5 cells/cm^2. The medium was changed every two days, and cells were used 14 days after confluence, when they expressed characteristics of enterocyte differentiation [30,31]. Caco-2 cells grown in media containing 5.6 and 25.2 mM glucose for 14 days after confluence were harvested by Trizol reagent (Thermo Fisher Scientific, NY, United States) for RNA isolation and real-time PCR reaction, and Cytobuster (EMD Millipore, Danvers, MA, United States) for Western blotting.

Caco-2 cells grown in 5.6 mM glucose were rinsed with 25 °C oxygenated bicarbonate buffer (128 mM NaCl, 4.7 mM KCl, 2.5 mM $CaCl_2$, 1.2 mM KH_2PO_4, 1.2 mM $MgSO_4$, and 20 mM $NaHCO_3$) with 10% FBS, 1% penicillin-streptomycin, and 1% nonessential amino acids. Cells were preincubated in gassed (95% O_2–5% CO_2) bicarbonate buffer containing 50 mM mannitol for 1 h at 37 °C. The buffer was then replaced with fresh bicarbonate buffer containing 50 mM glucose and 0.2 μCi/mL D-[^{14}C]glucose (GE Healthcare Bio-Sciences, Pittsburgh, PA, United States), with or without 0.1 μM to 2 mM niacin. In some experiments, 0.3 mM phlorizin or 0.1 mM phloretin was also present. Cells were washed quickly three times by stirring in ice-cold saline containing 0.3 mM phlorizin. The cells were digested with 0.3 M NaOH, and aliquots were added to scintillation fluid (Ultima Gold; Perkin-Elmer, Waltham, MA, United States). Glucose uptake was measured as disintegrations per min per well of a six-well plate containing a monolayer of Caco-2 cells.

2.8. siRNA Knockdown of GPR109a in Caco-2 Cells

Caco-2 cells grown on six wells plates reached 70% confluence at the time of transfection. One day before the transfection, the medium was changed to one containing no antibiotics. Stock Stealth™ RNA (ThermoFisher Scientific, Grand Island, NY, United States) was diluted to 40 nM with 50 μL Opti-MEM® I Reduced Serum Medium without serum. Lipofectamine®2000 (ThermoFisher Scientific, Grand Island, NY, United States) was diluted 50 times with Opti-MEM®I Reduced Serum Medium (ThermoFisher Scientific, Grand Island, NY, United States) and incubated 5 min at room temperature. The diluted Stealth™ RNA and Lipofectamine®2000 was mixed and incubated at room temperature for 10 min. The oligomer-Lipofectamine®2000 complexes were added to each well, followed by incubation of the cells at 37 °C in CO2 incubator for 72 h. The transfected cells were harvested for either protein detection or glucose uptake.

2.9. Statistical Analysis

All results were analyzed using Prism 3.0 software. The data were expressed as means ± standard error of the mean (SEM). Student's unpaired two-tailed *t*-test and One-Way Analysis of variance (ANOVA) (Tukey's post-hoc test) were employed to detect significant differences between two groups and among three or more groups, respectively. For all comparisons, $p < 0.05$ was considered statistically significant. For RT-PCR, the C_T value of the target gene of a sample was first corrected for the C_T value of β-actin, before being statistically analyzed [27].

3. Results

3.1. Enterocyte Expression of GPR109a

The real-time PCR analysis of mRNA expression of GPR109a normalized to β-actin revealed the presence of GPR109a mRNA in both *m+/db* and *db/db* mouse jejunal brush border (Figure 1A). Expression of GPR109a mRNA in enterocytes from 10-week-old *db/db* mice was higher than that seen in four-week-old *db/db* mice. At the age of 10 weeks, expression of GPR109a in *db/db* mouse jejunum was 2.96 folds greater than that of the control 10-week-old *m+/db* mouse jejunum. Consistently, Western blotting of enterocyte protein also revealed the presence of GPR109a protein in both *m+/db* and *db/db* mice (Figure 1B). Expression levels of GPR109a protein in enterocytes from 10-week-old diabetic *db/db* mice were 1.76 folds greater than their corresponding control 10-week-old *m+/db* mice.

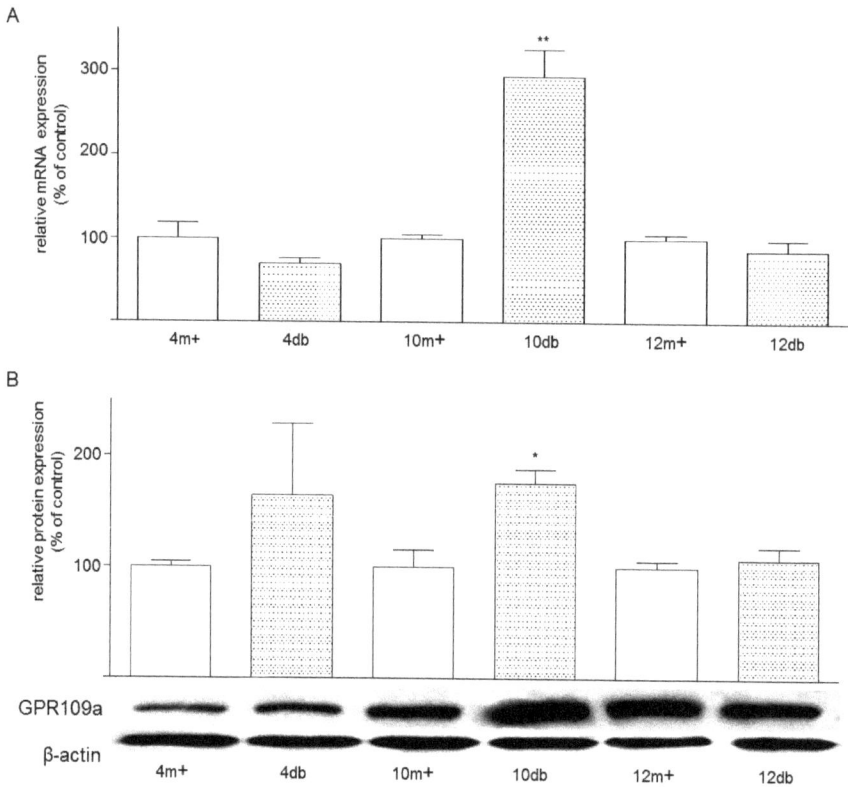

Figure 1. (**A**) Effects of age and Type 2 Diabetes Mellitus (T2DM) on the mRNA expression of GPR109a in jejunal mucosa. Mouse mRNA abundance was determined by real-time PCR using jejunal mucosa and data were calculated as the percentage of their corresponding m+ non-diabetic controls. All results are expressed relative to enterocytes of non-diabetic rats, and are given as mean ± standard error of the mean (SEM), $n = 3$–4; 10 db *vs.* 10 m+, ** $p < 0.01$; (**B**) Effects of age and T2DM on the protein expression of GPR109a in jejunal enterocytes. Western blot analysis showing the relative expression of GPR109a in homogenates of enterocytes prepared from jejuna of *m+/db* and *db/db* mice of 4, 10 or 12 weeks of age. Data were calculated as the percentage change compared to their corresponding *m+* non-diabetic control. Results are expressed as means ± SEM, $n = 3$–5, 10m+ *vs.* 10 db, * $p < 0.05$. 4m+, 8m+, 10m+ and 12m+ represent 4-, 8-, 10- and 12-week-old *m+/db* mice respectively; whereas 4 db, 8 db, 10 db and 12 db represent 4-, 8-, 10- and 12-week-old *db/db* mice, respectively.

3.2. Localization of GPR109a in Jejunal Mucosa of m+/db and db/db Mice, and Caco-2 Cells

Immunohistochemical results showed the localization of GPR109a at the level of the BBM along the entire jejunal villus length in both normal (*m+/db*) (Figure 2A–C) and diabetic (*db/db*) (Figure 2D–F) animals. However, expression of GPR109a was consistently higher in diabetic jejunum and this was particularly apparent at higher magnification (Figure 2H diabetic *vs.* Figure 2G normal). On the other hand, immunocytochemistry also revealed the presence of niacin receptors at the cell membrane of Caco-2 cells from the 14 days after confluence (Figure 2J–O). In examination, expression of niacin receptor was higher in cells grown in 25.2 mM glucose (Figure 2M) compared to those cultured in 5.6 mM glucose (Figure 2J).

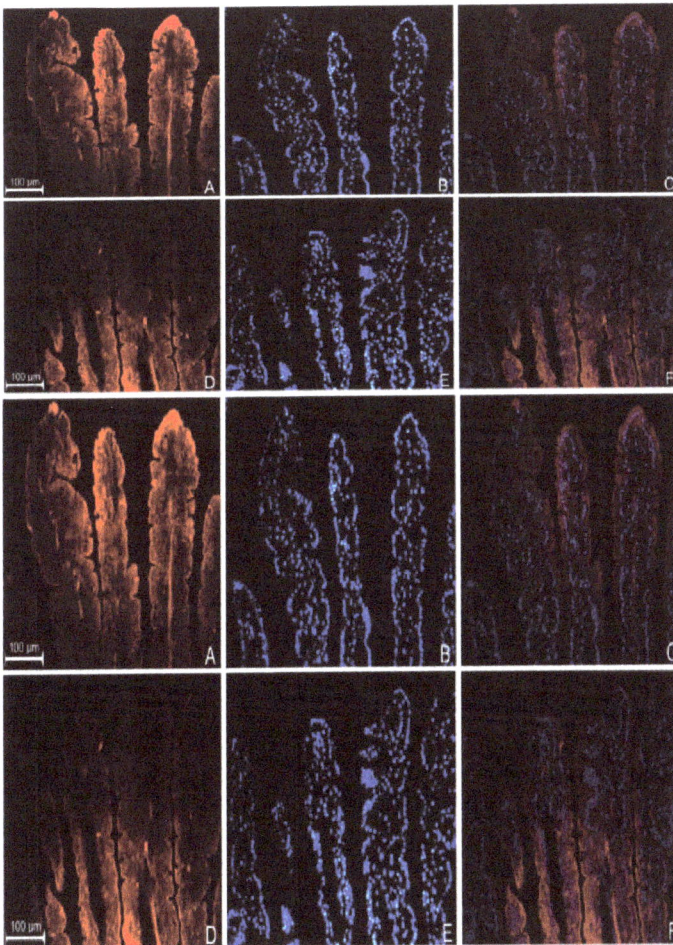

Figure 2. Immunodetection of GPR109a in jejunum of 10-week-old *m+/db* mice (**A**) and 10-week-old *db/db* mice (**D**). (**B,E**) are the nuclear DAPI staining of (**A,D**) respectively; (**C,F**) are their corresponding merged images. Higher magnification of niacin receptor staining of *m+/db* (**G**) and *db/db* (**H**); (**I**) shows jejunal sections prepared in the absence of primary antibodies (negative control). Immunodetection of niacin receptor in Caco-2 cells grown in 5.6 mM (**J**) and 25.2 mM glucose (**M**); (**K,N**) show nuclear 4′,6-diamidino-2-phenylindole (DAPI) staining of (**J**) and (**M**) respectively; (**L,O**) are the corresponding merged images.

3.3. Effects of Niacin on Jejunal Glucose Uptake

Next, we attempted to study the role of GPR109a in modulating jejunal glucose uptake. By using the intestine from non-diabetic (*m+/db*) mice, mucosal exposure to niacin for 10 min increased glucose uptake in a dose-dependent fashion (Figure 3). At 1 mM niacin, glucose uptake was increased by 26.8%.

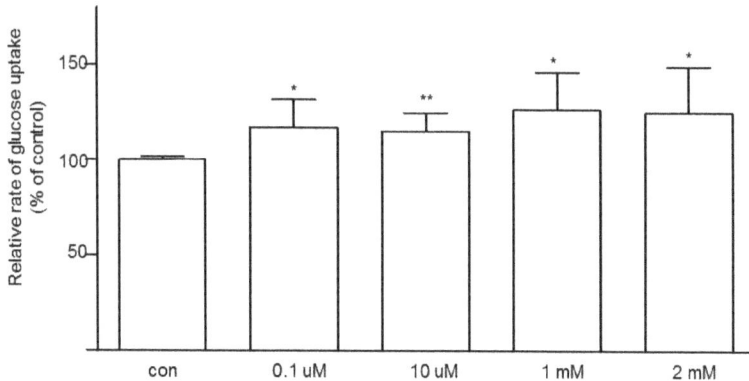

Figure 3. The dose-dependent effect of niacin on jejunal glucose uptake using 10-week-old *m+/db* mice. Data are expressed as relative percentage of glucose uptake relative to the control (con). *n* = 6 for each concentration of niacin. Data are given as means ± standard error of the mean (SEM), * $p < 0.05$ *vs.* control; ** $p < 0.01$ *vs.* control.

3.4. Effects of Glucose Concentrations on the Expression of GPR109a in Caco-2 Cells

Caco-2 cells were used to study the effects of glucose concentrations of the growth medium on the gene expression of GPR109a. GPR109a mRNA was expressed in Caco-2 cells grown in both low glucose and high glucose media. In comparison with the low glucose concentration (5.6 mM), it was observed that high glucose concentration (25.2 mM) increased both of the gene and protein levels of niacin receptor expression by 130.2% and 69%, respectively (Figure 4A, B).

3.5. Effects of Niacin and Glucose Transporter Inhibitors on Glucose Uptake in Caco-2 Cells

We also sought to study the role of the niacin receptor GPR109a in the modulation of glucose uptake in Caco-2 cells. Caco-2 cells grown on normal glucose (5.6 mM) and exposed to niacin for 10 min increased glucose uptake in a dose-dependent fashion (Figure 5A); at 1 mM niacin, glucose uptake was increased by 20.1%. On the other hand, the effects of the two glucose transporter inhibitors, the SGLT1 blocker phlorizin (0.3 mM) and GLUT2 blocker phloretin (0.1 mM), in the presence or absence, on the glucose uptake of Caco-2 cells grown in normal 5.6 mM glucose were also examined. As shown, 0.3 mM phlorizin and 0.1 mM phloretin inhibited glucose uptake by 23.3% and 62.5%, respectively.In addition, 1 mM niacin further increased glucose uptake when present with 0.3 mM phlorizin and 0.1 mM phloretin (Figure 5B). These data indicate that both SGLT1 and GLUT2 may be involved in the upregulation of niacin-induced glucose uptake.

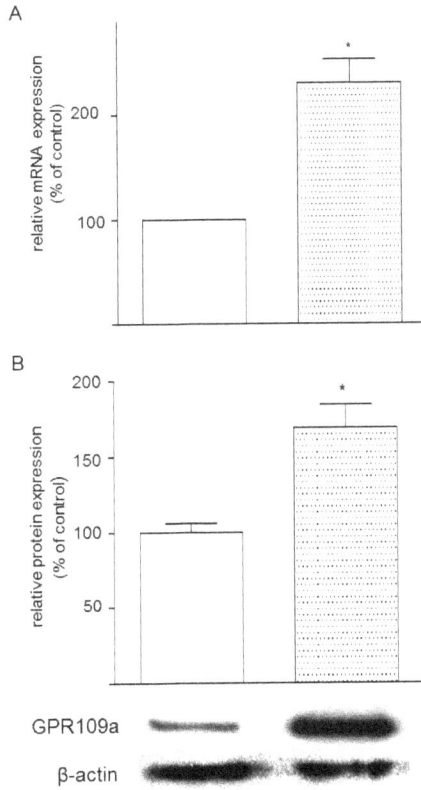

Figure 4. (**A**) Effects of high glucose concentration (25.2 mM) on the mRNA expression of GPR109a in Caco-2 cells *vs.* low glucose concentration (5.6 mM). Results are expressed as means ± standard error of the mean (SEM), $n = 3$, control = 5.6 mM glucose, control *vs.* 25.2 mM glucose, * $p < 0.05$; (**B**) Effects of high glucose (25.2 mM) on GPR109a protein expression in Caco-2 cells *vs.* control 5.6 mM glucose concentrations. Results are expressed as means ± SEM, $n = 6$, control = 5.6 mM *vs.* 25.2 mM, * $p < 0.05$.

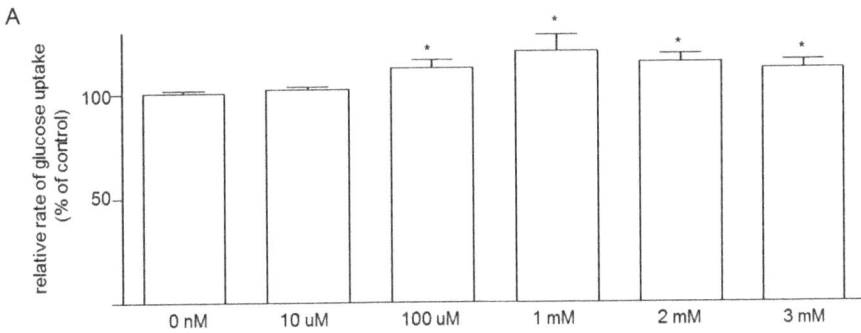

Figure 5. *Cont.*

B

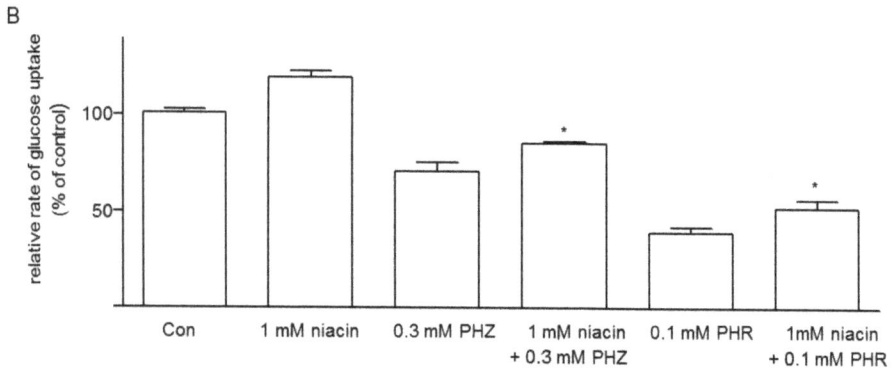

Figure 5. (**A**) Dose dependent effect of niacin on glucose uptake by Caco-2 cells grown in glucose (5.6 mM) (expressed as percentage of glucose uptake relative to their control). $n = 6$ for each concentration of niacin. Data are given as means ± standard error of the mean (SEM), 0 nM *vs.* treatment groups, * $p < 0.05$; (**B**) Glucose uptake by Caco-2 cells grown in 5.6 mM glucose showing effect of 1 mM niacin, with or without phlorizin (PHZ, 0.3 mM) and phloretin (PHR, 0.1 mM). Results are expressed relative to the respective control value (con). All data are given as means ± SEM, $n = 6$. 0.3 mM PHZ *vs.* 0.3 mM PHZ + 1 mM niacin and 0.1 mM PHR *vs.* 0.1 mM PHR + 1 mM niacin, * $p < 0.05$.

3.6. Effects of Knockdown of GPR109a on Glucose Uptake in Caco-2 Cells

Three different siRNA sequences (HSS155268, HSS155269 and HSS155270) were tried in the study of knockdown of niacin receptor in Caco-2 cells grown in 5.6 mM glucose. Western blot analysis showed that the knockdown experiments with siRNA HSS155269, HSS155270 and HSS155268 decreased protein expression of niacin receptors by 45.0%, 53.7%, and 32.5%, respectively as compared with the negative siRNA control group (Figure 6A). Therefore, we selected the siRNA HSS155270, the most effective knockdown sequence, which decreased the rate of glucose uptake of Caco-2 cells grown in 5.6 mM glucose by 30.2% (Figure 6B).

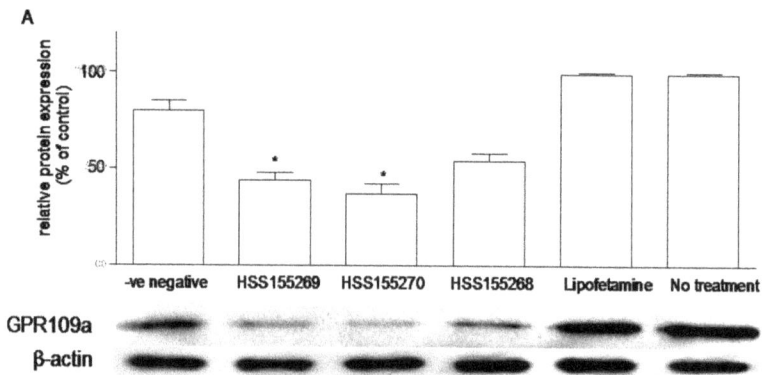

Figure 6. *Cont.*

B

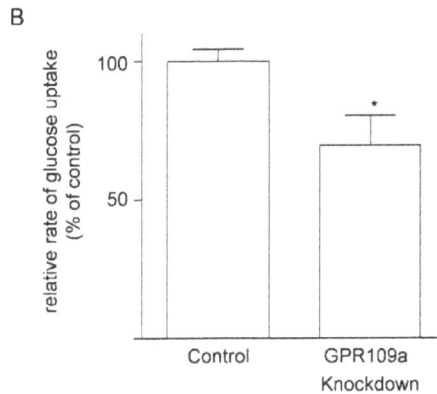

Figure 6. (**A**) Effects of siRNA knockdown of GPR109a on the expression of GPR109a protein in Caco-2 cells grown in 5.6 mM glucose. Western blot analysis showing the relative expression of niacin receptor in homogenates of cells prepared from the -ve negative (negative control siRNA, *Silencer*® Select Negative Control siRNA, non-targeting SiRNA with limited sequence similarity to known genes), and three different sequences of siRNA (HSS155269, HSS155270 and HSS155268). "Lipofetamine" contains only the lipofetamine transfection buffer, without any siRNA. "No treatment" contains neither the transfection buffer nor any siRNA. Results are expressed as means ± standard error of the mean (SEM), $n = 6$. HSS155269 *vs.* negative control, 45% decrease in expression, * $p < 0.05$; HSS155270 *vs.* negative control, 53.8% decrease in expression, * $p < 0.05$; (**B**) Effects of siRNA (HSS155270) knockdown of GPR109a on the glucose uptake of Caco-2 cells grown in 5.6 mM glucose. Knockdown of GPR109a decreased the rate of glucose uptake by 30.2%, $n = 5$, * $p < 0.05$.

4. Discussion

Niacin is a commonly employed anti-hyperlipidemia drug but it is also widely known to induce hyperglycemia during chronic and high-dose therapy [5,6]. Despite this, the mechanistic action of niacin and its receptor GPR109a in the regulation of glucose homeostasis, in particular with intestinal glucose uptake, remains ambiguous. The present study has shown, for the first time, that enterocyte GPR109a is expressed and functional in the local control of intestinal glucose absorption, and that type 2 diabetic and high glucose conditions upregulate the GPR109a expression, thus enhancing niacin-induced intestinal glucose uptake in the mice. Our laboratory has recently reported the novel role of niacin, via its activation of GPR109A, in pancreatic islets [10]. In that study, niacin was found to increase fasting glucose concentrations, reduce glucose-stimulated insulin secretion (GSIS) and insulin secretion, and impair glucose tolerance, thereby inducing pancreatic islet dysfunctions in high-fat diet (HFD) induced obese mice [10]. In this regard, the present study establishes a previously undiscovered role of niacin in local regulation of glucose homeostasis at the level of the small intestine in normal and diabetic states.

In the present study, we have first demonstrated that the mRNA and protein expression levels of the niacin receptor GPR109a were elevated in the diabetic *db/db* mice, as evidenced by real-time qPCR and Western blot, as well as further supported by the immunohistochemical results. Interestingly, an upregulated expression GPR109a was also observed in diabetic mouse and human retina, where GPR109a could serve as an anti-inflammatory receptor in retinal pigment epithelial cells and is closely associated with diabetic retinopathy [32]. It is well recognized that inflammatory process is a key causative factor in the pathogenesis of diabetes and GPR109a has been shown to be a potent anti-inflammatory receptor in various physiologically important organs, including but not limiting to, the colon [33], blood vessels [34], and pancreas [10]. In light of these findings, it prompts us to speculate that such an elevated GPR109a expression may be responsible for acting as a strategic counteractive mechanism against the inflammatory insults, as induced by hyperglycemia in diabetic states.

To address this issue, we sought to examine whether niacin could locally regulate glucose uptake across the small intestinal BBM. In fact, our laboratory has previously shown the functional existence of a local renin-angiotensin system (RAS) in the regulation of intestinal glucose uptake, where binding of the two physiologically active components of this system, angiotensin II, to its angiotensin type 1 receptor and the binding of angiotensin (1–7) to the Mas receptor at the jejunal BBM in enterocytes inhibit SGLT1-mediated glucose transport across this membrane in a dose-dependent fashion [23,35]. Therefore, we explore to investigate whether niacin is also able to regulate glucose uptake locally in the intestine. First of all, it is necessary to address if niacin arriving at the small intestine would be adequate to elicit its physiological function. Studies have shown that niacin is indeed equally absorbed by the stomach and the upper small intestine in human [36]. In fact, up to about four grams of niacin could be almost completely absorbed by adults. Intestinal luminal concentration of niacin under physiological conditions has been reported to lie in the micromolar but not in the millimolar range [37]. As a result, there should be sufficient amount of niacin reaching the jejunum for its physiological actions. Our results showed that niacin increased intestinal glucose uptake in *m+/db* mice significantly and dose-dependently; these data were further substantiated by the observed decrease in glucose uptake after GPR109a knockdown in Caco-2 cells. Our findings are in line with the observation that niacin treatment increases glucose uptake in adipocytes where such an effect of niacin on glucose uptake was antagonized by theophylline and isoprenaline, which are that agents that increase intracellular concentrations of $3',5'$-cyclic adenosine monophosphate (cAMP); in addition, niacin could further increase the maximum rate of glucose transport stimulated by insulin in adipocytes [38]. In adipocytes, niacin treatment significantly lowered the intracellular concentrations of cAMP in adipocytes, and a decrease in cAMP level upregulated glucose uptake [38,39]. However, cAMP has been shown to stimulate SGLT1 and thus mediated intestinal glucose uptake in enterocytes [40], thereby contradicting the findings in adipocytes. Not withstanding these findings, it might be plausible to postulate that cAMP is a downstream signaling molecule of GPR109a for its subsequent mediation of glucose uptake. Despite this, further investigations are warranted in order to confirm the precise role of cAMP in jejunal enterocytes.

Apart from the *in vivo* data, we further investigated the effects of high glucose treatment on the expression profiles of mRNA and protein of GPR109a in human Caco-2 cells. Our data revealed that 25.2 mM glucose concentration raised remarkably the mRNA and protein levels of GPR109a, when compared to those of the Caco-2 cells grown in 5.6 mM glucose. To address which glucose transporters are involved in GPR109a-mediated intestinal glucose uptake, we sought to add phlorizin (SGLT1 blocker) and phloretin (GLUT2 blocker) to examine whether the stimulatory effect of niacin on glucose uptake was mediated via SGLT1 and/or GLUT2. In this regard, we found both SGLT1 and GLUT2 were responsible for this regulatory process. In terms of SGLT1, cAMP has been shown to stimulate SGLT1 function in enterocytes as mentioned above [40] and involved in post-transcriptional stabilization of SGLT1 message [41]. Therefore, it is plausible to propose that cAMP may act as a downstream mediator for the action of niacin on SGLT1-mediated glucose uptake. In term of GLUT2, however, cAMP has been previously reported to prevent glucose-mediated stimulation of GLUT2 in hepatocytes [42], and thus a decrease in cAMP level in hepatocytes is supposed to upregulate GLUT2-mediated glucose uptake; however, this postulate is apparently contradictory with that of SGLT1. In view of this, the signaling molecules rather than GLUT2 might be involved in the regulation of niacin-stimulated GLUT2 activity, which merits intensive investigations in the future.

Besides, we also questioned whether there a crosstalk among GPR109A, SGLT1, and GLUT2 might exist. In this context, niacin binding to GPR109A has been shown to increase the Protein Kinase C (PKC) activity in CHO-K1 cells [43]. Furthermore, GLUT2 can be PKC-dependently translocated apically upon high glucose exposure [44]. In the pancreatic islet, activation of Protein Kinase A (PKA) by adenylyl cyclase inhibited the GLUT2 mediated initial rate of 3-O-methyl glucose uptake by 48% [45].

Also, activation of PKC has been shown to activate human SGLT1 [46]. In the apical GLUT2 model, SGLT1-mediated glucose transport promotes insertion of GLUT2 into the apical membrane within minutes, where the capacity of GLUT2 mediated glucose transport can be increased up to more than three fold [21]. On the grounds of the evidence, it might be possible that niacin binding to GPR109a inhibits the PKA activity, and activates PKC activity at the same time. The niacin binding might increase the translocation of GLUT2 to the apical membrane, thus GLUT2-mediated glucose uptake. Another possibility is that GPR109a activation by niacin effects the production of SGLT1. In the uptake experiment, the time of the niacin treatment lasted only few minutes. The time may not be long enough to induce the upregulation of SGLT1 expression. Since an increased SGLT1 activity would upregulate GLUT2 activity [21], the increase in GLUT2 activity by niacin binding to GPR109a might upregulate SGLT1 mediated glucose uptake.

5. Conclusions

In conclusion, the present study is the first to report that niacin is able to bind to the niacin receptor GPR109a to stimulate SGLT1- and GLUT2-mediated jejunal glucose uptake in hyperglycemia observed in diabetes. Given niacin is a crucial nutritional supplement that garners attention over the recent years, our results should provide a clinical implication that the niacin receptor GPR109a may serve as a potential therapeutic target for novel dietary or pharmacological approaches to controlling intestinal sugar delivery, thereby improving glycemic control for diabetes.

Acknowledgments: This work was fully supported by the General Research Fund of the Research Grants Council of the Hong Kong Special Administrative Region, China (Ref. No.: CUHK 14110314), awarded to P.S. Leung.

Author Contributions: Tung Po Wong performed the experiments, analyzed the data, and drafted the manuscript. Leo Ka Yu Chan contributed to the preparation of the manuscript and data analysis. Po Sing Leung conceived and designed the study and experiments, and compiled the manuscript. All authors approved the final version of the manuscript.

Conflicts of Interest: The authors declare no conflict of interest.

References

1. Sprafka, J.M.; Burke, G.L.; Folsom, A.R.; McGovern, P.G.; Hahn, L.P. Trends in prevalence of diabetes mellitus in patients with myocardial infarction and effect of diabetes on survival. The Minnesota Heart Survey. *Diabetes Care* **1991**, *14*, 537–543. [CrossRef]

2. Haffner, S.M.; Lehto, S.; Rönnemaa, T.; Pyörälä, K.; Laakso, M. Mortality from coronary heart disease in subjects with type 2 diabetes and in nondiabetic subjects with and without prior myocardial infarction. *N. Engl. J. Med.* **1998**, *339*, 229–234. [CrossRef]

3. Expert Panel on Detection. Evaluation, and Treatment of High Blood Cholesterol in Adults. Executive summary of the third report of the national cholesterol education program (NCEP) expert panel on detection, evaluation, and treatment of high blood cholesterol in adults (Adult Treatment Panel III). *JAMA* **2001**, *285*, 2486–2497.

4. Guyton, J.R.; Goldberg, A.C.; Kreisberg, R.A.; Sprecher, D.L.; Superko, H.R.; O'Connor, C.M. Effectiveness of once-nightly dosing of extended release niacin alone and in combination for hypercholesterolemia. *Am. J. Cardiol.* **1998**, *82*, 737–743. [CrossRef]

5. Phan, B.A.; Muñoz, L.; Shadzi, P.; Isquith, D.; Triller, M.; Brown, B.G.; Zhao, X.Q. Effects of niacin on glucose levels, coronary stenosis progression, and clinical events in subjects with normal baseline glucose levels (<100 mg/dL): A combined analysis of the Familial Atherosclerosis Treatment Study (FATS), HDL-Atherosclerosis Treatment Study (HATS), Armed Forces Regression Study (AFREGS), and Carotid Plaque Composition by MRI during lipid-lowering (CPC) study. *Am. J. Cardiol.* **2013**, *111*, 352–355.

6. Hochholzer, W.; Berg, D.D.; Giugliano, R.P. The facts behind niacin. *Ther. Adv. Cardiovasc. Dis.* **2011**, *5*, 227–240. [CrossRef]

7. Mcgovern, M.E. Use of nicotinic acid in patients with elevated fasting glucose, diabetes, or metabolic syndrome. *Br. J. Diabetes Vasc. Dis.* **2004**, *4*, 78. [CrossRef]

8. Victoria, C.R.; Meneghelli, U.G. Kinetics of jejunal glucose transport in niacin deficient rats. *Arq. Gastroenterol.* **1990**, *27*, 191–196.

9. Victoria, C.R. Jejunal electrogenic transport of glucose in rats with niacin deficiency. *Arq. Gastroenterol.* **1994**, *31*, 18–23.

10. Chen, L.; So, W.Y.; Li, Y.T.; Cheng, Q.; Boucher, B.J.; Leung, P.S. Niacin-induced hyperglycemia is partially mediated via niacin receptor GPR109a in pancreatic islets. *Mol. Cell. Endocrinol.* **2015**, *404*, 56–66. [CrossRef]

11. Soga, T.; Kamohara, M.; Takasaki, J.; Matsumoto, S.; Saito, T.; Ohishi, T.; Hiyama, H.; Matsuo, A.; Matsushime, H.; Furuichi, K. Molecular identification of nicotinic acid receptor. *Biochem. Biophys. Res. Commun.* **2003**, *303*, 364–369. [CrossRef]

12. Tunaru, S.; Kero, J.; Schaub, A.; Wufka, C.; Blaukat, A.; Pfeffer, K.; Offermanns, S. PUMA-G and HM74 are receptors for nicotinic acid and mediate its anti-lipolytic effect. *Nat. Med.* **2003**, *9*, 352–355. [CrossRef]

13. Wise, A.; Foord, S.M.; Fraser, N.J.; Barnes, A.A.; Elshourbagy, N.; Eilert, M.; Ignar, D.M.; Murdock, P.R.; Steplewski, K.; Green, A.; *et al.* Molecular identification of high and low affinity receptors for nicotinic acid. *J. Biol. Chem.* **2003**, *278*, 9869–9874. [CrossRef]

14. Offermanns, S. The nicotinic acid receptor GPR109A (HM74A or PUMA-G) as a new therapeutic target. *Trends Pharmacol. Sci.* **2006**, *7*, 384–390. [CrossRef]

15. Zellner, C.; Pullinger, C.R.; Aouizerat, B.E.; Frost, P.H.; Kwok, P.Y.; Malloy, M.J.; Kane, J.P. Variations in human HM74 (GPR109B) and HM74A (GPR109A) niacin receptors. *Hum. Mutat.* **2005**, *25*, 18–21. [CrossRef]

16. Cresci, G.A.; Thangaraju, M.; Mellinger, J.D.; Liu, K.; Ganapathy, V. Colonic gene expression in conventional and germ-free mice with a focus on the butyrate receptor GPR109A and the butyrate transporter SLC5A8. *J. Gastrointest. Surg.* **2010**, *14*, 449–461. [CrossRef]

17. Sharp, P.A.; Boyer, S.; Srai, S.K.; Baldwin, S.A.; Debnam, E.S. Early diabetes-induced changes in rat jejunal glucose transport and the response to insulin. *J. Endocrinol.* **1997**, *154*, 19–25. [CrossRef]

18. Kellett, G.L.; Helliwell, P.A. The diffusive component of intestinal glucose absorption is mediated by the glucose-induced recruitment of GLUT2 to the brush-border membrane. *Biochem. J.* **2000**, *350*, 155–162. [CrossRef]

19. Kellett, G.L. The facilitated component of intestinal glucose absorption. *J. Physiol.* **2001**, *531*, 585–595. [CrossRef]

20. Tobin, V.; le Gall, M.; Fioramonti, X.; Stolarczyk, E.; Blazquez, A.G.; Klein, C.; Prigent, M.; Serradas, P.; Cuif, M.H.; Magnan, C.; *et al.* Insulin internalizes GLUT2 in the enterocytes of healthy but not insulin-resistant mice. *Diabetes* **2008**, *57*, 55–62. [CrossRef]

21. Kellett, G.L.; Brot-Laroche, E. Apical GLUT2: A major pathway of intestinal sugar absorption. *Diabetes* **2005**, *54*, 3056–3062. [CrossRef]

22. Del Castillo, J.R. The use of hyperosmolar, intracellular-like solutions for the isolation of epithelial cells from guinea-pig small intestine. *Biochim. Biophys. Acta* **1987**, *901*, 201–208. [CrossRef]

23. Wong, T.P.; Debnam, E.S.; Leung, P.S. Involvement of an enterocyte renin-angiotensin system in the local control of SGLT1-dependent glucose uptake across the rat small intestinal brush border membrane. *J. Physiol.* **2007**, *584*, 613–623. [CrossRef]

24. Wong, T.P.; Debnam, E.S.; Leung, P.S. Diabetes mellitus and expression of the enterocyte renin-angiotensin system: Implications for control of glucose transport across the brush border membrane. *Am. J. Physiol. Cell Physiol.* **2009**, *297*, 601–610. [CrossRef]

25. Ip, S.P.; Wong, T.P.; Tsai, S.J.; Leung, P.S. The recovery of some components of the renin angiotensin system in the rat pancreas after chronic exposure to hypoxic condition. *J. Mol. Endocrinol.* **2003**, *3*, 563–571. [CrossRef]

26. Chu, K.Y.; Leung, P.S. Angiotensin II Type 1 receptor antagonism mediates uncoupling protein 2-driven oxidative stress and ameliorates pancreatic islet β-cell function in young Type 2 diabetic mice. *Antioxid. Redox. Signal.* **2007**, *9*, 869–878. [CrossRef]

27. Lau, T.; Carlsson, P.O.; Leung, P.S. Evidence for a local angiotensin-generating system and dose-dependent inhibition of glucose-stimulated insulin release by angiotensin II in isolated pancreatic islets. *Diabetologia* **2004**, *47*, 240–248. [CrossRef]

28. Debnam, E.S.; Smith, M.W.; Sharp, P.A.; Srai, S.K.; Turvey, A.; Keable, S.J. The effects of streptozotocin diabetes on sodium-glucose transporter (SGLT1) expression and function in rat jejunal and ileal villus-attached enterocytes. *Pflugers* **1995**, *430*, 151–159. [CrossRef]

29. Karasov, W.H.; Pond, R.S.; Solberg, D.H.; Diamond, J.M. Regulation of proline and glucose transport in mouse intestine by dietary substrate levels. *Proc. Natl. Acad. Sci. USA* **1983**, *80*, 7674–7677. [CrossRef]

30. Gilbert, T.; Rodriguez-Boulan, E. Induction of vacuolar apical compartments in the Caco-2 intestinal epithelial cell line. *J. Cell Sci.* **1991**, *100*, 451–458.

31. Jumarie, C.; Malo, C. Caco-2 cells cultured in serum-free medium as a model for the study of enterocytic differentiation *in vitro*. *J. Cell Physiol.* **1991**, *149*, 24–33. [CrossRef]

32. Gambhir, D.; Ananth, S.; Veeranan-Karmegam, R.; Elangovan, S.; Hester, S.; Jennings, E.; Offermanns, S.; Nussbaum, J.J.; Smith, S.B.; Thangaraju, M.; *et al.* GPR109A as an anti-inflammatory receptor in retinal pigment epithelial cells and its relevance to diabetic retinopathy. *Invest. Ophthalmol. Vis. Sci.* **2012**, *53*, 2208–2217. [CrossRef]

33. Singh, N.; Gurav, A.; Sivaprakasam, S.; Brady, E.; Padia, R.; Shi, H.; Thangaraju, M.; Prasad, P.D.; Manicassamy, S.; Munn, D.H.; *et al.* Activation of GPR109a, receptor for niacin and the commensal metabolite butyrate, suppresses colonic inflammation and carcinogenesis. *Immunity* **2014**, *40*, 128–139. [CrossRef]

34. Chai, J.T.; Digby, J.E.; Choudhury, R.P. GPR109A and Vascular inflammation. *Curr. Atheroscler. Rep.* **2013**, *15*, 325. [CrossRef]

35. Wong, T.P.; Ho, K.Y.; Ng, E.K.W.; Debnam, E.S.; Leung, P.S. Upregulation of ACE2-ANG-(1–7)-Mas axis in jejunal enterocytes of type 1 diabetic rats: Implications for glucose transport. *Am. J. Physiol. Endocrinol.* **2012**, *303*, E669–E681. [CrossRef]

36. Bechgaard, H.; Jespersen, S. GI absorption of niacin in humans. *J. Pharm. Sci.* **1977**, *66*, 871–872. [CrossRef]

37. Johnson, R.L.; Ghishan, F.K.; Kaunitz, J.D.; Merchant, J.L.; Said, H.M.; Wood, J.D. *Physiology of the Gastrointestinal Tract*, 5th ed.; Elsevier Inc.: San Diego, CA, USA, 2012; Volume 2.

38. Taylor, W.M.; Mak, M.L.; Halperin, M.L. Effect of 3′,5′-cyclic AMP on glucose transport in rat adipocytes. *Proc. Natl. Acad. Sci. USA* **1976**, *73*, 4359–4363. [CrossRef]

39. Taylor, W.M.; Halperin, M.L. Stimulation of glucose transport in rat adipocytes by insulin, adenosine, nicotinic acid and hydrogen peroxide. Role of adenosine 3′,5′-cyclic monophosphate. *Biochem. J.* **1979**, *178*, 381–389. [CrossRef]

40. Stümpel, F.; Scholtka, B.; Jungermann, K. A new role for enteric glucagon-37: Acute stimulation of glucose absorption in rat small intestine. *FEBS Lett.* **1997**, *410*, 515–519. [CrossRef]

41. Lee, W.Y.; Loflin, P.; Clancey, C.J.; Peng, H.; Lever, J.E. Cyclic nucleotide regulation of Na+/glucose cotransporter (SGLT1) mRNA stability. Interaction of a nucleocytoplasmic protein with a regulatory domain in the 3′-untranslated region critical for stabilization. *J. Biol. Chem.* **2000**, *275*, 33998–34008. [CrossRef]

42. Rencurel, F.; Waeber, G.; Bonny, C.; Antoine, B.; Maulard, P.; Girard, J.; Leturque, A. cAMP prevents the glucose-mediated stimulation of GLUT2 gene transcription in hepatocytes. *Biochem. J.* **1997**, *322*, 441–448. [CrossRef]

43. Li, G.; Deng, X.; Wu, C.; Zhou, Q.; Chen, L.; Shi, Y.; Huang, H.; Zhou, N. Distinct kinetic and spatial patterns of protein kinase C (PKC)- and epidermal growth factor receptor (EGFR)-dependent activation of extracellular signal-regulated kinases 1 and 2 by human nicotinic acid receptor GPR109A. *J. Biol. Chem.* **2011**, *286*, 31199–31212. [CrossRef]

44. Cohen, M.; Kitsberg, D.; Tsytkin, S.; Shulman, M.; Aroeti, B.; Nahmias, Y. Live imaging of GLUT2 glucose dependent trafficking and its inhibition in polarized epithelial cysts. *Open Biol.* **2014**, *4*. [CrossRef]

45. Thorens, B.; Dériaz, N.; Bosco, D.; DeVos, A.; Pipeleers, D.; Schuit, F.; Meda, P.; Porret, A. Protein kinase A-dependent phosphorylation of GLUT2 in pancreatic β cells. *J. Biol. Chem.* **1996**, *271*, 8075–8081.

46. Wright, E.M.; Hirsch, J.R.; Loo, D.D.; Zampighi, G.A. Regulation of Na+/glucose cotransporters. *J. Exp. Biol.* **1997**, *200*, 287–293.

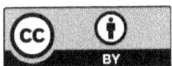

Section 2:
Diet and Mitochondrial Function

nutrients

MDPI

Article

Rutin Increases Muscle Mitochondrial Biogenesis with AMPK Activation in High-Fat Diet-Induced Obese Rats

Sangjin Seo [1,†], Mak-Soon Lee [1,†], Eugene Chang [1,†], Yoonjin Shin [1], Soojung Oh [1], In-Hwan Kim [2] and Yangha Kim [1,*]

[1] Department of Nutritional Science and Food Management, Ewha Womans University, Seoul 120-750, Korea; sjseo27@naver.com (S.J.S.); troph@hanmail.net (M.S.L.); eugenics77@hotmail.com (E.C.); yjin19@hotmail.com (Y.S.); ohsjmay@naver.com (S.O.)

[2] Department of Food and Nutrition, Korea University, Seoul 136-703, Korea; k610in@korea.ac.kr

* Correspondence: yhmoon@ewha.ac.kr; Tel.: +82-2-3277-3101; Fax: +82-2-3277-4425.

† These authors contributed equally to this work.

Received: 17 July 2015; Accepted: 14 September 2015; Published: 22 September 2015

Abstract: Decreased mitochondrial number and dysfunction in skeletal muscle are associated with obesity and the progression of obesity-associated metabolic disorders. The specific aim of the current study was to investigate the effects of rutin on mitochondrial biogenesis in skeletal muscle of high-fat diet-induced obese rats. Supplementation with rutin reduced body weight and adipose tissue mass, despite equivalent energy intake ($p < 0.05$). Rutin significantly increased mitochondrial size and mitochondrial DNA (mtDNA) content as well as gene expression related to mitochondrial biogenesis, such as peroxisome proliferator-activated receptor γ coactivator-1α (PGC-1α), nuclear respiratory factor-1 (NRF-1), transcription factor A (Tfam), and nicotinamide adenine dinucleotide (NAD)-dependent deacetylase, sirtulin1 (SIRT1) in skeletal muscle ($p < 0.05$). Moreover, rutin consumption increased muscle adenosine monophosphate-activated protein kinase (AMPK) activity by 40% ($p < 0.05$). Taken together, these results suggested at least partial involvement of muscle mitochondria and AMPK activation in the rutin-mediated beneficial effect on obesity.

Keywords: rutin; obesity; skeletal muscle; mitochondria; AMPK activity

1. Introduction

The rapidly increased prevalence of obesity has become a worldwide health epidemic due to its strong association with metabolic disorders, including type 2 diabetes, dyslipidemia, hypertension, and heart disease [1,2]. Skeletal muscle from obese humans shows increased intramuscular triglyceride content and decreased lipid oxidation [3,4]. In addition, decreased activities of enzymes indicative of muscle mitochondrial content and mitochondrial number in obese human skeletal muscle have also been reported [4–6]. Given the close association between obesity and skeletal muscle, the regulation of obesity-induced mitochondrial changes in skeletal muscle may be possible targets for the prevention and/or treatment of obesity and its associated comorbidities.

Mitochondrial dysfunction, including mitochondrial loss and decreased functional capacity of mitochondria, is associated with several transcriptional regulators and enzyme activities in obese skeletal muscle. Adenosine monophosphate-activated protein kinase (AMPK) stimulates mitochondrial biogenesis and β-oxidation by regulating a transcriptional regulation factor, peroxisome proliferator-activated receptor γ coactivator-1α (PGC-1α) [7–9]. PGC-1α directly increases the synthesis of nuclear respiratory factors (NRF1 and NRF2) and mitochondrial transcription factor A (Tfam), all of which increase mitochondrial DNA (mtDNA), an indicator of mitochondrial biogenesis and mitochondrial function [10,11]. In studies that investigated the association between mitochondrial biogenesis and obesity, genetic variation in the mtDNA demonstrates a close association with the severity of obesity [12,13]. A nicotinamide adenine dinucleotide (NAD)-dependent deacetylase, sirtulin1 (SIRT1) also interacts with PGC-1α, which plays a critical role in apoptosis, energy homeostasis, longevity, and mitochondrial function [14]. Another transcriptional candidate for mitochondrial function is carnitine palmitoyltransferase 1 (CPT1). CPT1 is a mitochondrial transmembrane enzyme that regulates the entry of long-chain fatty acids into mitochondria for fatty acid oxidation [15]. In obese human skeletal muscle, CPT1 activity and mitochondrial content are decreased, which in turn contribute to reduced fatty acid oxidation [4].

Rutin (rutoside, quercetin-3-*O*-rutinoside and sophorin) is a flavonol glycoside composed of quercetin and disaccharide rutinose and is present in many plants, including buckwheat [16]. *In vivo* and *in vitro* studies showed the anti-oxidant, anti-inflammatory, anti-hypertensive, and anti-platelet properties of rutin [17,18] by modulating oxidative stress, inflammation, lipogenesis, and glucose and lipid metabolism in liver and adipose tissue [19–22]. However, the favorable effect of rutin on obesity in relation to muscle mitochondrial changes has never been investigated. Thus, the purpose of our study was to determine the effect of rutin on obesity-induced mitochondrial loss and decreased functional capacity in skeletal muscle from high-fat diet-induced obese rats.

2. Experimental Section

2.1. Reagents

Trizol reagent and Moloney murine leukemia virus (M-MLV) reverse transcriptase were obtained from Invitrogen (Carlsbad, CA, USA). A universal SYBR Green polymerase chain reaction (PCR) Master Mix and Puregene DNA isolation kit were obtained from Qiagen (Valencia, CA, USA). Kits for the analysis of aspartate aminotransferase (AST), alanine aminotransferase (ALT), total cholesterol (TC), triglyceride (TG), and high density lipoprotein (HDL)-cholesterol were purchased from Asan Pharmaceutical Co. (Seoul, Korea). The AMPK Kinase Assay kit was obtained from MBL International Co. (Woburn, MA, USA). The BCA protein assay kit was purchased from Thermo Scientific (Waltham, MA, USA). Zoletil was provided by Virbac Laboratories (Carros, France). Rompun was supplied by Bayer Korea (Ansan, Korea). All other reagents including rutin were obtained from Sigma-Aldrich Inc. (St. Louis, MO, USA).

2.2. Animals and Experimental Design

Experimental protocols were approved by the Animal Experimentation Ethics Committee of Ewha Womans University in Seoul, Korea for the care and use of laboratory animals (permission number: 2012-02-080). A total of 24 male Sprague-Dawley rats (3 weeks old) were obtained from Daehan Experimental Animals (Eumseong, Korea), individually housed in stainless steel wire-mesh cages in a room maintained at $22 \pm 2\,°C$ with a 12-h light/dark cycle (light period: 6 am to 6 pm), and fed laboratory chow and water ad libitum for 1 week to stabilize their metabolic condition. After 1 week of acclimation, rats were randomly divided into groups ($n = 8$/group) and fed a normal diet (NOR), a high-fat diet (HFD) or a 0.1% (wt:wt) rutin-supplemented high-fat diet (HFD + Rutin) for 12 weeks. NOR was a commercial diet (Harlan 2018s; Harlan, Indianapolis, IN, USA) containing 18% crude protein, 6% fat, 44% carbohydrate, 18% fiber, and 5% ash. HFD (45% of energy) consisted of 23% fat, 17% casein, 12% sucrose, 20% starch, 15% dextrose, 6% cellulose, 4.3% minerals, and 1.2% vitamins (wt:wt), based on a modification of the AIN-93 diet [23]. Rutin was added to HFD. Body weight and food intake were monitored twice a week.

2.3. Sample Collection

At the end of 12 weeks, rats fasted overnight and were anesthetized with Zoletil:Rompun (4:1) at a dose of 0.1 mL/80 g body weight. Blood was collected by cardiac puncture, centrifuged at $1500\times g$ for 20 min at $4\,°C$ to obtain serum, and stored at $-20\,°C$ until analysis. Liver, white adipose tissue (epididymal and retroperitoneal), and skeletal muscle were dissected, immediately frozen in liquid nitrogen, and stored at −70°C until further analysis.

2.4. Blood Biochemical Measurements

Serum concentrations of AST, ALT, TC, TG and HDL-cholesterol were determined by enzymatic colorimetric methods using commercial kits (Asan Pharmaceutical Co., Ltd., Seoul, Korea). Low-density lipoprotein (LDL)-cholesterol was calculated using the Friedewald equation [24], and the atherogenic index (AI) was calculated using the Rosenfeld formula [25].

$$\text{LDL-cholesterol} = \text{TC} - \text{HDL-cholesterol} - (\text{TG}/5) \tag{1}$$

$$\text{AI} = (\text{TC} - \text{HDL-cholesterol})/\text{HDL-cholesterol} \tag{2}$$

2.5. Hepatic and Fecal Lipids Analyses

Hepatic and fecal lipids were extracted using the method described by Bligh and Dyer [26]. Briefly, 500 mg of tissues or feces was homogenized in 1.5 mL of 0.9% saline and 7.5 mL of methanol:chloroform (2:1, v:v). After the addition of 2.5 mL of chloroform, the mixture was shaken horizontally for 10 min and centrifuged at $2000 \times g$ for 10 min. The lower chloroform phase was collected into a fresh tube and subsequently dried and weighed. TC and TG concentrations were determined by enzymatic colorimetric methods using commercial kits as described above.

2.6. Histological Analysis

Dissected epididymal adipose tissue samples were fixed in 10% (v/v) formalin for 24 h. Tissues were then embedded in paraffin, sliced into 5-μm-thick sections, and stained with hematoxylin-eosin (H&E). H&E-stained sections were observed under a microscope (Olympus, Tokyo, Japan) and digital images were captured at 200× magnification.

2.7. Electron Microscopic Analysis

Skeletal muscle was prefixed with 2% glutaraldehyde plus 2% paraformaldehyde in 0.1 M phosphate buffer. Glutaraldehyde-fixed samples were treated with 2% osmium tetroxide, dehydrated, and embedded in epoxy resin. Selected 1-μm-thick sections were stained with toluidine blue and then cut into approximately 60- to 70-μm ultra-thin sections using an Ultramicrotome (Richert-Jung, Buffalo, NY, USA) using a diamond knife. Thin sections were stained with 1%–2% aqueous uranyl acetate, followed by 1% lead citrate. Stained sections were examined using an H-7650 transmission electron microscope (Hitachi, Japan) at the accelerating voltage of 80 kV.

2.8. Real-time Quantitative Reverse-transcription Polymerase Chain Reaction (qRT-PCR)

The isolation of RNA from epididymal adipose tissue and skeletal muscle was performed using Trizol reagent. Complementary DNA (cDNA) was synthesized from 4 μg of total RNA using a M-MLV Reverse Transcriptase Kit. Primers used are shown in Table 1. Real-time quantitative reverse-transcription polymerase chain reaction (qRT-PCR) was carried out using Universal SYBR Green PCR Master Mix on a fluorometric thermal cycler (Rotor-GeneTM 2000; Corbett Research, Mortlake, NSW, Australia). Data were analyzed using the ΔΔCt method for relative quantification [27]. The expression of each target was normalized to the average of β-actin as a control and expressed as the fold change related to the HFD group.

Table 1. Primers used for quantitative real-time polymerase chain reaction (PCR).

Name	GeneBank No.	Primer sequence (5′-3′)	Amplicon Size (bp)
aP2	NM_053365	F: TCACCCCAGATGACAGGAAA R: CATGACACATTCCACCACCA	140
β-actin	NM_031144	F: GGCACCACACTTTCTACAAT R: AGGTCTCAAACATGATCTGG	123
CPT-1	NM_031559	F: TCGGCAGACCTATTTTGCAC R: ATTTGGCGTAGCTGTCGATG	143
NRF1	NM_001100708	R: ATGGCTTGAGGATCTGGGAG F: CTGTGGCTGATGGAGAGGTG R: CACTGTTAAGGGCCATGGTG	189
PGC-1α	NM_031347	F: GCACCAGAAAACAGCTCCAA R: TTACTGAAGTTGCCATCCCG	130
SIRT1	XM_003751934.1	F: GTTCTGACTGGAGCTGGGGT R: ATGGCTTGAGGATCTGGGAG	119
SREBP-1c	AF286470	F: AGGAGGCCATCTTGTTGCTT R: GTTTTGACCCTTAGGGCAGC	134
PPAR-γ	NM_001145366	F: TGTGGGGATAAAGCATCAGC R: CAAGGCACTTCTGAAACCGA	175
Tfam	NM_031326	F: TGGGCTTAGAGAAGGAAGCC R: TGCTGACCGAGGTCTTTTTG	107

aP2, fatty acid-binding protein 2; CPT-1, carnitine palmitoyltransferase 1; NRF1, nuclear respiratory factor 1; PGC-1α, peroxisome proliferative activated receptor gamma coactivator 1 alpha; PPAR-γ, peroxisome proliferator-activated receptor-γ; SIRT1, sirtuin 1; SREBP-1c, sterol regulatory element-binding protein-1c; Tfam, mitochondrial transcription factor A.

2.9. Mitochondrial DNA (mtDNA) Content Analysis

Total DNA was extracted from muscle using a Puregene DNA isolation kit. The mtDNA content was calculated using real-time quantitative PCR by measuring the mitochondrial gene (Cox1, subunit 1 of cytochrome oxidase) *vs.* nuclear gene (GAPDH, glyceraldehyde 3-phosphate dehydrogenase).

2.10. AMPK Activity Assay

AMPK activity was evaluated using an AMPK Kinase Assay kit as described previously [28]. Using a semi-quantitative method, AMPK activity was detected by measuring the phosphorylation of Ser789 on IRS-1 with anti-mouse phospho-Ser789 IRS-1 monoclonal antibody and peroxidase-coupled anti-mouse IgG, which catalyzes the conversion of the chromogenic substrate tetramethylbenzidine. Protein was determined using a BCA protein assay kit. AMPK activity was normalized to protein concentration and expressed as the fold change compared to the HFD group.

2.11. Statistical Analysis

Data are expressed as the mean ± standard error of the mean (SEM). Differences among groups were determined by Student's *t*-test for the comparison of two groups or one-way analysis of variance (ANOVA) following Tukey's multiple comparison using SPSS software (version 17; IBM Corporation, Armonk, NY, USA). Statistical significance was defined as $p < 0.05$.

3. Results

3.1. Effect of Rutin Supplementation on Body Weight, Energy Intake, and Fat Accumulation

At the beginning of the experiment, the initial body weight was not significantly different among groups. After 12 weeks of rutin consumption, final body weight was significantly decreased by 8.5% compared to the HFD group ($p < 0.05$) (Figure 1A and Table 2). The HFD + Rutin group showed a significantly lower total weight of epididymal and retroperitoneal adipose tissues by 24% than total adipose tissue weight of HFD group ($p < 0.05$) (Table 2). As shown in Figure 1C, the size of epididymal adipocytes was smaller in the HFD + Rutin group than in the HFD group. The food intake and energy efficiency ratio were not significantly different between HFD and HFD + Rutin, which indicate that the beneficial effects of rutin on body weight and the mass of white adipose tissue were not caused by reduced energy consumption (Figure 1B and Table 2).

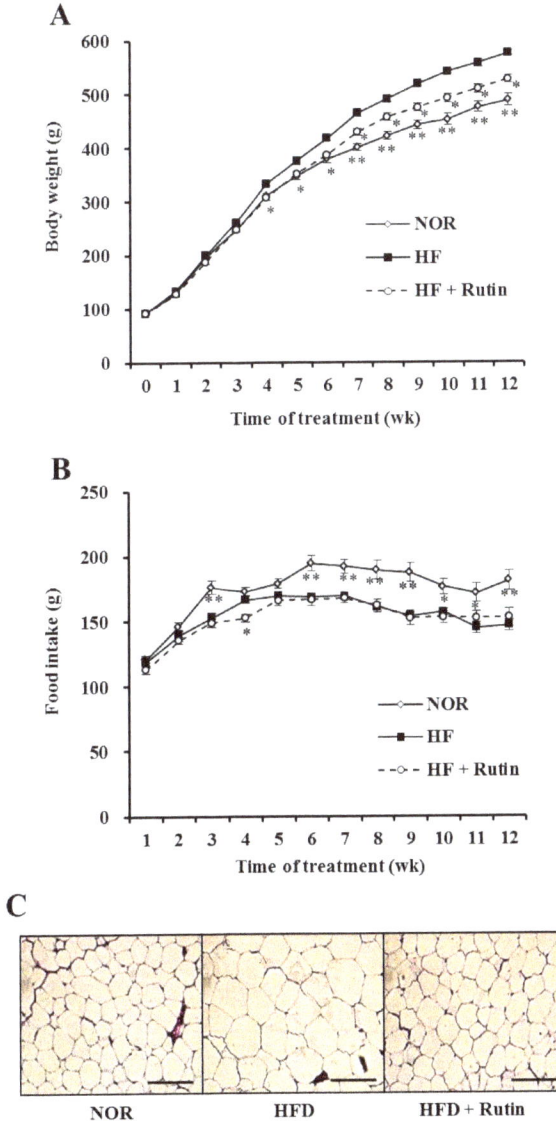

Figure 1. Effect of rutin on diet-induced obesity. Changes in body weight (**A**) and food intake (**B**). Representative histological sections (**C**) of epididymal adipose tissue (hematoxylin and eosin stain, scale bar = 50 µm). The data are expressed as the mean ± standard error of the mean (SEM) (n = 8 per group). * $p < 0.05$; ** $p < 0.01$ compared to the high-fat diet (HFD; 45% of energy) group. NOR, normal diet; HFD, high-fat diet; HFD + Rutin, rutin-supplemented high-fat diet.

Nutrients **2015**, *7*, 8152–8169

Table 2. Effect of rutin on body weight, food intake, and tissue weight.

Variables	NOR	HFD	HFD + Rutin
Initial body weight (g)	92.36 ± 1.41	91.10 ± 1.76	92.12 ± 1.68
Final body weight (g)	487.40 ± 12.59 [c]	573.64 ± 7.22 [a]	528.54 ± 9.05 [b]
Food intake (g/day)	24.97 ± 0.57 [a]	21.96 ± 0.30 [b]	21.63 ± 0.38 [b]
Total food intake (kg/12 weeks)	2.02 ± 0.05 [a]	1.78 ± 0.02 [b]	1.75 ± 0.03 [b]
Food efficiency (g gain/g consumed)	0.19 ± 0.002 [c]	0.27 ± 0.003 [a]	0.25 ± 0.006 [b]
Energy intake (kcal/day)	77.42 ± 1.77 [b]	101.99 ± 1.40 [a]	100.45 ± 1.79 [a]
Total energy intake (kcal/12 weeks)	6271 ± 144 [b]	8261 ± 113 [a]	8137 ± 145 [a]
Energy efficiency (g gain/kcal consumed)	0.06 ± 0.001 [a]	0.06 ± 0.001 [a]	0.05 ± 0.001 [b]
Liver weight (g/100 g body weight)	2.65 ± 0.06	2.44 ± 0.03	2.54 ± 0.09
Adipose tissue weight (g/100 g body weight)			
Epididymal	2.30 ± 0.18 [b]	3.84 ± 0.16 [a]	3.28 ± 0.18 [a]
Retroperitoneal	2.28 ± 0.16 [b]	4.29 ± 0.19 [a]	2.94 ± 0.26 [b]
Total	4.58 ± 0.33 [b]	8.14 ± 0.29 [a]	6.22 ± 0.33 [b]

The data are expressed as the mean ± standard error of the mean (SEM) ($n = 8$). [a, b, c] Different letters indicate a significant difference among groups according to Tukey's multiple comparison test ($p < 0.05$). NOR, normal diet; HFD, high-fat diet.

3.2. Effect of Rutin on Serum Lipid Profiles

HFD-increased serum concentrations in TG and LDL-cholesterol showed 43% and 55% reduction in the rutin-supplemented group, respectively ($p < 0.05$). Rutin consumption significantly increased the serum HDL-cholesterol level by 62% compared to HFD group ($p < 0.05$), resulting in a significant decrease of the atherogenic index (AI) (Table 3).

Table 3. Effect of rutin on serum lipid profiles.

Serum Lipid Profiles	NOR	HFD	HFD + Rutin
Serum lipids (mmol/L)			
Triglyceride	1.03 ± 0.12 [a,b]	1.25 ± 0.09 [a]	0.71 ± 0.04 [b]
Total cholesterol	2.32 ± 0.14 [a,b]	2.65 ± 0.12 [a]	2.16 ± 0.15 [a,b]
HDL cholesterol	1.45 ± 0.21 [b]	1.3 ± 0.13 [b]	2.1 ± 0.32 [a]
LDL cholesterol	0.7 ± 0.17 [a,b]	1.09 ± 0.12 [a]	0.49 ± 0.22 [b]
Atherogenic index (AI)	0.91 ± 0.27 [a,b]	1.7 ± 0.36 [a]	0.51 ± 0.24 [b]
AST (IU/L)	65.8 ± 4.0	69.7 ± 4.1	66.0 ± 2.5
ALT (IU/L)	8.8 ± 3.1	6.2 ± 2.4	7.2 ± 2.9

Values are shown as the mean ± standard error of the mean (SEM) ($n = 8$). [a, b] Different letters indicate a significant difference among groups according to Tukey's multiple comparison test ($p < 0.05$). NOR, normal diet; HFD, high-fat diet; HDL, high-density lipoprotein; LDL, low-density lipoprotein; AST, aspartate aminotransferase; ALT, alanine aminotransferase; IU, international unit.

3.3. Alterations in Hepatic and Fecal Lipid Profiles by Rutin Supplementation

Twelve weeks of rutin supplementation significantly reduced the hepatic total lipid, TG, and TC by 27%, 37%, and 35%, respectively, compared to the HFD group ($p < 0.05$) (Table 4). The amount of fecal lipid in the HFD + Rutin group was significantly increased by 33% compared to the HFD group ($p < 0.05$). There was an increasing trend of fecal TG levels in the HFD + Rutin group, but there was no significance.

3.4. Influence of Rutin on Liver Weight and Serum AST and ALT Activities

Liver weight was not altered by rutin supplementation (Table 2). In addition, serum levels of AST and ALT were not significantly different among groups (Table 3). The data indicated that rutin did not induce hepatic toxicity.

Table 4. Effect of rutin on hepatic and fecal lipid profiles.

Hepatic and Fecal Lipid Profiles	NOR	HFD	HFD + Rutin
Hepatic lipids (μmol/g)			
Total lipid	26.7 ± 1.3 [b]	42.2 ± 1.3 [a]	30.9 ± 1.9 [b]
Triglyceride	3.79 ± 0.69 [c]	11.70 ± 1.76 [a]	7.33 ± 1.36 [b]
Total cholesterol	1.26 ± 0.10 [b]	2.70 ± 0.21 [a]	1.75 ± 0.13 [b]
Fecal lipids (μmol/g)			
Total lipid	23.9 ± 1.6 [b]	28.5 ± 1.0 [a,b]	38.0 ± 3.8 [a,*]
Triglyceride	0.36 ± 0.04 [b]	0.47 ± 0.04 [a,b]	0.66 ± 0.09 [a]

Values are expressed as the mean ± standard error of the mean (SEM) ($n = 8$). [a, b, c] Different letters indicate a significant difference among groups according to Tukey's multiple comparison test ($p < 0.05$). Asterisks (*) indicate a significant difference from HF diet, $p < 0.05$. NOR, normal diet; HFD, high-fat diet.

3.5. Effect of Rutin on Expression of Adipogenic Genes and AMPK Activity in Adipose Tissue

The mRNA levels of adipogenic genes such as peroxisome proliferator activated receptor-γ (PPAR-γ), sterol regulatory element binding protein-1c (SREBP-1c), and adipocyte protein 2 (aP2) were significantly decreased by rutin in epididymal white adipose tissue ($p < 0.05$) (Figure 2A). AMPK activation, which regulates body fat accumulation by modulating adipogenic or fatty acid oxidation-related genes, was measured by a semi-quantitative analysis. As shown in Figure 2B, the HFD + Rutin group exhibited significantly increased AMPK activity by 50% in adipose tissue compared to the HFD group ($p < 0.05$). Therefore, the favorable effects of rutin on body weight and adipose tissue mass may be associated with a decrease of adipogenesis in adipose tissue.

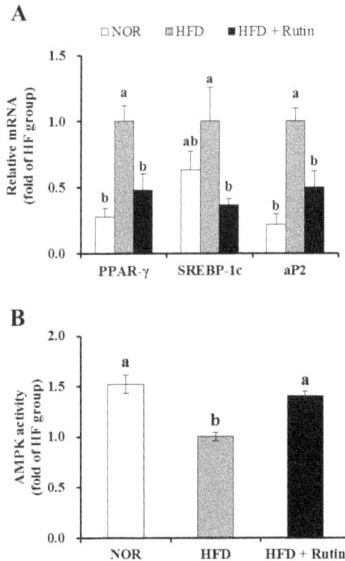

Figure 2. Effect of rutin on adipogenic gene expression and adenosine monophosphate-activated protein kinase (AMPK) activity in adipose tissue. The messenger RNA (mRNA) levels of peroxisome proliferator activated receptor-γ (PPAR-γ), sterol regulatory element binding protein-1c (SREBP-1c) and adipocyte protein 2 (aP2) were determined by real-time polymerase chain reaction (RT-PCR) and normalized for all samples to β-actin (**A**). AMPK activity was measured using an AMPK kinase kit and normalized to protein levels (**B**). The results are expressed as the fold change compared to the HFD group (mean ± standard error of the mean (SEM), $n = 8$ per group). Bars with different letters (a, b) are significantly different according to Tukey's multiple comparison test at $p < 0.05$.

3.6. Effect of Rutin on Mitochondrial Morphology and Content (mtDNA) in Skeletal Muscle

To investigate the effect of rutin on changes in muscle mitochondria, transmission electron microscopy (TEM) was used. The HFD group showed a smaller size and number of skeletal muscle mitochondria, which was reversed by rutin administration (Figure 3A). In addition, Figure 3B showed that mtDNA content was significantly increased by rutin supplementation, which served as evidence of enlargement and increased mitochondria number ($p < 0.05$).

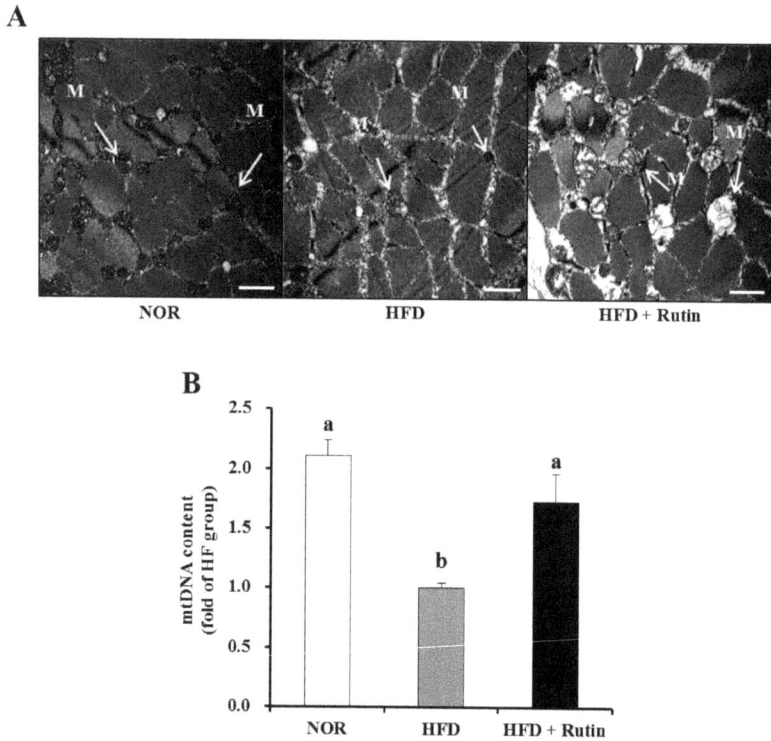

Figure 3. Effect of rutin on muscle mitochondrial morphology and mitochondrial DNA (mtDNA) content. Electron microscopy of muscle (magnification of 20,000; scale bars = 2 μm) (**A**). Arrows indicate the position of mitochondria (M). The mtDNA content was quantified by real-time PCR (**B**). Values are expressed as the mean ± standard error of the mean (SEM) (*n* = 8 per group). Bars with different letters (a, b) indicate significant differences compared to the HFD group according to Tukey's multiple comparison test ($p < 0.05$).

3.7. Effect of Rutin on Mitochondrial Gene Expression and AMPK Activity in Skeletal Muscle

Rutin administration significantly increased mRNA expression of NRF1, Tfam, PGC-1α, SIRT1, and CPT1 involved in muscle mitochondrial biogenesis and function ($p < 0.05$) (Figure 4A). Next, we determined AMPK activity, which affects muscle mitochondrial biogenesis and oxidative capacity for β-oxidation. Rutin-supplemented HFD significantly increased AMPK activity by 40% in muscle compared to the HFD group (Figure 4B). The data indicated that the beneficial effect of rutin on obesity may be due to an increase in mitochondrial biogenesis and capacity in skeletal muscle.

A

B

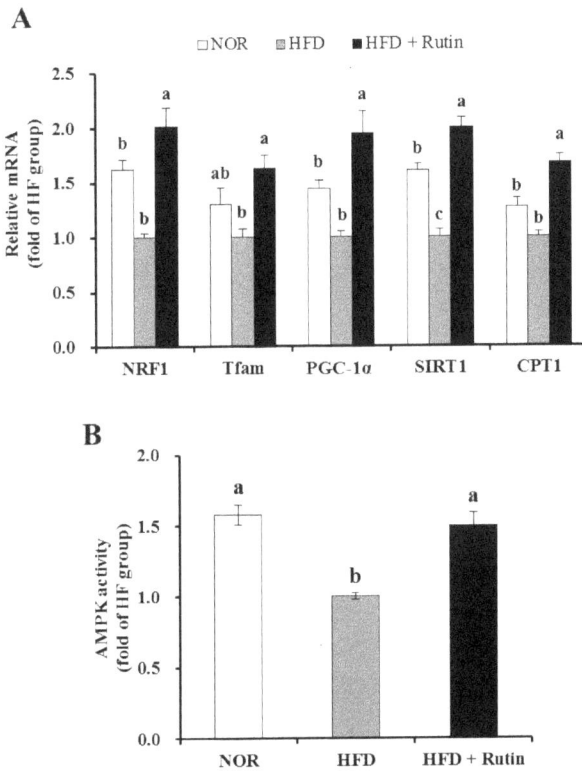

Figure 4. Effect of rutin on mitochondrial gene expression of genes related to mitochondrial biogenesis and function in skeletal muscle. The levels of nuclear respiratory factor 1 (NRF1), transcription factor A (Tfam), peroxisome proliferator-activated receptor γ coactivator-1α (PGC-1α), sirtulin1 (SIRT1) and arnitine palmitoyltransferase 1 (CPT1) mRNA were analyzed by real-time PCR and normalized to β-actin (**A**). adenosine monophosphate-activated protein kinase (AMPK) activity was measured using an AMPK kinase kit and normalized to protein levels (**B**). The results are expressed as the fold change compared to the HFD group (mean ± standard error of the mean (SEM), $n = 8$ per group). Bars with different letters (a, b) indicate a statistically significant difference according to Tukey's multiple comparison test ($p < 0.05$).

4. Discussion

Mitochondrial changes and dysfunction, including decreased mtDNA content, mitochondrial size, and functional capacity of mitochondria, manifest in the skeletal muscle of obese human subjects and rodents [4–6,29–31]. Beneficial effects of rutin supplementation on obesity have been reported [19,20,22,32]. The favorable role of rutin in glucose and lipid metabolism and its associated metabolic disorders led us to investigate the effects of rutin on obesity-induced mitochondrial changes in skeletal muscle.

In the present study, we evaluated the influence of rutin on the HFD-decreased mitochondrial content, mitochondrial gene expression, and AMPK activity, which is involved in mitochondrial biogenesis and function. Using three groups of rats fed a NOR, HFD and HFD + Rutin, we found that rutin supplementation led to significant increases in the HFD-decreased size and number of mitochondria, mtDNA and gene expression and enzyme activity related to mitochondrial biogenesis and function in skeletal muscle, together with reductions in HFD-induced weight gain and the enlargement of adipose tissue.

In the present study, rutin-fed rats showed a significant decrease in body weight without changing food intake, consistent with other previous results [21,32]. Moreover, rutin consumption decreased adipose size, adipogenic gene expression of PPAR-γ, SREBP-1c, and aP2, and AMPK activity in epididymal adipose tissue, indicating the anti-obesity property of rutin. PPAR-γ and SREBP-1c are critical transcription factors that regulate adipocyte differentiation and lipogenesis [33,34]. In addition, aP2 is highly expressed in adipose tissue and regarded as a marker of obesity, reflecting the magnitude of fat accumulation [35]. In adipocyte energy homeostasis, AMPK regulates body fat deposition by decreasing adipogenic genes such as SREBP-1c and PPAR-γ [36]. Adipogenic gene expression and adipose tissue hypertrophy were inhibited *in vitro* in 3T3-L1 cells treated with rutin and animals fed with rutin supplemented with a high-fat diet [19,20]. Therefore, our findings demonstrated that the beneficial effect of rutin on obesity was at least partially due to anti-adipogenic activity in adipose tissue.

The currently used rutin dosage was determined as described in previous studies [21,37]. A concentration of 0.1% rutin in the diet was well tolerated by rats in the present study, as demonstrated by the results showing that liver weight and serum ALT and AST levels were unaffected by rutin supplementation. In rodent animal models, HFD generally does not induce liver damage. When fed with 60% HFD, 16 weeks period of HFD significantly increases hepatic expression involved in inflammation [38]. In addition, high-fat liquid diet including 71% of energy derived from fat induces hepatic inflammation after 4 weeks [39] or 6 weeks [40]. However, 42% HFD for 12 weeks dose not induce any liver changes in Sprague-Dawely rats which were similar as our current study design [41]. Similar to published data showing the beneficial effects of rutin on diet-induced dyslipidemia [21], 12 weeks of rutin supplementation in the present study significantly attenuated HFD-increased serum and hepatic lipid parameters and decreased the atherogenic index. Moreover, total fecal lipids were increased in the HFD + Rutin group, implying that increased total fecal lipid excretion may contribute to a reduction in body weight and serum lipids in the HFD + Rutin group.

Concerning the association between rutin and muscle, studies have shown that rutin improves glucose transport in isolated soleus muscles from rats [42,43]. However, the effect of rutin on mitochondrial changes in skeletal muscle during the progression of obesity has never been elucidated. Obesity is closely associated with mitochondrial dysfunction (*i.e.*, decreased oxidation capacity and fatty acid oxidation), reduced expression in a cluster of nuclear genes responsible for oxidative metabolism (PGC-1α), and decreased mitochondrial biogenesis (*i.e.*, the generation of new mtDNA and proteins) in skeletal muscle [5,6]. Indeed, HFD-induced obesity reduced the number and size of muscle mitochondria observed by TEM, mtDNA content, and AMPK activation, all of which were improved by rutin supplementation in the present study. Therefore, we suggest that rutin plays a preventive role in obesity-induced mitochondrial changes in skeletal muscle.

Mitochondrial dysfunction, including decreased mitochondrial biogenesis and functional capacity, is associated with several transcriptional regulators and enzyme activities in obese skeletal muscle. As a regulator of mitochondrial biogenesis and function, AMPK promotes mitochondrial biogenesis by direct phosphorylation and interaction with PGC-1α, which up-regulates the synthesis of NRF1 and Tfam. PGC-1α activity is increased by SIRT1-induced deacetylation. AMPK also regulates energy metabolism by increasing the gene expression of PGC-1α and SIRT1, which are involved in fatty acid oxidation [7–10,44]. All key regulators of muscle mitochondrial biogenesis and function, such as NRF1, Tfam, PGC-1α, and SIRT1, were significantly decreased by HFD and then were fully recovered by rutin supplementation in our current study. NRF1 stimulates the expressions of Tfam, a key nuclear-encoded transcription factor of mtDNA transcription [45,46]. Another mitochondrial enzyme involved in fatty acid oxidation [15], CPT-1, was also significantly increased with rutin. Increased transcription of mtDNA initiates mitochondrial biosynthesis, ultimately leading to mitochondrial abundance in size and number [11,47]. However, rutin-modified mitochondrial size and number were not directly measured in the present study. Using more precise and direct methods such as digital imaging software and stereological principles of point sampling in a blind fashion needs to be taken into consideration to evaluate the role of rutin on muscle mitochondrial size and volume density in the future study [5,48,49]. In addition, molecular mechanisms by which rutin improves mitochondrial function in muscle of obese rats have not been fully determined. Abnormalities in both mitochondrial biogenesis and mitochondrial function including ATP synthesis, oxidative respiration, and intracellular calcium and nitric oxide production are involved in increased reactive oxygen species (ROS) production and endoplasmic reticulum (ER) stress in aging, heart failure, insulin resistance, and obesity [50–53]. Therefore, further investigation is needed to determine whether rutin affects mitochondrial contents of ATP, calcium, ROS, and ER stress. Given association between SIRT1 and muscle mitochondrial biogenesis and function, actions of rutin-induced quercetin cannot be ruled out. Indeed, rutin supplemented diet significantly increases plasma quercetin concentration [54–56], which is involved in the activation of SIRT1, a NAD-dependent deacetlyase [57]. In human fecal microbiota, rutin is involved in bacterial metabolism and action in the gut in relation to fat uptake [58]. In this regard, there is a possibility that rutin-decreased body weight gain in HF-diet fed rats may be associated with direct effect of gut fat uptake and/or indirect influence of rutin-increased blood quercetin on SIRT1 activation. A following study might be necessary to investigate direct and indirect effects of rutin on obesity.

Taken together, the prevention of obesity-induced muscle mitochondrial loss and the improvement of high diet-reduced mitochondrial gene expression in skeletal muscle may demonstrate the favorable effect of rutin on obesity.

5. Conclusions

Our study demonstrated that rutin supplementation decreases high-fat diet-induced weight gain and adipose tissue mass, accompanied by increased mtDNA and mitochondrial gene expression involved in mitochondrial biogenesis and function and AMPK activation in skeletal muscle. These results suggested anti-obesity property of rutin may possibly be associated with rutin-mediated muscle mitochondrial changes. Further studies are warranted to delineate more precise mechanisms by which rutin affects muscle fibers, mitochondrial biogenesis, oxidative capacity and function, and its associated health outcomes. To the best our knowledge, this is the first study to suggest that rutin may be partially associated with increased mitochondrial biogenesis and function in muscle of obese rats.

Acknowledgments: This work was supported by the National Research Foundation of Korea (2013R1A1A2009522 and 2014R1A1A3050953) and BK 21 plus (22A20130012143).

Author Contributions: Sangjin Seo and Mak-Soon Lee conducted experiments and performed data analysis. Eugene Chang wrote and edited the manuscript and contributed to the discussion. Yoonjin Shin conducted statistical analysis. In-Hwan Kim contributed to the discussion. Yangha Kim conceived, designed and directed the study and revised the manuscript. All authors reviewed the final manuscript.

Conflicts of Interest: The authors declare no conflicts of interest.

References

1. Caballero, B. The global epidemic of obesity: An overview. *Epidemiol. Rev.* **2007**, *29*, 1–5. [PubMed]
2. Mokdad, A.H.; Ford, E.S.; Bowman, B.A.; Dietz, W.H.; Vinicor, F.; Bales, V.S.; Marks, J.S. Prevalence of obesity, diabetes, and obesity-related health risk factors, 2001. *JAMA* **2003**, *289*, 76–79. [CrossRef] [PubMed]
3. Bonen, A.; Parolin, M.L.; Steinberg, G.R.; Calles-Escandon, J.; Tandon, N.N.; Glatz, J.F.; Luiken, J.J.; Heigenhauser, G.J.; Dyck, D.J. Triacylglycerol accumulation in human obesity and type 2 diabetes is associated with increased rates of skeletal muscle fatty acid transport and increased sarcolemmal FAT/CD36. *FASEB J.* **2004**, *18*, 1144–1146. [CrossRef] [PubMed]
4. Kim, J.Y.; Hickner, R.C.; Cortright, R.L.; Dohm, G.L.; Houmard, J.A. Lipid oxidation is reduced in obese human skeletal muscle. *Am. J. Physiol. Endocrinol. Metab.* **2000**, *279*, E1039–E1044. [PubMed]

5. Kelley, D.E.; He, J.; Menshikova, E.V.; Ritov, V.B. Dysfunction of mitochondria in human skeletal muscle in type 2 diabetes. *Diabetes* **2002**, *51*, 2944–2950. [CrossRef] [PubMed]
6. Boudina, S.; Sena, S.; O'Neill, B.T.; Tathireddy, P.; Young, M.E.; Abel, E.D. Reduced mitochondrial oxidative capacity and increased mitochondrial uncoupling impair myocardial energetics in obesity. *Circulation* **2005**, *112*, 2686–2695. [CrossRef] [PubMed]
7. Bergeron, R.; Ren, J.M.; Cadman, K.S.; Moore, I.K.; Perret, P.; Pypaert, M.; Young, L.H.; Semenkovich, C.F.; Shulman, G.I. Chronic activation of AMP kinase results in NRF-1 activation and mitochondrial biogenesis. *Am. J. Physiol. Endocrinol. Metab.* **2001**, *281*, E1340–E1346. [PubMed]
8. Jager, S.; Handschin, C.; St-Pierre, J.; Spiegelman, B.M. AMP-activated protein kinase (AMPK) action in skeletal muscle via direct phosphorylation of PGC-1alpha. *Proc. Natl. Acad. Sci. U.S.A.* **2007**, *104*, 12017–12022. [CrossRef] [PubMed]
9. Reznick, R.M.; Shulman, G.I. The role of AMP-activated protein kinase in mitochondrial biogenesis. *J. Physiol.* **2006**, *574*, 33–39. [CrossRef] [PubMed]
10. Wu, Z.; Puigserver, P.; Andersson, U.; Zhang, C.; Adelmant, G.; Mootha, V.; Troy, A.; Cinti, S.; Lowell, B.; Scarpulla, R.C.; et al. Mechanisms controlling mitochondrial biogenesis and respiration through the thermogenic coactivator PGC-1. *Cell* **1999**, *98*, 115–124. [CrossRef]
11. Ekstrand, M.I.; Falkenberg, M.; Rantanen, A.; Park, C.B.; Gaspari, M.; Hultenby, K.; Rustin, P.; Gustafsson, C.M.; Larsson, N.G. Mitochondrial transcription factor a regulates mtDNA copy number in mammals. *Hum. Mol. Genet.* **2004**, *13*, 935–944. [CrossRef] [PubMed]
12. Okura, T.; Koda, M.; Ando, F.; Niino, N.; Tanaka, M.; Shimokata, H. Association of the mitochondrial DNA 15497G/A polymorphism with obesity in a middle-aged and elderly Japanese population. *Hum. Genet.* **2003**, *113*, 432–436. [CrossRef] [PubMed]
13. Liguori, R.; Mazzaccara, C.; Pasanisi, F.; Buono, P.; Oriani, G.; Finelli, C.; Contaldo, F.; Sacchetti, L. The mtDNA 15497 G/A polymorphism in cytochrome b in severe obese subjects from Southern Italy. *Nutr. Metab. Cardiovasc. Dis.* **2006**, *16*, 466–470. [CrossRef] [PubMed]
14. Gerhart-Hines, Z.; Rodgers, J.T.; Bare, O.; Lerin, C.; Kim, S.H.; Mostoslavsky, R.; Alt, F.W.; Wu, Z.; Puigserver, P. Metabolic control of muscle mitochondrial function and fatty acid oxidation through SIRT1/PGC-1alpha. *EMBO J.* **2007**, *26*, 1913–1923. [CrossRef] [PubMed]
15. McGarry, J.D.; Brown, N.F. The mitochondrial carnitine palmitoyltransferase system from concept to molecular analysis. *Eur. J. Biochem.* **1997**, *244*, 1–14. [CrossRef] [PubMed]
16. Kurisawa, M.; Chung, J.E.; Uyama, H.; Kobayashi, S. Enzymatic synthesis and antioxidant properties of poly (rutin). *Biomacromolecules* **2003**, *4*, 1394–1399. [CrossRef] [PubMed]
17. La Casa, C.; Villegas, I.; de la Lastra, C.A.; Motilva, V.; Calero, M.M. Evidence for protective and antioxidant properties of rutin, a natural flavone, against ethanol induced gastric lesions. *J. Ethnopharmacol.* **2000**, *71*, 45–53. [CrossRef]
18. Sheu, J.R.; Hsiao, G.; Chou, P.H.; Shen, M.Y.; Chou, D.S. Mechanisms involved in the antiplatelet activity of rutin, a glycoside of the flavonol quercetin, in human platelets. *J. Agric. Food Chem.* **2004**, *52*, 4414–4418. [CrossRef] [PubMed]
19. Choi, I.; Park, Y.; Choi, H.; Lee, E.H. Anti-adipogenic activity of rutin in 3T3-L1 cells and mice fed with high-fat diet. *Biofactors* **2006**, *26*, 273–281. [CrossRef] [PubMed]
20. Hsu, C.L.; Yen, G.C. Effects of flavonoids and phenolic acids on the inhibition of adipogenesis in 3T3-L1 adipocytes. *J. Agric. Food Chem.* **2007**, *55*, 8404–8410. [CrossRef] [PubMed]
21. Panchal, S.K.; Poudyal, H.; Arumugam, T.V.; Brown, L. Rutin attenuates metabolic changes, nonalcoholic steatohepatitis, and cardiovascular remodeling in high-carbohydrate, high-fat diet-fed rats. *J. Nutr.* **2011**, *141*, 1062–1069. [CrossRef] [PubMed]
22. Wu, C.H.; Lin, M.C.; Wang, H.C.; Yang, M.Y.; Jou, M.J.; Wang, C.J. Rutin inhibits oleic acid induced lipid accumulation via reducing lipogenesis and oxidative stress in hepatocarcinoma cells. *J. Food Sci.* **2011**, *76*, T65–T72. [CrossRef] [PubMed]
23. Reeves, P.G. Components of the AIN-93 diets as improvements in the AIN-76A diet. *J. Nutr.* **1997**, *127*, 838S–841S. [PubMed]
24. Friedewald, W.T.; Levy, R.I.; Fredrickson, D.S. Estimation of the concentration of low-density lipoprotein cholesterol in plasma, without use of the preparative ultracentrifuge. *Clin. Chem.* **1972**, *18*, 499–502. [PubMed]

Nutrients **2015**, *7*, 8152–8169

25. Rosenfeld, L. Lipoprotein analysis. Early methods in the diagnosis of atherosclerosis. *Arch. Pathol. Lab Med.* **1989**, *113*, 1101–1110. [PubMed]

26. Bligh, E.G.; Dyer, W.J. A rapid method of total lipid extraction and purification. *Can. J. Biochem. Physiol.* **1959**, *37*, 911–917. [CrossRef] [PubMed]

27. Livak, K.J.; Schmittgen, T.D. Analysis of relative gene expression data using real-time quantitative PCR and the 2(-Delta Delta C(T)) method. *Methods* **2001**, *25*, 402–408. [CrossRef] [PubMed]

28. Lee, M.S.; Kim, I.H.; Kim, C.T.; Kim, Y. Reduction of body weight by dietary garlic is associated with an increase in uncoupling protein mRNA expression and activation of AMP-activated protein kinase in diet-induced obese mice. *J. Nutr.* **2011**, *141*, 1947–1953. [CrossRef] [PubMed]

29. Kelley, D.E.; Goodpaster, B.; Wing, R.R.; Simoneau, J.A. Skeletal muscle fatty acid metabolism in association with insulin resistance, obesity, and weight loss. *Am. J. Physiol.* **1999**, *277*, E1130–E1141. [PubMed]

30. Turner, N.; Bruce, C.R.; Beale, S.M.; Hoehn, K.L.; So, T.; Rolph, M.S.; Cooney, G.J. Excess lipid availability increases mitochondrial fatty acid oxidative capacity in muscle: Evidence against a role for reduced fatty acid oxidation in lipid-induced insulin resistance in rodents. *Diabetes* **2007**, *56*, 2085–2092. [CrossRef] [PubMed]

31. Koves, T.R.; Ussher, J.R.; Noland, R.C.; Slentz, D.; Mosedale, M.; Ilkayeva, O.; Bain, J.; Stevens, R.; Dyck, J.R.; Newgard, C.B.; *et al.* Mitochondrial overload and incomplete fatty acid oxidation contribute to skeletal muscle insulin resistance. *Cell Metab.* **2008**, *7*, 45–56. [CrossRef] [PubMed]

32. Hsu, C.L.; Wu, C.H.; Huang, S.L.; Yen, G.C. Phenolic compounds rutin and o-coumaric acid ameliorate obesity induced by high-fat diet in rats. *J. Agric. Food Chem.* **2009**, *57*, 425–431. [CrossRef] [PubMed]

33. Rosen, E.D.; Walkey, C.J.; Puigserver, P.; Spiegelman, B.M. Transcriptional regulation of adipogenesis. *Genes Dev.* **2000**, *14*, 1293–1307. [PubMed]

34. White, U.A.; Stephens, J.M. Transcriptional factors that promote formation of white adipose tissue. *Mol. Cell Endocrinol.* **2010**, *318*, 10–14. [CrossRef] [PubMed]

35. Xu, A.; Wang, Y.; Xu, J.Y.; Stejskal, D.; Tam, S.; Zhang, J.; Wat, N.M.; Wong, W.K.; Lam, K.S. Adipocyte fatty acid-binding protein is a plasma biomarker closely associated with obesity and metabolic syndrome. *Clin. Chem.* **2006**, *52*, 405–413. [CrossRef] [PubMed]

36. Rossmeisl, M.; Flachs, P.; Brauner, P.; Sponarova, J.; Matejkova, O.; Prazak, T.; Ruzickova, J.; Bardova, K.; Kuda, O.; Kopecky, J. Role of energy charge and amp-activated protein kinase in adipocytes in the control of body fat stores. *Int. J. Obes. Relat. Metab. Disord.* **2004**, *28* (Suppl. 4), S38–S44. [CrossRef] [PubMed]

37. Park, S.Y.; Bok, S.H.; Jeon, S.M.; Park, Y.B.; Lee, S.J.; Jeong, T.S.; Choi, M.S. Effect of rutin and tannic acid supplements on cholesterol metabolism in rats. *Nutr. Res.* **2002**, *22*, 283–295. [CrossRef]

38. Lee, Y.S.; Li, P.; Huh, J.Y.; Hwang, I.J.; Lu, M.; Kim, J.I.; Ham, M.; Talukdar, S.; Chen, A.; Lu, W.J.; *et al.* Inflammation is necessary for long-term but not short-term high-fat diet-induced insulin resistance. *Diabetes* **2011**, *60*, 2474–2483. [CrossRef] [PubMed]

39. Esposito, E.; Iacono, A.; Bianco, G.; Autore, G.; Cuzzocrea, S.; Vajro, P.; Canani, R.B.; Calignano, A.; Raso, G.M.; Meli, R. Probiotics reduce the inflammatory response induced by a high-fat diet in the liver of young rats. *J. Nutr.* **2009**, *139*, 905–911. [CrossRef] [PubMed]

40. Wang, Y.; Ausman, L.M.; Russell, R.M.; Greenberg, A.S.; Wang, X.D. Increased apoptosis in high-fat diet-induced nonalcoholic steatohepatitis in rats is associated with c-Jun NH2-terminal kinase activation and elevated proapoptotic Bax. *J. Nutr.* **2008**, *138*, 1866–1871. [PubMed]

41. Gauthier, M.S.; Favier, R.; Lavoie, J.M. Time course of the development of non-alcoholic hepatic steatosis in response to high-fat diet-induced obesity in rats. *Br. J. Nutr.* **2006**, *95*, 273–281. [CrossRef] [PubMed]

42. Kappel, V.D.; Cazarolli, L.H.; Pereira, D.F.; Postal, B.G.; Zamoner, A.; Reginatto, F.H.; Silva, F.R. Involvement of GLUT-4 in the stimulatory effect of rutin on glucose uptake in rat soleus muscle. *J. Pharm. Pharmacol.* **2013**, *65*, 1179–1186. [CrossRef] [PubMed]

43. Kappel, V.D.; Zanatta, L.; Postal, B.G.; Silva, F.R. Rutin potentiates calcium uptake via voltage-dependent calcium channel associated with stimulation of glucose uptake in skeletal muscle. *Arch. Biochem. Biophys.* **2013**, *532*, 55–60. [CrossRef] [PubMed]

44. Canto, C.; Auwerx, J. PGC-1alpha, SIRT1 and AMPK, an energy sensing network that controls energy expenditure. *Curr. Opin. Lipidol.* **2009**, *20*, 98–105. [CrossRef] [PubMed]

45. Gleyzer, N.; Vercauteren, K.; Scarpulla, R.C. Control of mitochondrial transcription specificity factors (TFB1M and TFB2M) by nuclear respiratory factors (NRF-1 and NRF-2) and PGC-1 family coactivators. *Mol. Cell Biol.* **2005**, *25*, 1354–1366. [CrossRef] [PubMed]

46. Kelly, D.P.; Scarpulla, R.C. Transcriptional regulatory circuits controlling mitochondrial biogenesis and function. *Genes Dev.* **2004**, *18*, 357–368. [CrossRef] [PubMed]
47. Manach, C.; Morand, C.; Texier, O.; Favier, M.L.; Agullo, G.; Demigne, C.; Regerat, F.; Remesy, C. Quercetin metabolites in plasma of rats fed diets containing rutin or quercetin. *J. Nutr.* **1995**, *125*, 1911–1922. [PubMed]
48. Toledo, F.G.; Watkins, S.; Kelley, D.E. Changes induced by physical activity and weight loss in the morphology of intermyofibrillar mitochondria in obese men and women. *J. Clin. Endocrinol. Metab.* **2006**, *91*, 3224–3227. [CrossRef] [PubMed]
49. Toledo, F.G.; Menshikova, E.V.; Ritov, V.B.; Azuma, K.; Radikova, Z.; DeLany, J.; Kelley, D.E. Effects of physical activity and weight loss on skeletal muscle mitochondria and relationship with glucose control in type 2 diabetes. *Diabetes* **2007**, *56*, 2142–2147. [CrossRef] [PubMed]
50. Umanskaya, A.; Santulli, G.; Xie, W.; Andersson, D.C.; Reiken, S.R.; Marks, A.R. Genetically enhancing mitochondrial antioxidant activity improves muscle function in aging. *Proc. Natl. Acad. Sci. U.S.A.* **2014**, *111*, 15250–15255. [CrossRef] [PubMed]
51. Santulli, G.; Xie, W.; Reiken, S.R.; Marks, A.R. Mitochondrial calcium overload is a key determinant in heart failure. *Proc. Natl. Acad. Sci. U.S.A.* **2015**. [CrossRef] [PubMed]
52. Kim, J.A.; Wei, Y.; Sowers, J.R. Role of mitochondrial dysfunction in insulin resistance. *Circ. Res.* **2008**, *102*, 401–414. [CrossRef] [PubMed]
53. Santulli, G.; Pagano, G.; Sardu, C.; Xie, W.; Reiken, S.; D'Ascia, S.L.; Cannone, M.; Marziliano, N.; Trimarco, B.; Guise, T.A.; *et al.* Calcium release channel RyR2 regulates insulin release and glucose homeostasis. *J. Clin. Investig.* **2015**, *125*, 1968–1978. [CrossRef] [PubMed]
54. Manach, C.; Morand, C.; Demigne, C.; Texier, O.; Regerat, F.; Remesy, C. Bioavailability of rutin and quercetin in rats. *FEBS Lett.* **1997**, *409*, 12–16. [CrossRef]
55. Escande, C.; Nin, V.; Price, N.L.; Capellini, V.; Gomes, A.P.; Barbosa, M.T.; O'Neil, L.; White, T.A.; Sinclair, D.A.; Chini, E.N. Flavonoid apigenin is an inhibitor of the NAD+ ase CD38: Implications for cellular NAD+ metabolism, protein acetylation, and treatment of metabolic syndrome. *Diabetes* **2013**, *62*, 1084–1093. [CrossRef] [PubMed]
56. Dong, J.; Zhang, X.; Zhang, L.; Bian, H.X.; Xu, N.; Bao, B.; Liu, J. Quercetin reduces obesity-associated ATM infiltration and inflammation in mice: A mechanism including AMPKα1/SIRT1. *J. Lipid Res.* **2014**, *55*, 363–374. [CrossRef] [PubMed]
57. Howitz, K.T.; Bitterman, K.J.; Cohen, H.Y.; Lamming, D.W.; Lavu, S.; Wood, J.G.; Zipkin, R.E.; Chung, P.; Kisielewski, A.; Zhang, L.L.; *et al.* Small molecule activators of sirtuins extend saccharomyces cerevisiae lifespan. *Nature* **2003**, *425*, 191–196. [CrossRef] [PubMed]
58. Aura, A.M.; Martin-Lopez, P.; O'Leary, K.A.; Williamson, G.; Oksman-Caldentey, K.M.; Poutanen, K.; Santos-Buelga, C. In vitro metabolism of anthocyanins by human gut microflora. *Eur. J. Nutr.* **2005**, *44*, 133–142. [CrossRef] [PubMed]

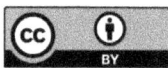

nutrients

MDPI

Article

Alternate-Day High-Fat Diet Induces an Increase in Mitochondrial Enzyme Activities and Protein Content in Rat Skeletal Muscle

Xi Li [1,†], Kazuhiko Higashida [2,3,4,*,†], Takuji Kawamura [1] and Mitsuru Higuchi [2,3]

[1] Graduate School of Sport Sciences, Waseda University, 2-579-15, Mikajima, Tokorozawa city,
     Saitama 359-1192, Japan; linokoto@akane.waseda.jp (X.L.); takuji@toki.waseda.jp (T.K.)
[2] Faculty of Sport Sciences, Waseda University, 2-579-15, Mikajima, Tokorozawa city, Saitama 359-1192, Japan;
     mhiguchi@waseda.jp
[3] Institute of Advanced Active Aging Research, Waseda University, 2-579-15, Mikajima, Tokorozawa city,
     Saitama 359-1192, Japan
[4] Department of Food Science and Nutrition, The University of Shiga Prefecture, 2500 Hassaka-Cho,
     Hikone city, Shiga 522-8533, Japan
*   Correspondence: higashida.k@shc.usp.ac.jp; Tel.: +81-749-28-8258
†   These authors contributed equally to this work.

Received: 13 January 2016; Accepted: 30 March 2016; Published: 6 April 2016

Abstract: Long-term high-fat diet increases muscle mitochondrial enzyme activity and endurance performance. However, excessive calorie intake causes intra-abdominal fat accumulation and metabolic syndrome. The purpose of this study was to investigate the effect of an alternating day high-fat diet on muscle mitochondrial enzyme activities, protein content, and intra-abdominal fat mass in rats. Male Wistar rats were given a standard chow diet (CON), high-fat diet (HFD), or alternate-day high-fat diet (ALT) for 4 weeks. Rats in the ALT group were fed a high-fat diet and standard chow every other day for 4 weeks. After the dietary intervention, mitochondrial enzyme activities and protein content in skeletal muscle were measured. Although body weight did not differ among groups, the epididymal fat mass in the HFD group was higher than those of the CON and ALT groups. Citrate synthase and beta-hydroxyacyl CoA dehydrogenase activities in the plantaris muscle of rats in HFD and ALT were significantly higher than that in CON rats, whereas there was no difference between HFD and ALT groups. No significant difference was observed in muscle glycogen concentration or glucose transporter-4 protein content among the three groups. These results suggest that an alternate-day high-fat diet induces increases in mitochondrial enzyme activities and protein content in rat skeletal muscle without intra-abdominal fat accumulation.

Keywords: high-fat diet; alternate-day; mitochondria; skeletal muscle; rat

1. Introduction

Endurance exercise training induces an increase in mitochondrial content in skeletal muscle [1], resulting in increased capacity of muscles to regenerate ATP. The increase in muscle mitochondrial content also results in a change in substrate utilization—with increased fat oxidation and decreased utilization of muscle glycogen [2,3]. Since the performance of endurance exercise is directly related to the muscle glycogen concentration prior to exercise, these biochemical adaptations of skeletal muscle lead to enhanced exercise performance after exercise training.

Aforementioned muscle adaptation is also caused by a high-fat diet feeding. Miller *et al.* [4] demonstrated that a 5-week high-fat diet in rats elevated mitochondrial enzyme activities in skeletal muscle. This biochemical adaptation in skeletal muscle has been reported by other groups in rodents and human subjects [5–8], although other groups reported opposite results, which high-fat diet feeding results in down-regulation of mitochondrial genes [9] or skeletal muscle from over-feeding-induced obese subject has impaired mitochondrial oxidative capacity [10,11]. Interestingly, in contrast to exercise training [12], the biochemical adaptation to high-fat diet in skeletal muscle occurs slowly, over at least 3–4 weeks [13]. Recent studies have shown the possible mechanisms by which a high-fat diet induces an increase in mitochondrial biogenesis in skeletal muscle [13–16], e.g., peroxisome proliferator activated receptor (PPAR) δ activation by raising plasma free fatty acids (FFA) and induction of PPAR γ coactivator-1α (PGC-1α).

It is well known that a long-term high-fat diet causes intra-abdominal fat accumulation, insulin resistance, and obesity. Miller *et al.* [4] reported that high-fat diet-fed rats gained more body weight than did the control diet-fed rats, despite a significant increase in mitochondrial enzyme activities. This observation might be the reason why a high-fat diet is not adopted by the endurance athlete, although it has some merit in that there is an increase in mitochondrial enzyme activities and a concomitant decrease in utilization of glycogen during endurance exercise. Thus, the dietary regimen that induces increases in mitochondrial oxidative capacities in skeletal muscle without intra-abdominal fat accumulation and body weight gain will offer many advantages. In this context, the present study aimed to determine whether the repeated increase in FFA caused by an alternate-day high-fat diet results in an increase in the mitochondrial oxidative capacity without accumulation of intra-abdominal fat mass. Here, we report that an alternate-day high-fat diet, comprising a high-fat diet and standard diet every other day, has a significant effect on muscle mitochondrial enzymes—it increases mitochondrial enzyme activities and protein content without causing excess body weight gain and intra-abdominal fat accumulation.

2. Methods

2.1. Materials

Reagents for SDS-PAGE were obtained from Bio-Rad (Hercules, CA, USA). Monoclonal long-chain acyl CoA dehydrogenase antibody and horseradish peroxidase (HRP)-conjugated secondary antibodies were obtained from Sigma (St. Louis, MO, USA) and Cell Signaling Technologies (Danvers, MA, USA), respectively. Anti-PGC-1α antibody was obtained from Calbiochem (San Diego, CA, USA). Polyclonal antiserum specific for GLUT-4 was a generous gift from Mike Mueckler (Washington University, St. Louis, MO, USA). Enhanced chemiluminescence (ECL) reagent was purchased from Millipore (Temecula, CA, USA). All other chemicals were obtained from Sigma.

2.2. Treatment of Animals

Four-week-old male Wistar rats (70–90 g body weight) were obtained from CLEA Japan (Tokyo, Japan). All rats were housed in rooms lighted from 9:00 a.m. to 9:00 p.m. The room temperature was maintained at 22–24 °C. Rats were separated into those receiving a control diet (CON: $n = 6$), high-fat diet (HFD: $n = 6$), and an alternate-day high-fat diet (ALT: $n = 6$). The high-fat diet was prepared using lard, corn oil, sucrose, and casein (32%, 18%, 27%, and 23%, respectively, of total calories), supplemented with minerals (51 g/kg, AIN93G mineral mix: CLEA Japan), vitamins (22 g/kg, AIN93 vitamin mix: CLEA Japan), and methionine (4.4 g/kg: Wako Pure Chemical). The standard diet, CE-2 was obtained from CLEA Japan; it contained as percentage of calories, 59% carbohydrate, 12% fat, and 29% protein. The energy content of the high-fat diet was 5.1 kcal/g, whereas that of the standard diet was 3.4 kcal/g. The rats were provided with food and water *ad libitum*. Rats in the CON and HFD groups were fed the control diet and the high-fat diet for 4 weeks, respectively. Rats in the ALT group were fed the control diet alternated with the high-fat diet every other day. The ALT animals were fed the high-fat diet on the day before sacrifice. Food was removed at 9:00 p.m. the day before muscle dissection. Between 9:00 and 12:00 a.m. on the next day, rats were anesthetized with an intraperitoneal injection of pentobarbital sodium (50 mg/kg) and blood samples were drawn from the abdominal aorta. After the blood sampling, plantaris muscle and epididymal fat pads were removed.

This experimental protocol was approved by the Committee for Animal Experimentation in the School of Sport Sciences at Waseda University (No. 2014-A096).

2.3. Measurement of Mitochondrial Enzyme Activities

For enzyme activity measurements, a portion of plantaris muscles were homogenized in ice-cold buffer containing 175 mM KCl, 10 mM GSH, and 2 mM EDTA, pH 7.4. The homogenates were frozen and thawed three times and mixed thoroughly before enzyme activities were measured. For the β-hydroxyacyl-CoA dehydrogenase (β-HAD) assay, an aliquot of the homogenate was centrifuged at $700\times g$ for 10 min at 4 °C. Citrate synthase (CS), a marker of oxidative enzymes, and β-HAD activities were measured using Srere's [17] and Bass's [18] methods, respectively.

2.4. Western Blot Analysis

A portion of frozen plantaris muscles were homogenized in ice-cold RIPA buffer containing 50 mM Tris-HCl, pH 7.4, 150 mM NaCl, 0.25% deoxycholic acid, 1% NP-40, 1 mM EDTA, and a protease inhibitor cocktail (Cell Signaling Technologies, Danvers, CA, USA). Protein concentrations were measured using a BCA protein assay kit (Pierce, Rockford, IL, USA) according to the manufacturer's instruction. Samples were diluted in 4× sample buffer (Invitrogen, Camarillo, CA, USA). Equal amounts of sample protein were subjected to SDS-PAGE (10% resolving gels) and then transferred to PVDF membranes at 200 mA for 90 min. After transfer, the membranes were washed in Tris-buffered saline with 0.1% Tween 20 (TBST; 20 mM Tris base, 137 mM NaCl, pH 7.6), and then membranes were blocked with TBST supplemented with 5% skimmed powdered milk for 1 h at room temperature. After blocking, the membranes were incubated overnight at 4 °C with antibodies specific for long chain acyl CoA dehydrogenase (LCAD), glucose transporter-4 (GLUT-4) and PGC-1α at concentrations of 1:2000–5000. The HRP-conjugated secondary antibody (goat anti-rabbit IgG) was used at a concentration of 1:10,000. Bands were visualized by ECL and scanned using a chemiluminescence detector (LAS 3000, FUJIFILM). The membranes were stained with Coomassie Brilliant Blue (CBB) to verify and normalize the protein loading [19]. Band intensities were quantified using ImageJ (NIH).

2.5. Analytical Procedure

Concentrations of plasma glucose, FFA, and triglyceride were determined using kits (Glucose C2 Test Wako, NEFA-C Test Wako, Triglyceride E Test Wako, respectively) according to the manufacturer's instructions. Plasma insulin concentration was measured using an enzyme-linked immunospecific assay kit according to the manufacturer's instruction (Mercodia AB, Uppsala, Sweden).

2.6. Succinate Dehydrogenase (SDH) Staining

For histological analysis, plantaris muscles were frozen in isopentane, which had been cooled in liquid nitrogen. Serial cross-sections (5 μm thick) were cut in a cryostat at −20 °C. Sections were stained for succinate dehydrogenase (SDH) activity, complex II of the mitochondrial respiratory chain, as follows. Sections were first allowed to reach room temperature before they were then incubated in a solution containing nitro blue tetrazolium (0.5 mg/mL), sodium succinate (50 mM), and phosphate buffer (0.12 M potassium dihydrogenphosphate, 0.88 M disodium hydrogen phosphate) for 25 min at 37 °C. Cross-sections were then washed three times in distilled water, dehydrated in 70% (1 min), 80% (1 min), 90% (1 min), and 100% (1 min) ethanol, and then cover-slipped using an aqueous mounting medium.

2.7. Muscle Glycogen Concentration

Glycogen concentration in plantaris muscles was determined by using the method of Lowry and Passonneau [20] after acid hydrolysis.

2.8. Statistical Analysis

The data are presented as the mean ± standard error of the mean (SEM). Statistical analysis was performed using analysis of variance (ANOVA). The Tukey's test was used for *post hoc* analysis when the ANOVA test indicated significant differences. When the normality (Shapiro–Wilk test) was not met, variables were analyzed using the Kruskal–Wallis test and the Steel–Dwass *post hoc* test was used as needed. Statistical significance accepted at $p < 0.05$.

3. Results

3.1. Body Weight, Epididymal Fat Weight, and Plasma Parameters

Table 1 shows the body weight and epididymal fat weight. The 4-week high-fat diet resulted in an increase in epididymal fat weight in the HFD group (CON *vs.* HFD, $p < 0.05$). However, at 4 weeks, epididymal fat weight in the ALT group was not significantly different from that in CON group.

Table 1. Effects of alternate-day high-fat diet feeding on body weight, epididymal fat mass, plasma glucose, free fatty acids, and insulin concentrations in rats.

	CON	HFD	ALT
Initial body weight (g)	87 ± 1	86 ± 5	87 ± 1
Final body weight (g)	298 ± 5	297 ± 9	298 ± 3
Epididymal fat mass (g)	3.1 ± 0.2	5.1 ± 0.3 *	3.8 ± 0.1
Plasma glucose (mg/mL)	96.9 ± 2.6	96.8 ± 6.3	81.1 ± 2.6 #
Plasma FFA (mEq/L)	0.28 ± 0.02	0.44 ± 0.05 *	0.44 ± 0.06 *
Plasma insulin (µg/L)	0.39 ± 0.3	0.42 ± 0.4	0.39 ± 0.3

CON, control group; HFD, high-fat diet group; ALT, alternate-day high-fat diet group. Values are mean ± SEM of 6 animals per group. * indicates significant difference at a level of $p < 0.05$ *vs.* CON. # indicates significant difference at a level of $p < 0.05$ *vs.* CON and HFD.

Plasma FFA concentration in the HFD and ALT groups was significantly higher than that in the CON group (CON *vs.* HFD and ALT, $p < 0.05$). Although the precise mechanism is not clear, plasma glucose concentration in the ALT group was significantly lower than those of CON and HFD (ALT *vs.* CON and HFD, $p < 0.05$). There was no significant difference in plasma insulin concentration among the three groups (Table 1).

3.2. Mitochondrial Enzymes Activities and PGC-1α Protein Content

Citrate synthase activities in the plantaris muscle of the HFD and ALT rats were significantly higher than in the same muscle of the CON rats (Figure 1A) (CON *vs.* HFD, $p < 0.01$; CON *vs.* ALT, $p < 0.05$). After the 4-week dietary intervention, the β-HAD activity in the HFD and ALT groups was significantly higher than that in the CON group (Figure 1B) (CON *vs.* HFD and ALT, $p < 0.05$). Protein content of PGC-1α in HFD group was significantly higher than that of the CON group ($p < 0.05$, Figure 2A). Furthermore, PGC-1α protein content was increased by 4-week alternate-day high-fat diet feeding ($p < 0.05$. Figure 2A). Both HFD and ALT induced a significant increase in LCAD protein content in plantaris muscle (Figure 2B) (CON *vs.* HFD and ALT, $p < 0.05$).

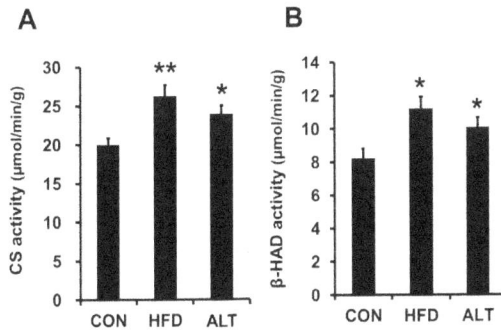

Figure 1. Effects of alternate-day high-fat diet feeding on citrate synthase (**A**) and β-HAD (**B**) enzyme activities in rat skeletal muscle. Values are mean ± SEM of 6 animals per group. * and ** indicate significant differences at levels of $p < 0.05$ and $p < 0.01$ *vs.* CON, respectively.

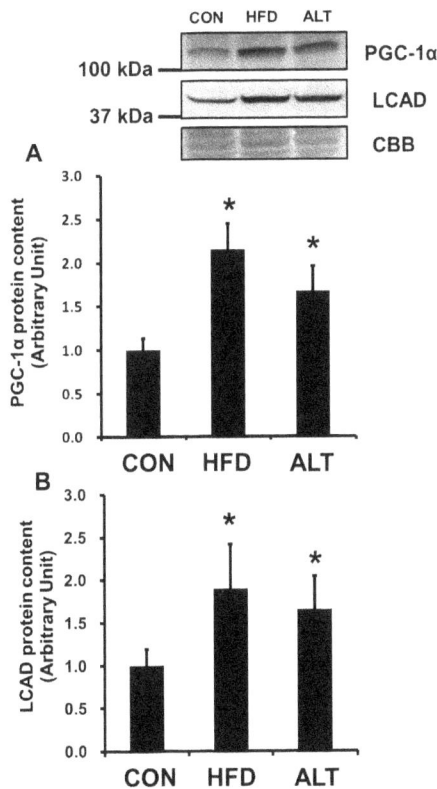

Figure 2. Effects of alternate-day high-fat diet feeding on PGC-1α (**A**) and LCAD (**B**) protein content in rat skeletal muscle. Values are mean ± SEM of 6 animals per group. * indicates significant difference at a level of $p < 0.05$ *vs.* CON.

3.3. SDH Activity

Next, we assessed the effect of an alternate-day high-fat diet on the oxidative capacity in skeletal muscles using histochemistry. Figure 3 shows representative images of SDH staining of the plantaris muscle from CON, HFD, and ALT groups. Succinate dehydrogenase activity staining was increased in HFD and ALT groups compared to the CON group.

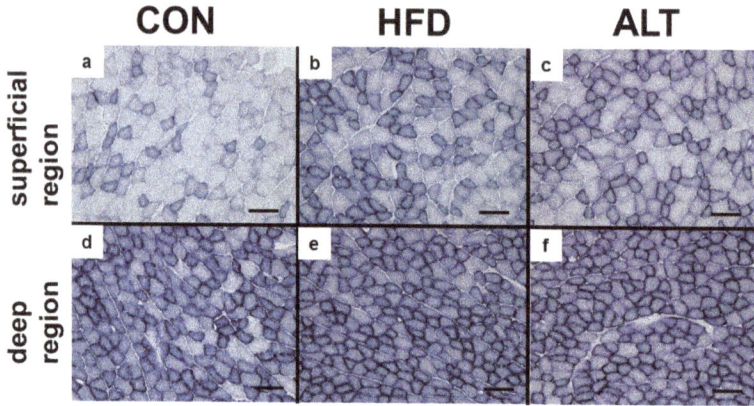

Figure 3. Effect of alternate-day high-fat diet feeding on succinate dehydrogenase (SDH) staining in plantaris muscle. Representative SDH-stained images are presented. SDH staining of superficial region of plantaris muscle from CON (**a**), HFD (**b**) and ALT (**c**) and deep region from CON (**d**), HFD (**e**) and ALT (**f**). Plantaris muscle of both HFD and ALT showed relatively dark staining for SDH compare to that of CON. Scale bar, 100 μm.

3.4. Muscle Glycogen Concentration and Glucose Transporter-4 Protein Content

Previous studies reported that long term high-fat diet feeding reduces muscle glycogen concentration [4,6,8]. Since GLUT-4-mediated glucose transport across the plasma membrane is one of the rate-limiting step of glycogen synthesis in skeletal muscle [21], we measured muscle glycogen concentration and GLUT-4 protein content. As shown in Figure 4, we observed no significant difference in glycogen concentration (Figure 4A) or GLUT-4 content (Figure 4B) in plantaris muscles among the three groups.

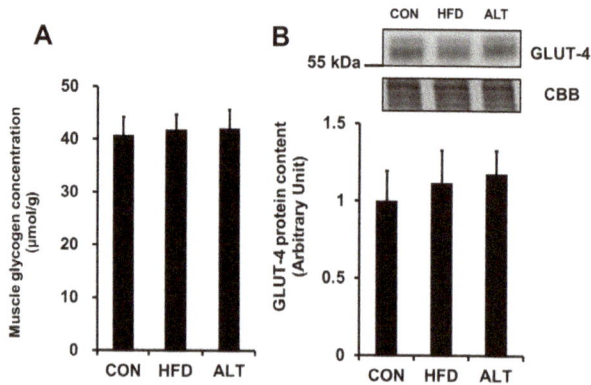

Figure 4. Effects of alternate-day high-fat diet feeding on glycogen concentration (**A**) and GLUT-4 protein content (**B**) in rat skeletal muscle. Values are mean ± SEM of 6 animals per group.

4. Discussion

The main findings of the present study were that an alternate-day high-fat diet induces increases in mitochondrial enzyme activities and protein content in rat skeletal muscle, without causing intra-abdominal fat accumulation.

It was first reported by Holloszy [1] that endurance exercise training increases mitochondrial enzyme activities in rat skeletal muscle, and this finding was confirmed by other research groups assessing human skeletal muscle [22]. The most important physiological effect of an increase in mitochondrial content in skeletal muscle is the sparing of muscle glycogen during submaximal exercise. The glycogen-sparing effect mediated by a smaller decrease in creatine phosphate and ATP, and a smaller increase in inorganic phosphate, stimulates glycogenolysis [2,23]. Miller *et al.* [4] reported that rats, which were fed a high-fat diet for 5 weeks ran for a longer duration than those fed a high-carbohydrate diet. The improvement in endurance performance is concomitant with an increase in skeletal muscle citrate synthase (a key enzyme of the tricarboxylic acid cycle) and β-HAD enzyme activity (a major index of the β-oxidation) and lower utilization of muscle glycogen concentration. This result suggests that a high-fat diet induces an increase in mitochondrial biogenesis, muscle glycogen sparing during exercise, which thereby prolongs submaximal endurance exercise performance. In agreement with this finding, our results also showed that a 4-week high-fat diet induces an increase in key mitochondrial enzyme activities in rat skeletal muscle, and that an alternate-day high-fat diet induces an increase in mitochondrial enzymes in rat skeletal muscle to a level comparable to that observed after a daily high-fat diet (Figure 1A,B). This result suggests that an alternate-day high-fat diet is sufficient to increase mitochondrial enzyme activities and protein content in skeletal muscle.

The main disadvantage of a long-term high-fat diet is the huge accumulation of intra-abdominal fat and increasing body weight. In the present study, intra-abdominal fat mass in HFD rats was about 60% higher than that of CON rats (Table 1). Since there is a strong correlation between intra-abdominal fat mass and insulin resistance [24,25], it is difficult to adopt the long term high-fat diet for endurance athletes. Not only is it particularly unhealthy, but also will it result in an increase in body weight, which negatively affects endurance exercise performance. However, an alternate-day high-fat diet induced muscle adaptation, but did not cause excessive intra-abdominal fat accumulation. Results from the present investigation suggest that it is possible that dietary intervention with a high-fat diet can induce increases in mitochondrial oxidative capacities in skeletal muscle, while reducing health risk. However, in the present study, the diet intervention period was only 4 weeks to determine the effect of alternate-day high-fat diet feeding on intra-abdominal fat accumulation. If a longer period of dietary intervention is performed, an increase in body fat might be observed. It should be investigated whether time course changes of accumulation of intra-abdominal fat by an alternate-day high-fat diet.

Recently, the possible mechanisms involved in this high-fat diet-induced increase in mitochondrial protein content in skeletal muscle have been studied. It has been reported that raising plasma FFA results in an increase in PPAR δ activation and mitochondrial biogenesis [13]. In this study, plasma concentration of FFA is higher in both HFD and ALT groups than in the CON group. Therefore, it is likely that there is a similar activation of PPARδ by raising plasma FFA in both the HFD and ALT groups resulting in an increase in mitochondrial enzyme activities in skeletal muscle. The transcriptional coactivator PGC-1α is known to induce mitochondrial biogenesis by activation of transcription factors and coordinated expression of a large number of proteins [26]. In this study, PGC-1α protein content in HFD was significantly higher than that of CON. Furthermore, the ALT group had an elevated protein content of PGC-1α (Figure 2A). It was reported that PGC-1α proteins significantly increase after 4 weeks of HFD, without an increase in the rate of transcription [13]. The finding that PGC-1α mRNA expression does not increase in skeletal muscle of rat fed a high-fat diet [13], suggested a hypothesis that high-fat diet results in an increase in PGC-1α protein content through post-translational mechanisms, such as decrease in degradation of PGC-1α protein. Although the precise mechanisms by which high-fat diet increases PGC-1α protein content through post-translational mechanisms are not clear, our findings suggested that repeated stimulation of HFD by ALT is sufficient to elevate PGC-1α protein content and mitochondrial proteins.

Several studies reported that rats fed a high-fat diet are capable of intense exercise despite a limited muscle glycogen stores [4,6,8]. In the present study, we did not find differences in muscle glycogen concentration among the different groups. Furthermore, the protein content of GLUT-4, a predominant form of glucose transporter in skeletal muscle, was not different among the three groups (Figure 4A,B). The difference in glycogen concentration in response to a high-fat diet between our study and previous studies might be due to the fat content of the diet. The diet used in this study comprised 50% of calories from fat, whereas rats in the previous studies were fed diets comprising 78% fat [4,8]. This extremely low carbohydrate diet may result in lower glycogen concentrations in skeletal muscle.

In contrast to animal studies, human studies have failed to demonstrate a beneficial effect of a high-fat diet on endurance exercise performance [5,27]. The difference in results between animal and human studies may be because of fat composition in diet. The control diet used in most of the animal studies comprised approximately 10% of calories from fat, whereas a typical Japanese and American diet consists of about 25% [28] and 34% fat [29], respectively. It might be difficult to detect a high-fat diet-induced increase in endurance performance in humans, because the fat content in the diet of humans is higher than that used in experimental animals. However, because a high-fat diet, containing 62% calories from fat, induces increases in mitochondrial enzymes in human skeletal muscle [7], human skeletal muscle is capable of adaptation responses to a high-fat diet. Therefore, it will be interesting in future studies to determine whether manipulation of dietary fat, not using a high-fat diet, induces an increase in mitochondrial oxidative enzyme capacity in human skeletal muscle and enhance endurance exercise performance.

Recent works by Shortreed *et al.* demonstrated that high-fat diet feeding for 8 weeks impaired oxidative capacity in mice skeletal muscle [30]. In contrast, Sadler *et al.* reported that 2-week high-fat diet feeding in mice down-regulated citrate synthase activity, but it gradually increased at 16 weeks [31]. While it is difficult to be certain why the adaptations to high-fat diet differ from the studies, the time course of development of mitochondrial impairment by over-feeding or high-fat diet, and the differences of animal model (mouse or rat), should be investigated carefully in future studies. Furthermore, although the increase in mitochondrial volume, enzyme activity, and changes in organelle composition is referred to as mitochondrial biogenesis, we assessed the limited numbers of mitochondrial proteins, including β-oxidation enzymes (β-HAD and LCAD) and citrate cycle enzyme (citrate synthase) in this study. In addition, recent studies showed the functional role of mitochondrial reactive oxygen species, which affecting calcium handling proteins involved in muscle contractility [32,33]. Future extensive investigations are expected to directly measure the mtDNA copy number, mitochondrial volume, and calcium handling capacity of mitochondria to examine whether the alternate-day high-fat diet feeding induces an increase in functional mitochondria in skeletal muscle.

5. Conclusions

In conclusion, we found that provision of an alternate-day high-fat diet for 4 weeks induces increases in mitochondrial enzyme activities and protein content in rat skeletal muscle without intra-abdominal fat accumulation.

Author Contributions: Kazuhiko Higashida and Mitsuru Higuchi conceived and designed the experiments. Xi Li, Kazuhiko Higashida and Takuji Kawamura performed research. Kazuhiko Higashida and Mitsuru Higuchi wrote the paper, Xi Li and Takuji Kawamura revised intellectual and critically the manuscript. All authors approved the final manuscript.

Conflicts of Interest: The authors declare no conflict of interest.

References

1. Holloszy, J.O. Biochemical adaptations in muscle. Effects of exercise on mitochondrial oxygen uptake and respiratory enzyme activity in skeletal muscle. *J. Biol. Chem.* **1967**, *242*, 2278–2282. [PubMed]

2. Constable, S.H.; Favier, R.J.; McLane, J.A.; Fell, R.D.; Chen, M.; Holloszy, J.O. Energy metabolism in contracting rat skeletal muscle: Adaptation to exercise training. *Am. J. Physiol.* **1987**, *253*, C316–C322. [PubMed]

3. Martin, W.H.; Dalsky, G.P.; Hurley, B.F.; Matthews, D.E.; Bier, D.M.; Hagberg, J.M.; Rogers, M.A.; King, D.S.; Holloszy, J.O. Effect of endurance training on plasma free fatty acid turnover and oxidation during exercise. *Am. J. Physiol.* **1993**, *265*, E708–E714. [PubMed]

4. Miller, W.C.; Bryce, G.R.; Conlee, R.K. Adaptations to a high-fat diet that increase exercise endurance in male rats. *J. Appl. Physiol. Respir. Environ. Exerc. Physiol.* **1984**, *56*, 78–83. [PubMed]

5. Phinney, S.D.; Bistrian, B.R.; Evans, W.J.; Gervino, E.; Blackburn, G.L. The human metabolic response to chronic ketosis without caloric restriction: Preservation of submaximal exercise capability with reduced carbohydrate oxidation. *Metabolism* **1983**, *2*, 769–776. [CrossRef]

6. Simi, B.; Sempore, B.; Mayet, M.H.; Favier, R.J. Additive effects of training and high-fat diet on energy metabolism during exercise. *J. Appl. Physiol.* **1991**, *71*, 197–203. [PubMed]

7. Helge, J.W.; Kiens, B. Muscle enzyme activity in humans: Role of substrate availability and training. *Am. J. Physiol.* **1997**, *272*, R1620–R1624. [PubMed]

8. Lee, J.S.; Bruce, C.R.; Spriet, L.L.; Hawley, J.A. Interaction of diet and training on endurance performance in rats. *Exp. Physiol.* **2001**, *86*, 499–508. [PubMed]

9. Sparks, L.M.; Xie, H.; Koza, R.A.; Mynatt, R.; Hulver, M.W.; Bray, G.A.; Smith, S.R. A high-fat diet coordinately downregulates genes required for mitochondrial oxidative phosphorylation in skeletal muscle. *Diabetes* **2005**, *54*, 1926–1933. [CrossRef] [PubMed]

10. Tanner, C.J.; Barakat, H.A.; Dohm, G.L.; Pories, W.J.; MacDonald, K.G.; Cunningham, P.R.; Swanson, M.S.; Houmard, J.A. Muscle fiber type is associated with obesity and weight loss. *Am. J. Physiol. Endocrinol. Metab.* **2002**, *282*, E1191–E1196. [CrossRef] [PubMed]

11. Hickey, M.S.; Carey, J.O.; Azevedo, J.L.; Houmard, J.A.; Pories, W.J.; Israel, R.G.; Dohm, G.L. Skeletal muscle fiber composition is related to adiposity and *in vitro* glucose transport rate in humans. *Am. J. Physiol.* **1995**, *268*, E453–E457. [PubMed]

12. Higashida, K.; Kim, S.H.; Higuchi, M.; Holloszy, J.O.; Han, D.H. Normal adaptations to exercise despite protection against oxidative stress. *Am. J. Physiol. Endocrinol. Metab.* **2011**, *301*, E779–E784. [CrossRef] [PubMed]

13. Hancock, C.R.; Han, D.H.; Chen, M.; Terada, S.; Yasuda, T.; Wright, D.C.; Holloszy, J.O. High-fat diets cause insulin resistance despite an increase in muscle mitochondria. *Proc. Natl. Acad. Sci. USA* **2008**, *105*, 7815–7820. [CrossRef] [PubMed]

14. Garcia-Roves, P.; Huss, J.M.; Han, D.H.; Hancock, C.R.; Iglesias-Gutierrez, E.; Chen, M.; Holloszy, J.O. Raising plasma fatty acid concentration induces increased biogenesis of mitochondria in skeletal muscle. *Proc. Natl. Acad. Sci. USA* **2007**, *104*, 10709–10713. [CrossRef] [PubMed]

15. Turner, N.; Bruce, C.R.; Beale, S.M.; Hoehn, K.L.; So, T.; Rolph, M.S.; Cooney, G.J. Excess Lipid Availability Increases Mitochondrial Fatty Acid Oxidative Capacity in Muscle. Evidence against a Role for Reduced Fatty Acid Oxidation in Lipid-Induced Insulin Resistance in Rodents. *Diabetes* **2007**, *56*, 2085–2092. [CrossRef] [PubMed]

16. Fillmore, N.; Jacobs, D.L.; Mills, D.B.; Winder, W.W.; Hancock, C.R. Chronic AMP-activated protein kinase activation and a high-fat diet have an additive effect on mitochondria in rat skeletal muscle. *J. Appl. Physiol.* **2010**, *109*, 511–520. [CrossRef] [PubMed]

17. Srere, P.A. Citrate synthase. *Methods Enzymol.* **1969**, *13*, 3–5.

18. Bass, A.; Brdiczka, D.; Eyer, P.; Hofer, S.; Pette, D. Metabolic differentiation of distinct muscle types at the level of enzymatic organization. *Eur. J. Biochem.* **1968**, *10*, 198–206. [CrossRef]

19. Welinder, C.; Ekblad, L. Coomassie staining as loading control in Western blot analysis. *J. Proteome Res.* **2011**, *10*, 1416–1419. [CrossRef] [PubMed]

20. Lowry, O.H.; Passonneau, J.V. *A Flexible System of Enzymatic Analysis*; Academic Press: New York, NY, USA, 1972.

21. Fisher, J.S.; Nolte, L.A.; Kawanaka, K.; Han, D.H.; Jones, T.E.; Holloszy, J.O. Glucose transport rate and glycogen synthase activity both limit skeletal muscle glycogen accumulation. *Am. J. Physiol. Endocrinol. Metab.* **2002**, *282*, E1214–E1221. [CrossRef] [PubMed]
22. Morgan, T.E.; Cobb, L.A.; Short, F.A.; Ross, R.; Gunn, D.R. Effects of Long-Term Exercise on Human Muscle Mitochondria. *Adv. Exp. Med. Biol.* **1971**, *11*, 87–95.
23. Favier, R.J.; Constable, S.H.; Chen, M.; Holloszy, J.O. Endurance exercise training reduces lactate production. *J. Appl. Physiol.* **1986**, *61*, 885–889. [PubMed]
24. Kim, J.Y.; Nolte, L.A.; Hansen, P.A.; Han, D.H.; Ferguson, K.; Thompson, P.A.; Holloszy, J.O. High-fat diet-induced muscle insulin resistance: Relationship to visceral fat mass. *Am. J. Physiol. Regul. Integr. Comp. Physiol.* **2000**, *279*, R2057–R2065. [PubMed]
25. Racette, S.B.; Evans, E.M.; Weiss, E.P.; Hagberg, J.M.; Holloszy, J.O. Abdominal adiposity is a stronger predictor of insulin resistance than fitness among 50–95 years old. *Diabetes Care* **2006**, *29*, 673–678. [CrossRef] [PubMed]
26. Handschin, C.; Spiegelman, B.M. Peroxisome proliferator-activated receptor gamma coactivator 1 coactivators, energy homeostasis, and metabolism. *Endocr. Rev.* **2006**, *27*, 728–735. [CrossRef] [PubMed]
27. Helge, J.W.; Wulff, B.; Kiens, B. Impact of a fat-rich diet on endurance in man: Role of the dietary period. *Med. Sci. Sports Exerc.* **1998**, *30*, 456–461. [CrossRef] [PubMed]
28. Ministry of Health, Labour and Welfare. *The National Health and Nutrition Survey*; Ministry of Health, Labour and Welfare: Tokyo, Japan, 2013.
29. US Department of Agriculture/Agricultural Research Service. *Nutrient Intake from Food: Percentages of Energy from Protein, Carbohydrate, Fat, and Alcohol, by Gender and Age, in the United States, 2011–2012*; USDA: Wahington, DC, USA, 2014. Available online: http://www.ars.usda.gov/SP2UserFiles/Place/80400530/pdf/1112/Table_5_EIN_GEN_11.pdf (accessed on 30 March 2016).
30. Shortreed, K.E.; Krause, M.P.; Huang, J.H.; Dhanani, D.; Moradi, J.; Ceddia, R.B.; Hawke, T.J. Muscle-specific adaptations, impaired oxidative capacity and maintenance of contractile function characterize diet-induced obese mouse skeletal muscle. *PLoS ONE* **2009**, *4*, e7293. [CrossRef] [PubMed]
31. Sadler, N.C.; Angel, T.E.; Lewis, M.P.; Pederson, L.M.; Chauvigné-Hines, L.M.; Wiedner, S.D.; Zink, E.M.; Smith, R.D.; Wright, A.T. Activity-based protein profiling reveals mitochondrial oxidative enzyme impairment and restoration in diet-induced obese mice. *PLoS ONE* **2012**, *7*, e47996. [CrossRef] [PubMed]
32. Umanskaya, A.; Santulli, G.; Xie, W.; Andersson, D.C.; Reiken, S.R.; Marks, A.R. Genetically enhancing mitochondrial antioxidant activity improves muscle function in aging. *Proc. Natl. Acad. Sci. USA* **2014**, *111*, 15250–15255. [CrossRef] [PubMed]
33. Santulli, G.; Xie, W.; Reiken, S.R.; Marks, A.R. Mitochondrial calcium overload is a key determinant in heart failure. *Proc. Natl. Acad. Sci. USA* **2015**, *112*, 11389–11394. [CrossRef] [PubMed]

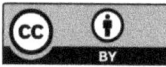

Section 3:
Glucose Homeostasis and Dyslipidemia

nutrients

MDPI

Article

Nigerian Honey Ameliorates Hyperglycemia and Dyslipidemia in Alloxan-Induced Diabetic Rats

Omotayo O. Erejuwa [1,*], Ndubuisi N. Nwobodo [1], Joseph L. Akpan [1], Ugochi A. Okorie [1], Chinonyelum T. Ezeonu [2], Basil C. Ezeokpo [3], Kenneth I. Nwadike [4], Erhirhie Erhiano [5], Mohd S. Abdul Wahab [6] and Siti A. Sulaiman [6]

[1] Department of Pharmacology and Therapeutics, Faculty of Medicine, Ebonyi State University, Abakaliki 480214, Ebonyi State, Nigeria; nnwobodo@yahoo.com (N.N.N.); etejoe2006@gmail.com (J.L.A.); ugoochi94@gmail.com (U.A.O.)

[2] Department of Pediatrics, Faculty of Medicine, Ebonyi State University, Abakaliki 480214, Ebonyi State, Nigeria; ctezeonu@gmail.com

[3] Department of Internal Medicine, Faculty of Medicine, Ebonyi State University, Abakaliki 480214, Ebonyi State, Nigeria; ezeokpo_bc@yahoo.co.uk

[4] Department of Pharmacology and Therapeutics, College of Medicine, University of Nigeria, Enugu 400211, Enugu State, Nigeria; kenneth.nwadike@unn.edu.ng

[5] Department of Physiology, College of Health Sciences, Usmanu Danfodiyo University, Sokoto 840212, Sokoto State, Nigeria; erhianoefe@yahoo.com

[6] Department of Pharmacology, School of Medical Sciences, Universiti Sains Malaysia, Kubang Kerian 16150, Kelantan, Malaysia; msuhaimikb@usm.my (M.S.A.W.); sbsamrah@usm.my (S.A.S.)

* Correspondence: erejuwa@gmail.com; Tel.: +234-8022526381

Received: 20 November 2015; Accepted: 31 December 2015; Published: 24 February 2016

Abstract: Diabetic dyslipidemia contributes to an increased risk of cardiovascular disease. Hence, its treatment is necessary to reduce cardiovascular events. Honey reduces hyperglycemia and dyslipidemia. The reproducibility of these beneficial effects and their generalization to honey samples of other geographical parts of the world remain controversial. Currently, data are limited and findings are inconclusive especially with evidence showing honey increased glycosylated hemoglobin in diabetic patients. It was hypothesized that this deteriorating effect might be due to administered high doses. This study investigated if Nigerian honey could ameliorate hyperglycemia and hyperlipidemia. It also evaluated if high doses of honey could worsen glucose and lipid abnormalities. Honey (1.0, 2.0 or 3.0 g/kg) was administered to diabetic rats for three weeks. Honey (1.0 or 2.0 g/kg) significantly ($p < 0.05$) increased high density lipoprotein (HDL) cholesterol while it significantly ($p < 0.05$) reduced hyperglycemia, triglycerides (TGs), very low density lipoprotein (VLDL) cholesterol, non-HDL cholesterol, coronary risk index (CRI) and cardiovascular risk index (CVRI). In contrast, honey (3.0 g/kg) significantly ($p < 0.05$) reduced TGs and VLDL cholesterol. This study confirms the reproducibility of glucose lowering and hypolipidemic effects of honey using Nigerian honey. However, none of the doses deteriorated hyperglycemia and dyslipidemia.

Keywords: honey; diabetes mellitus; hyperglycemia; hyperlipidemia; dyslipidemia; lipid profile; alloxan; rats

1. Introduction

Diabetes mellitus is a metabolic disorder associated with an increased risk of cardiovascular disease (CVD), a main cause of mortality in diabetes [1]. Although several factors account for increased CVD risk in diabetes, abnormalities of lipid metabolism are important contributors [2]. Hence, in addition to controlling hyperglycemia, treatment of dyslipidemia is inevitable to reduce cardiovascular events in diabetes [3]. While the current agents employed for the treatment of dyslipidemia are effective, these drugs are not easily affordable to many patients [4]. Besides, the use of some of these agents is associated with undesirable side effects. Some of these factors compel patients to seek alternative and complementary medicines. Even though complementary and alternative medicines are easily accessible and more affordable, their use is not without drawback. These agents are of unproven efficacy, and there are great concerns for safety and risk of untoward adverse effects [5].

One such complementary medicine that has gained wide attention in the past decade is honey. The anecdotal use of honey dates back to 2100–2000 BC [6]. Research in the past few years has provided convincing evidence in support of antioxidant, antibacterial and the wound healing properties of honey [7–9]. With regard to other reported beneficial effects, especially metabolic and cardiovascular effects such as antihypertensive, hypolipidemic, hypoglycemic and antidiabetic effects of honey, data are limited and the findings remain inconclusive particularly in clinical studies. At the moment, due to paucity of data, it remains unclear if these reported beneficial metabolic effects of honey can be reproduced using any honey sample or is restricted to a specific honey or certain honeys. Evidence has revealed that there is variation in the composition of honey. This variation depends on certain factors including geographical origin and botanical sources of the nectar [10]. Other factors such as climate, environment and processing techniques also contribute to variation in honey composition [10,11]. The variation in honey composition may influence the pharmacological effects derived from the honey samples. This leads to another uncertainty as to whether findings obtained with a honey sample from a particular geographical origin or floral source can be generalized to honey samples from other geographical parts or botanical sources of the world [12].

More worrisome is the evidence from a study which showed that honey increased glycosylated hemoglobin in diabetic patients [13]. This finding appears to suggest a potential deteriorating effect of honey on glycemic control. However, it was later explained that this particular finding should not be generalized to all honey samples as a result of two factors. These factors are: the administered high doses and the high glucose content of the administered honey [14]. In that particular study, graded doses of honey were administered orally to diabetic patients for eight weeks. The initial dose (1.0 g/kg/day) was increased by 0.5 g/kg/day every two weeks till the end of the study. Besides, the honey in question had a considerably higher glucose content than that found in most honey samples [15]. It was suggested that these two factors would invariably enhance glycosylation and contribute to increased glycosylated hemoglobin in diabetic patients [14]. This potential deterioration of glycemic control resulting from honey administration may also aggravate dyslipidemia in diabetes. Therefore, this study was carried out to investigate if Nigerian honey could reduce hyperglycemia and ameliorate lipid abnormalities in alloxan-induced diabetic rats. It also aimed to evaluate if high doses of honey could deteriorate glucose and lipid derangements in alloxan-induced diabetic rats.

2. Materials and Methods

2.1. Chemicals

Alloxan and glucose were purchased from Sigma-Aldrich, MO, USA. All other reagents used were of analytical grade.

2.2. Animals

The Wistar rats were purchased from animal house unit, Nsukka, Nigeria. The animals were acclimatized for at least 2 weeks. Two rats were housed per cage and maintained in a well ventilated animal room with temperature of 25–27 °C and 12-h light/dark cycle. The rats had free access to rat chow and portable water *ad libitum*. The animals were handled with humane care and in accordance with institutional guidelines of Ethics Committee of Ebonyi State University (EBSU/UREC/15/FCM/004) and international guidelines on the Use and Handling of Experimental Animals [16].

2.3. Honey

Honey was purchased from a bee farm in Ebonyi State, Nigeria. The honey had a NAFDAC (National Agency for Food and Drug Administration Control) registered number. The honey was dissolved in drinking water and prepared freshly each time it was administered.

2.4. Induction of Diabetes Mellitus

Diabetes mellitus was induced in overnight fasted male Wistar rats (180–220 g) via intraperitoneal administration of 150 mg/kg body weight (BW) of alloxan dissolved in normal saline. Another group of fasted rats was administered normal saline without alloxan. The rats were given 20% (w/v) glucose solution to prevent fatal post-alloxan hypoglycemia. Forty-eight hours (48 h) post-alloxan administration, rats with elevated fasting blood glucose (BG) concentrations $\geqslant$250 mg/dL were considered diabetic and included in the study.

2.5. Treatment

The animals were randomly divided into five groups. All the groups (except group 5) consisted of 6 rats. Group 5 comprised 5 rats because a rat died few days to the end of the treatment period. Using oral canula, the rats were administered drinking water or honey once daily between 8:00 and 9:00 a.m. for 3 weeks as follows:

- Group 1: Non-diabetic rats administered 1 mL/kg BW of drinking water
- Group 2: Diabetic rats administered 1 mL/kg BW of drinking water
- Group 3: Diabetic rats treated with 1.0 g/kg BW of honey
- Group 4: Diabetic rats treated with 2.0 g/kg BW of honey
- Group 5: Diabetic rats treated with 3.0 g/kg BW of honey

Before the commencement of treatment, body weight and fasting blood glucose concentrations were measured using weighing scale and Accu-Chek Active glucometer (Roche, Germany), respectively. After treatment for 3 weeks, the rats were fasted overnight for at least 16 h (4 p.m.–8 a.m.). The body weight and blood glucose concentrations were measured. The animals were then sacrificed under light diethyl ether anesthesia. Blood samples were collected in plain tubes and allowed to clot at room temperature. The blood samples were centrifuged at 1500 rpm for 10 min. The supernatants (sera) were collected and stored at $-20\,^{\circ}$C till further analysis.

2.6. Biochemical Analysis

The serum concentrations of total cholesterol (TC), triglycerides (TGs) and high density lipoprotein (HDL) cholesterol were determined using Agappe kits (Agappe Diagnostics, Knonauerstrasse, Cham, Switzerland) on EMP-168 Biochemical Analyzer according to the manufacturer's instructions. Serum low density lipoprotein (LDL) and very low density lipoprotein (VLDL) cholesterol were estimated using the Friedewald equations [17].

$$LDL\,cholesterol\,=\,TC-[HDL\,cholesterol\,+\,(TG/5)] \tag{1}$$

$$VLDL\,cholesterol\,=\,TG/5 \tag{2}$$

Non-HDL cholesterol was calculated by the formula:

$$Non\text{-}HDL\,cholesterol\,=\,TC-HDL\,cholesterol \tag{3}$$

2.7. Determination of Atherogenic Index (AI), Coronary Risk Index (CRI) and Cardiovascular Risk Index (CVRI)

The AI, CRI and CVRI were calculated using the formulae ([18,19]):

$$AI = LDL\,cholesterol/HDL\;cholesterol \tag{4}$$

$$CRI = TC/HDL\,cholesterol \tag{5}$$

$$CVRI = TGs/HDL\,cholesterol \tag{6}$$

2.8. Statistical Analysis

The results were analyzed using SPSS version 14. Data are expressed as mean $\pm$ SEM. Each group consisted of 6 rats (except the diabetic + 3.0 g/kg BW honey group which comprised 5 rats). Differences among treated groups were assessed by one way analysis of variance (ANOVA) followed by Tukey's *post hoc* test. The results of initial and final blood glucose concentrations were analyzed using paired *t* test. $p \leqslant 0.05$ was considered statistical significant.

3. Results

3.1. Effect of Honey on Percentage (%) Change in Body Weight (BW) of Diabetic Rats

The % change in BW was significantly reduced ($p < 0.01$ or $p < 0.001$) in diabetic rats including those treated with honey (Figure 1). Honey treatment did not improve % change in BW in diabetic rats.

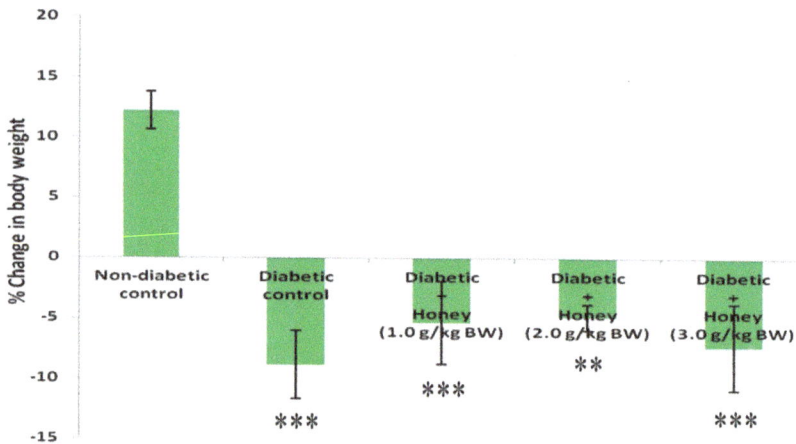

Figure 1. Effect of honey on % change in BW of diabetic rats. Data are expressed as mean $\pm$ SEM. ** & *** A significant decrease ($p < 0.01$ & $p < 0.001$) when compared with non-diabetic control.

3.2. Effects of Honey on Blood Glucose (BG) Concentrations and Percentage (%) Change in BG of Diabetic Rats

Figure 2 shows the effect of honey on BG concentrations of diabetic rats. The initial and final BG concentrations in non-diabetic and diabetic control groups did not differ. Compared with the initial BG concentrations, final BG levels were significantly ($p < 0.05$) lower in diabetic rats administered 1.0 or 2.0 g/kg BW of honey. Compared with diabetic control rats, only 1.0 or 2.0 g/kg BW of honey significantly ($p < 0.05$) reduced % change in BG in diabetic rats (Figure 3). The 3.0 g/kg BW of honey did decrease % change in BG but was not statistically significant.

Nutrients **2016**, *8*, 95

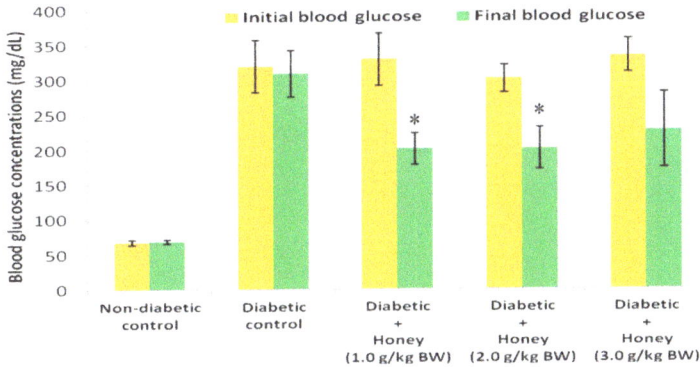

Figure 2. Effect of honey on BG concentrations of diabetic rats. Data are expressed as mean $\pm$ SEM. * A significant decrease ($p < 0.05$) when compared with initial BG concentrations within the same group.

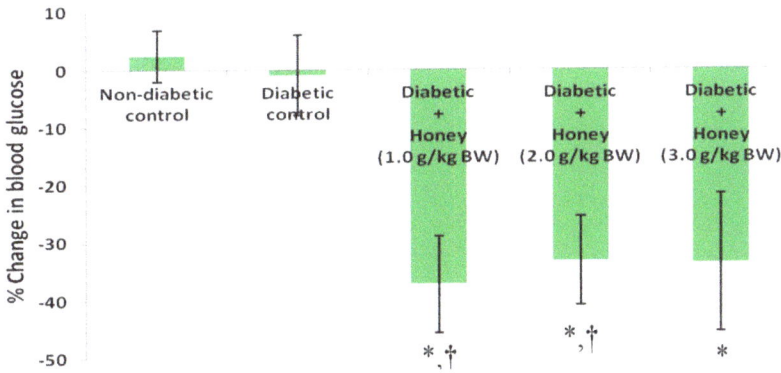

Figure 3. Effect of honey on % change in BG of diabetic rats. Data are expressed as mean $\pm$ SEM. * A significant decrease ($p < 0.05$) when compared with non-diabetic control; † A significant decrease ($p < 0.05$) when compared with diabetic control.

3.3. Effects of Honey on Triglycerides (TG), High Density Lipoprotein (HDL), Non-HDL and Very Low Density Lipoprotein (VLDL) Cholesterol of Diabetic Rats

The data on the effects of honey on TG, HDL, non-HDL and VLDL cholesterol in diabetic rats are presented in Figures 4–7 respectively. The diabetic control group had significantly ($p < 0.05$) elevated levels of TG compared with non-diabetic rats. All the three doses of honey significantly ($p < 0.05$) reduced TG levels in diabetic rats (Figure 4). Though not statistically significant ($p > 0.05$), HDL cholesterol was reduced in diabetic control group (Figure 5). The 2.0 g/kg BW of honey significantly ($p < 0.05$) increased HDL cholesterol in diabetic rats. The diabetic control rats had significantly ($p < 0.05$) elevated levels of non-HDL cholesterol (Figure 6). Compared with diabetic control, the non-HDL cholesterol level was significantly ($p < 0.05$) reduced in diabetic rats administered 1.0 or 2.0 g/kg BW of honey. The reduction of non-HDL cholesterol produced by 3.0 g/kg BW of honey was not statistically significant. The diabetic control group had significantly ($p < 0.05$) elevated levels of VLDL cholesterol compared with non-diabetic rats (Figure 7). All the three doses of honey significantly ($p < 0.05$) reduced VLDL cholesterol levels in diabetic rats.

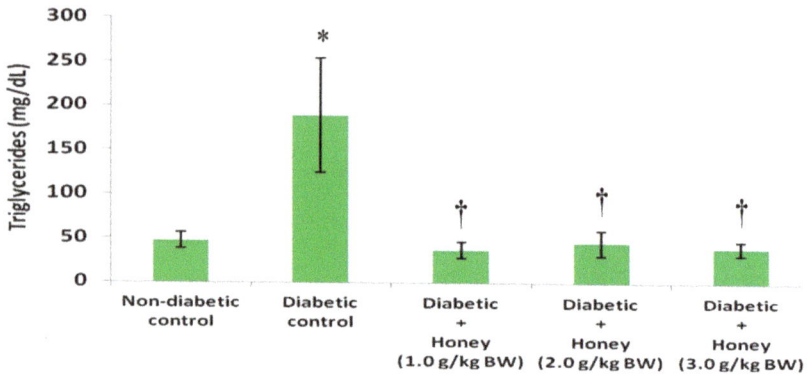

Figure 4. Effect of honey on triglycerides of diabetic rats. Data are expressed as mean ± SEM. * A significant increase ($p < 0.05$) when compared with non-diabetic control; † A significant decrease ($p < 0.05$) when compared with diabetic control.

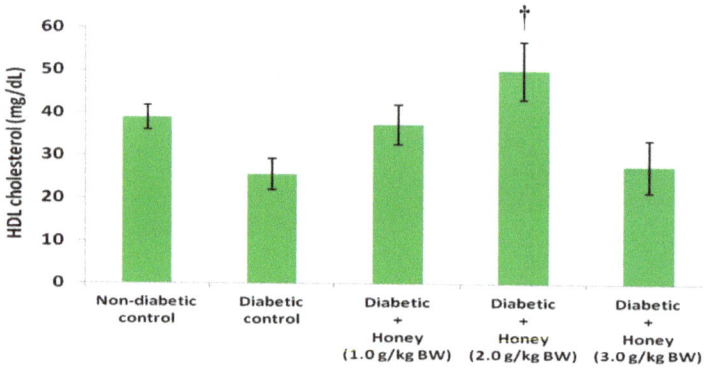

Figure 5. Effect of honey on HDL cholesterol of diabetic rats. Data are expressed as mean ± SEM. † A significant increase ($p < 0.05$) when compared with diabetic control.

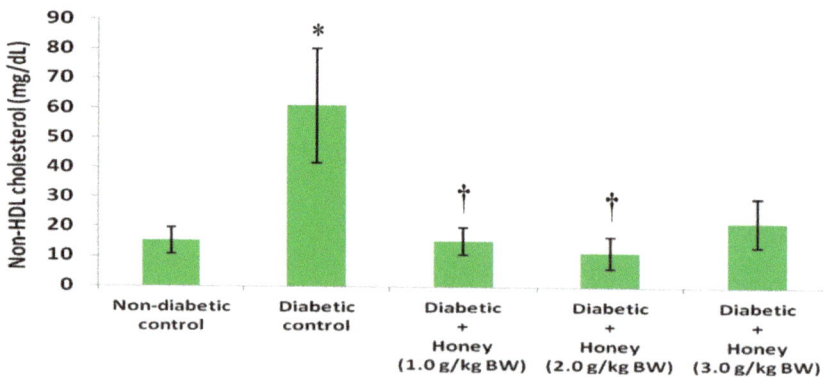

Figure 6. Effect of honey on non-HDL cholesterol of diabetic rats. Data are expressed as mean ± SEM. * A significant increase ($p < 0.05$) when compared with non-diabetic control; † A significant decrease ($p < 0.05$) when compared with diabetic control.

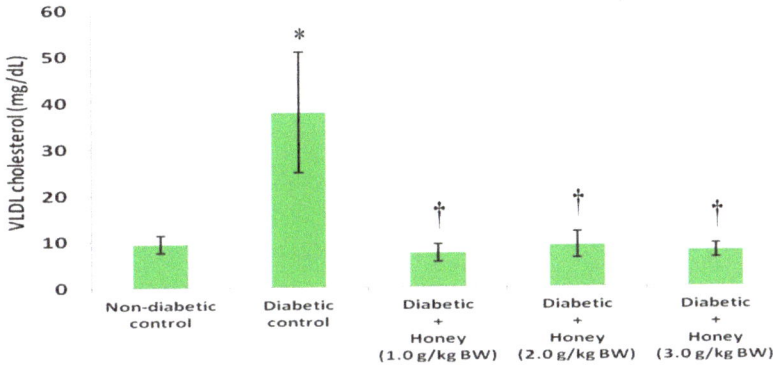

Figure 7. Effect of honey on VLDL cholesterol of diabetic rats. Data are expressed as mean ± SEM.
* A significant increase ($p < 0.05$) when compared with non-diabetic control; † A significant decrease
($p < 0.05$) when compared with diabetic control.

3.4. Effects of Honey on Coronary and Cardiovascular Risk Indices of Diabetic Rats

Figure 8 shows the effect of honey on coronary risk index (CRI) in diabetic rats. The diabetic control rats had significantly ($p < 0.05$) higher levels of CRI compared with non-diabetic control. Administration of 1.0 or 2.0 g/kg BW of honey significantly ($p < 0.05$) reduced CRI in diabetic rats. The 3.0 g/kg BW of honey did reduce coronary risk index but not statistically significant. The effect of honey on cardiovascular risk index (CVRI) in diabetic rats is presented in Figure 9. The diabetic control rats had significantly ($p < 0.05$) higher CVRI compared with non-diabetic control. With the exception of 3.0 g/kg BW of honey, honey treatment significantly ($p < 0.05$) reduced CVRI in diabetic rats.

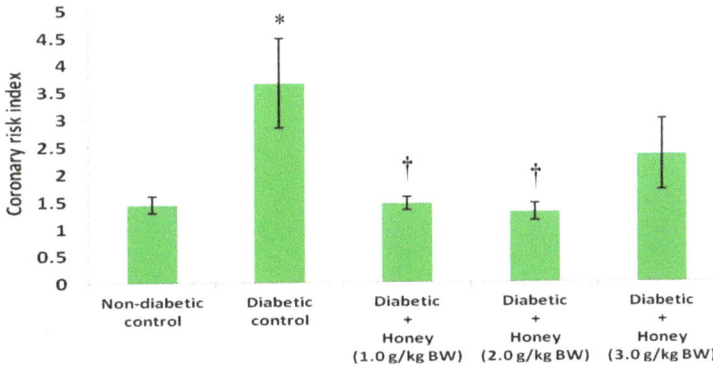

Figure 8. Effect of honey on coronary risk index of diabetic rats. Data are expressed as mean ± SEM.
* A significant increase ($p < 0.05$) when compared with non-diabetic control; † A significant decrease
($p < 0.05$) when compared with diabetic control.

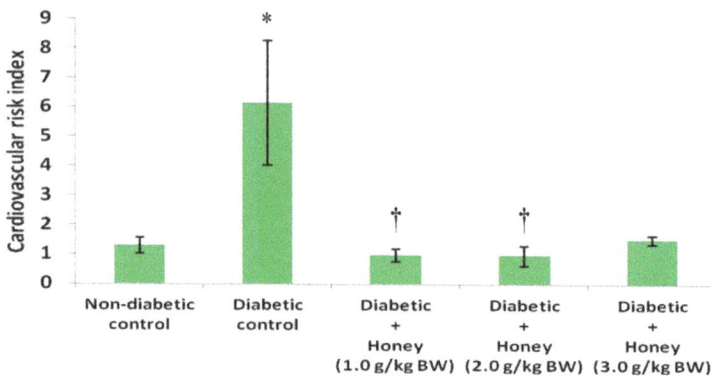

Figure 9. Effect of honey on cardiovascular risk index of diabetic rats. Data are expressed as mean ± SEM. * A significant increase ($p < 0.05$) when compared with non-diabetic control; † A significant decrease ($p < 0.05$) when compared with diabetic control.

3.5. Effects of Honey on Total Cholesterol (TC), LDL Cholesterol and Atherogenic Index of Diabetic Rats

Table 1 shows the data on the effects of honey on TC, LDL cholesterol and atherogenic index. Though not statistically significant, the diabetic control rats had elevated levels of TC, LDL cholesterol and atherogenic index compared with non-diabetic rats. Although honey treatment (especially 1.0 or 2.0 g/kg BW of honey) reduced these parameters towards those of the non-diabetic rats, the reductions were not statistically significant ($p > 0.05$).

Table 1. Effects of honey on total cholesterol (TC), low density lipoprotein (LDL) cholesterol and atherogenic index.

Group	TC (mg/dL)	LDL Cholesterol (mg/dL)	Atherogenic Index
Non-diabetic control	54.3 ± 2.4	8.0 ± 3.7	0.2 ± 0.1
Diabetic control	86.7 ± 18.1	23.2 ± 13.0	1.1 ± 0.7
Diabetic + Honey (1.0 g/kg BW)	52.6 ± 5.4	7.9 ± 2.9	0.2 ± 0.1
Diabetic + Honey (2.0 g/kg BW)	61.6 ± 5.6	4.4 ± 2.8	0.1 ± 0.1
Diabetic + Honey (3.0 g/kg BW)	49.4 ± 3.0	21.6 ± 7.5	1.0 ± 0.6

Data are expressed as mean ± SEM.

4. Discussion

In this study, a model of alloxan-induced diabetes was utilized to investigate the potential glucose lowering and hypolipidemic effect of Nigerian honey and also to evaluate if high doses of honey would deteriorate hyperglycemia and dyslipidemia. The three doses used in this study were selected based on previous findings as reported for Malaysian honey [7,20]. The lowest dose (1.0 g/kg BW) was shown to improve glycemic control and hyperlipidemia in streptozotocin-induced diabetic rats [21]. Two additional higher doses of honey (2.0 and 3.0 g/kg BW) were chosen as a follow-up to a study that reported exacerbating effect of honey on glycemic control in diabetic patients [13]. It was suggested that the administered high doses of honey might contribute to such deteriorating effect of honey [14].

The study found that alloxan-induced diabetic rats exhibited significant % reduction in body weight. Decreased body weight is commonly observed in alloxan-induced diabetic rodents [22]. This is attributed to break down of adipose tissue lipids and skeletal muscle protein [23]. Honey treatment did not improve % change in body weight in diabetic rats. This is in contrast with previous reports which found improved body weight following honey supplementation in streptozotocin-induced diabetic rats [7,20]. In the present study, honey treatment (1.0 or 2.0 g/kg BW) significantly reduced blood glucose levels in diabetic rats. These findings concur with previous results which demonstrated glucose lowering effect of honey in diabetic rats [7,20,22] and diabetic patients [24]. The potential mechanisms by which honey mediates its glucose lowering effect have been elaborated [25]. Fructose, oligosaccharides, antioxidants and mineral elements are some of the numerous honey constituents that may contribute to its glucose lowering effect [25–27]. Besides these individual constituents with glucose-lowering properties, their synergistic interactions will contribute considerably to glucose lowering effect of honey.

The results showed that, unlike 1.0 or 2.0 g/kg BW dose, 3.0 g/kg BW dose did not produce significant reduction in blood glucose concentrations. In a previous study, 0.2 g/kg BW of honey did not produce significant reduction in blood glucose level but 1.2 or 2.4 g/kg BW significantly decreased hyperglycemia [20]. As reported in that study, there was no additional benefit of doubling the dose of honey from 1.2 to 2.4 g/kg BW on hyperglycemia. Likewise in this study, there was no significant difference in the glucose lowering effect of 1.0 or 2.0 g/kg BW of honey. However, there is a clear disparity in the findings of these two studies. While the previous study revealed a dose-dependent glucose lowering response [20], this new study did not show that. In order to harmonize these inconsistencies, it is imperative to consider all the doses in these two studies in a context. The doses are 0.2, 1.0, 1.2, 2.0, 2.4 and 3.0 g/kg BW. While the 0.2 g/kg BW dose did not elicit glucose lowering effect most probably as a result of insufficient dose, the reason for the lack of significant glucose lowering response of 3.0 g/kg BW dose remains unknown. An analysis of these doses and their glycemic responses reveals a trend whereby honey at a particular dose (sub-therapeutic dose) did not exert glucose lowering effect. However, as the dose was increased, it produced glucose lowering effect. Additional dose increments also resulted in glucose lowering responses but with no additional glucose-lowering benefit. It then reached a dose at which further dose increment resulted in a loss of glucose lowering effect. Further studies are necessary to reveal if additional doses beyond 3.0 g/kg BW of honey will eventually deteriorate hyperglycemia.

Considering that 0.2 g/kg BW and 3.0 g/kg BW of honey did not elicit significant glucose lowering effect, based on existing studies, it can be inferred that the therapeutic doses of honey range between 1.0 and 2.4 g/kg BW. In view of the fact that any dose of honey selected between 1.0 and 2.4 g/kg BW will exert glucose lowering effect without further glucose-lowering benefit, it would be plausible to propose 1.0 g/kg BW as the optimal dose of honey. This dose (1.0 g/kg BW) of honey has been investigated in several other studies involving various diseases and therapeutic effects have been reported [28–33]. It is worth mentioning that even if 3.0 g/kg BW of honey had elicited considerable glucose lowering response, considering the lack of additional glucose-lowering response compared with 1.0 g/kg BW dose, it would still not be pharmacologically acceptable to utilize this dose or other higher doses for therapeutic purposes in diabetes studies especially clinical research. In view of the fact that 3.0 g/kg BW of honey neither reduced considerably nor increased blood glucose concentrations, it is uncertain if administration of this dose to diabetic rats over a longer period of time will alter hyperglycemic level. This could not be observed in this study, which was terminated at three weeks because of increased mortality in the diabetic control group. Another limitation is the fact that glycosylated hemoglobin (which was found to be increased in honey-supplemented diabetic patients [13]) was not measured in this study though it will not be valid.

Diabetic dyslipidemia constitutes an important modifiable risk factor for cardiovascular disorders. Consequently, the treatment of dyslipidemia is an important strategy in diabetes management [34]. The diabetic control rats had significantly elevated serum levels of TGs, non-HDL and VLDL cholesterol similar to what was reported previously [35]. The serum concentrations of TC and LDL cholesterol in diabetic rats were also increased but not statistically significant. In contrast, HDL cholesterol level was non-significantly lower in the diabetic control group than in the non-diabetic group. The findings on TC, LDL and HDL cholesterol in alloxan-induced diabetic control rats are comparable to those reported in a previous study [36]. Alloxan-induced diabetes is associated with reduced insulin level resulting from destruction of β-cells following alloxan administration [37]. This low level of insulin promotes hypertriglyceridemia and secretion of VLDL cholesterol [38,39]. Elevated levels of TGs in turn displace protein content of VLDL and LDL. This disproportionate imbalance of protein and triglyceride content of lipoproteins leads to decreased uptake of these lipoproteins by lipoprotein receptors [40]. The accumulation of these lipoproteins and TGs is implicated in many vascular disorders. LDL cholesterol is an independent risk factor for the development of coronary heart disease (CHD) [41]. The TGs, unlike LDL cholesterol, are not directly atherogenic, but it is an important risk factor for the development of cardiovascular disease (CVD) [25]. Administration of honey to diabetic rats markedly reduced TGs, non-HDL and VLDL cholesterol. However, honey (3.0 g/kg BW) did not significantly reduce non-HDL cholesterol. While the lowest dose of honey (1.0 g/kg BW) increased the HDL level towards that of the non-diabetic rats, the highest dose (3.0 g/kg BW) produced no such effect. In contrast, 2.0 g/kg BW of honey significantly increased HDL cholesterol. In previous studies, honey at a dose of 1.0 g/kg BW was found to significantly reduce TGs and VLDL cholesterol while it increased HDL cholesterol in diabetic rats [21,32]. Similar beneficial effects of honey on lipid abnormalities were also reported in both type 1 and type 2 diabetic patients [13,24,42]. The ameliorative effects of honey as observed in this study as well as those of the previous studies clearly demonstrate the benefits of honey in the treatment of dyslipidemia.

Even though honey supplementation of diabetic rats was associated with non-significant reduction of LDL cholesterol, it is noteworthy that honey administration significantly reduced elevated levels of both TGs and non-HDL cholesterol (which consists of the LDL, intermediate density lipoprotein (IDL) and VLDL cholesterol fractions). This is important because increased non-HDL cholesterol level together with hypertriglyceridemia in the presence of abnormal glucose metabolism increases risk of CVD [43]. Therefore, the marked ameliorative effects of honey on TGs and non-HDL cholesterol indicate honey can reduce risk of CVD. In this study, the effect of honey on lipid ratios (such as LDL/HDL cholesterol, TC/HDL cholesterol and TG/HDL cholesterol) in diabetic rats was evaluated. Assessment of lipid ratios is better than individual lipid parameters in predicting risk of atherogenicity, CHD and CVD [44]. Non-significant increase in LDL/HDL cholesterol was observed in diabetic control group. LDL/HDL cholesterol reflects atherogenic index (AI) [44]. Increased AI has also been reported in alloxan-induced diabetic rats [35]. Honey administration (especially 1.0 or 2.0 g/kg BW) tended to reduce atherogenic index. The data indicated TC/HDL cholesterol was markedly increased in diabetic control rats. The TC/HDL cholesterol is an index of CHD and is designated as coronary risk index (CRI) [45]. Honey supplementation (except the 3.0 g/kg BW dose) considerably reduced CRI which indicates honey can decrease the risk of CHD in diabetic rats. On the other hand, the TG/HDL cholesterol predicts the development of CVD and serves as cardiovascular risk index (CVRI) [46]. Recent evidence has also shown that TG/HDL cholesterol is an important predictor of cardiac disease mortality [47]. The results showed that the diabetic control rats had significantly elevated CVRI. However, some researchers reported non-significant elevation of this lipid ratio in alloxan-induced diabetic control mice [48]. Honey therapy (except the 3.0 g/kg BW dose) significantly reduced CVRI in diabetic rats. This finding therefore suggests that honey is capable of reducing risk of CVD in diabetic rats. Increased TG/HDL-C ratio is also a reflection of elevated levels of small and dense subclass of LDL cholesterol (sdLDL), which contribute to increased cardiovascular risk [49]. Hence, the decreased TG/HDL cholesterol in honey-treated diabetic rats suggests that honey supplementation reduced sdLDL in diabetic rats.

In view of the role of insulin in lipid metabolism and prevention of hypertriglyceridemia [50], it is plausible to propose a role of insulin in the hypolipidemic effect of honey. Based on the current literature, honey may ameliorate dyslipidemia in part via enhanced release of insulin from the remnant pancreatic β-cells. This proposition is supported by compelling evidence from previous studies. Some beneficial effects of honey on insulin have been reported in human subjects [42,51]. Similarly, honey has been shown to increase serum insulin level in streptozotocin-induced diabetic rats [21] and C-peptide (a peptide released from the β-cells during cleavage of insulin from proinsulin) in diabetic patients [24].

Histological examination of pancreata from honey-treated diabetic rats has also revealed less severe injury, incomplete restoration of cellular population as well as bigger size of the islets of Langerhans compared with pancreata from untreated diabetic rats [52]. Besides, honey has been shown to protect the pancreas against oxidative stress [53]. This may, in turn, contribute to protection of β-cells against hyperglycemia-induced oxidative damage [52–54]. All these pancreatic protective effects of honey will help to preserve the β-cells which invariably will contribute to increased serum insulin levels as reported [21]. Increased secretion of insulin will enhance lipogenesis and inhibit lipolysis leading to amelioration of hyperlipidemia [55].

It is worthy of note that, compared to the other two doses, the 3.0 g/kg BW of honey ameliorated dyslipidemia to a less extent or partially. This is evident by the lack of significant effect of this dose on serum levels of HDL, non-HDL cholesterol, TC/HDL cholesterol and TG/HDL cholesterol. Furthermore, an analysis of the data presented in Table 1 reveals the values of LDL cholesterol and atherogenic risk index in the diabetic rats treated with 3.0 g/kg BW of honey were elevated towards those of the diabetic control rats. These data on the lipid parameters and lipid ratios seem to suggest that honey at 3.0 g/kg BW lost its hypolipidemic effect. Interestingly, this reduced or loss of hypolipidemic effect of 3.0 g/kg BW of honey is in agreement with its loss of glucose lowering effect. Additional studies involving higher doses or the same dose but for a longer duration of treatment may help to reveal if honey can worsen dyslipidemia.

5. Conclusions

This study shows that, using comparable doses as reported for Malaysian honey, Nigerian honey ameliorates hyperglycemia and dyslipidemia in alloxan-induced diabetic rats. Thus, this study adds to the limited available evidence that the glucose lowering and hypolipidemic effects of honey are not restricted to honey samples of a particular geographical origin. In addition, the study extends previous findings by reporting that the beneficial effects of honey on glucose and lipid metabolism as well as lipid ratios may be lost at high doses of honey. The study, however, did not find any deteriorating effect of the highest dose of honey (3.0 g/kg BW) on hyperglycemia and dyslipidemia. Considering that the therapeutic benefits of honey on metabolic derangements tended to be lost or reduced at the highest dose, it remains unclear if 3.0 g/kg BW of honey or higher doses administered over a longer duration of time would worsen hyperglycemia and dyslipidemia in diabetes.

Acknowledgments: This study was supported in part by a grant from Universiti Sains Malaysia (Grant No.: 203/PPSP/617186).

Author Contributions: O.O.E. conceived, designed and carried out the study. O.O.E analyzed the data and wrote the manuscript. All authors contributed to acquisition of funding, and reviewed and approved the final version of the manuscript.

Conflicts of Interest: The authors have no conflicts of interest concerning the work described in this manuscript. The company that produced the honey was not involved at any stage of the study, neither did it support financially the research. In addition, none of the authors have any affiliation directly or indirectly with the company.

Abbreviations

The following abbreviations are used in this manuscript:

CVD	cardiovascular disease
CHD	coronary heart disease
NAFDAC	National Agency for Food and Drug Administration Control
BW	body weight
BG	blood glucose
TC	total cholesterol
TGs	triglycerides
LDL	low density lipoprotein

VLDL	very low density lipoprotein
HDL	high density lipoprotein
Non-HDL	non-high density lipoprotein
AI	atherogenic index
CRI	coronary risk index
CVRI	cardiovascular risk index
SEM	standard error of mean
ANOVA	analysis of variance

References

1. Laing, S.P.; Swerdlow, A.J.; Slater, S.D.; Burden, A.C.; Morris, A.; Waugh, N.R.; Gatling, W.; Bingley, P.J.; Patterson, C.C. Mortality from heart disease in a cohort of 23,000 patients with insulin-treated diabetes. *Diabetologia* **2003**, *46*, 760–765. [CrossRef] [PubMed]
2. Susanti, E.; Donosepoetro, M.; Patellongi, I.; Arif, M. Differences between several atherogenic parameters in patients with controlled and uncontrolled type 2 diabetes mellitus. *Med. J. Indones.* **2010**, *19*, 103–108. [CrossRef]
3. Ballantyne, C.M. Treatment of dyslipidemia to reduce cardiovascular risk in patients with multiple risk factors. *Clin. Cornerstone* **2007**, *8*, S6–S13. [CrossRef]
4. Williams, J.; Steers, W.N.; Ettner, S.L.; Mangione, C.M.; Duru, O.K. Cost-related nonadherence by medication type among medicare part D beneficiaries with diabetes. *Med. Care* **2013**, *51*, 193–198. [CrossRef] [PubMed]
5. Singh, D.; Gupta, R.; Saraf, S.A. Herbs-are they safe enough? An overview. *Crit. Rev. Food Sci. Nutr.* **2012**, *52*, 876–898. [CrossRef] [PubMed]
6. Crane, E. History of honey. In *Honey, a Comprehensive Survey*; Crane, E., Ed.; William Heinemann: London, UK, 1975; pp. 439–488.
7. Erejuwa, O.O.; Sulaiman, S.A.; Wahab, M.S.; Sirajudeen, K.N.; Salleh, S.; Gurtu, S. Effects of Malaysian tualang honey supplementation on glycemia, free radical scavenging enzymes and markers of oxidative stress in kidneys of normal and streptozotocin-induced diabetic rats. *Int. J. Cardiol.* **2009**, *137*, S45. [CrossRef]
8. Erejuwa, O.O.; Sulaiman, S.A.; Abdul Wahab, M.S. Honey: A novel antioxidant. *Molecules* **2012**, *17*, 4400–4423. [CrossRef] [PubMed]
9. Tan, H.T.; Rahman, R.A.; Gan, S.H.; Halim, A.S.; Hassan, S.A.; Sulaiman, S.A.; Kirnpal-Kaur, B. The antibacterial properties of Malaysian tualang honey against wound and enteric microorganisms in comparison to manuka honey. *BMC Complement. Altern. Med.* **2009**, *9*, 1–8. [CrossRef] [PubMed]
10. Gheldof, N.; Wang, X.H.; Engeseth, N.J. Identification and quantification of antioxidant components of honeys from various floral sources. *J. Agric. Food Chem.* **2002**, *50*, 5870–5877. [CrossRef] [PubMed]
11. Wang, J.; Li, Q.X. Chemical composition, characterization, and differentiation of honey botanical and geographical origins. *Adv. Food Nutr. Res.* **2011**, *62*, 89–137. [PubMed]
12. Erejuwa, O.O. Effect of honey in diabetes mellitus: Matters arising. *J. Diabetes Metab. Disord.* **2014**, *13*, 23. [CrossRef] [PubMed]
13. Bahrami, M.; Ataie-Jafari, A.; Hosseini, S.; Foruzanfar, M.H.; Rahmani, M.; Pajouhi, M. Effects of natural honey consumption in diabetic patients: An 8-week randomized clinical trial. *Int. J. Food Sci. Nutr.* **2009**, *60*, 618–626. [CrossRef] [PubMed]
14. Erejuwa, O.O. The use of honey in diabetes mellitus: Is it beneficial or detrimental? *Int. J. Endocrinol. Metab.* **2012**, *10*, 444–445. [CrossRef]
15. Bogdanov, S.; Jurendic, T.; Sieber, R.; Gallmann, P. Honey for nutrition and health: A review. *J. Am. Coll. Nutr.* **2008**, *27*, 677–689. [CrossRef] [PubMed]
16. United States Department of Health and Human Services, Public Health Service, National Institutes of Health. *Guide for the Care and Use of Laboratory Animals*; NIH Publication No. 85-23; National Institutes of Health: Bethesda, MD, USA, 1985.
17. Friedewald, W.T.; Levy, R.I.; Fredrickson, D.S. Estimation of the concentration of low-density lipoprotein cholesterol in plasma, without use of the preparative ultracentrifuge. *Clin. Chem.* **1972**, *18*, 499–502. [PubMed]

18. Abbott, R.D.; Wilson, P.W.; Kannel, W.B.; Castelli, W.P. High density lipoprotein cholesterol, total cholesterol screening and myocardial infarction. The Framingham Study. *Arteriosclerosis* **1988**, *8*, 207–211. [CrossRef] [PubMed]

19. Alladi, S.; Khada, A.; Shanmugan, M. Induction of hypercholesterolemia by simple soil protein with acetate generating amino acid. *Nutr. Rep. Int.* **1989**, *40*, 893–894.

20. Erejuwa, O.O.; Gurtu, S.; Sulaiman, S.A.; Wahab, M.S.; Sirajudeen, K.N.; Salleh, M.S. Hypoglycemic and antioxidant effects of honey supplementation in streptozotocin-induced diabetic rats. *Int. J. Vitam. Nutr. Res.* **2010**, *80*, 74–82. [PubMed]

21. Erejuwa, O.O.; Sulaiman, S.A.; Wahab, M.S.; Sirajudeen, K.N.; Salleh, M.S.; Gurtu, S. Glibenclamide or metformin combined with honey improves glycemic control in streptozotocin-induced diabetic rats. *Int. J. Biol. Sci.* **2011**, *7*, 244–252. [CrossRef] [PubMed]

22. Fasanmade, A.A.; Alabi, O.T. Differential effect of honey on selected variables in alloxan-induced and fructose-induced diabetic rats. *Afr. J. Biomed. Res.* **2008**, *11*, 191–196.

23. Pamela, C.C.; Richard, A.H. *Biochemistry*, 2nd ed.; JP Lippincott: Philadelphia, PA, USA, 1994; pp. 248–251.

24. Abdulrhman, M.M.; El-Hefnawy, M.H.; Aly, R.H.; Shatla, R.H.; Mamdouh, R.M.; Mahmoud, D.M.; Mohamed, W.S. Metabolic effects of honey in type 1 diabetes mellitus: A randomized crossover pilot study. *J. Med. Food* **2013**, *16*, 66–72. [CrossRef] [PubMed]

25. Erejuwa, O.O.; Sulaiman, S.A.; Wahab, M.S. Honey—A novel antidiabetic agent. *Int. J. Biol. Sci.* **2012**, *8*, 913–934. [CrossRef] [PubMed]

26. Erejuwa, O.O.; Sulaiman, S.A.; Wahab, M.S. Oligosaccharides might contribute to the antidiabetic effect of honey: A review of the literature. *Molecules* **2011**, *17*, 248–266. [CrossRef] [PubMed]

27. Erejuwa, O.O.; Sulaiman, S.A.; Wahab, M.S. Fructose might contribute to the hypoglycemic effect of honey. *Molecules* **2012**, *17*, 1900–1915. [CrossRef] [PubMed]

28. Erejuwa, O.O.; Sulaiman, S.A.; Wahab, M.S. Effects of honey and its mechanisms of action on the development and progression of cancer. *Molecules* **2014**, *19*, 2497–2522. [CrossRef] [PubMed]

29. Erejuwa, O.O.; Sulaiman, S.A.; Wahab, M.S.; Sirajudeen, K.N.; Salleh, S.; Gurtu, S. Honey supplementation in spontaneously hypertensive rats elicits antihypertensive effect via amelioration of renal oxidative stress. *Oxid. Med. Cell. Longev.* **2012**, *2012*, 374037. [CrossRef] [PubMed]

30. Kadir, E.A.; Sulaiman, S.A.; Yahya, N.K.; Othman, N.H. Inhibitory effects of tualang honey on experimental breast cancer in rats: A preliminary study. *Asian Pac. J. Cancer Prev.* **2013**, *14*, 2249–2254. [CrossRef] [PubMed]

31. Mohamed, M.; Sulaiman, S.A.; Jaafar, H.; Sirajudeen, K.N. Antioxidant protective effect of honey in cigarette smoke-induced testicular damage in rats. *Int. J. Mol. Sci.* **2011**, *12*, 5508–5521. [CrossRef] [PubMed]

32. Nasrolahi, O.; Heidari, R.; Rahmani, F.; Farokhi, F. Effect of natural honey from ilam and metformin for improving glycemic control in streptozotocin-induced diabetic rats. *Avicenna J. Phytomed.* **2012**, *2*, 212–221. [PubMed]

33. Zaid, S.S.; Sulaiman, S.A.; Sirajudeen, K.N.; Othman, N.H. The effects of tualang honey on female reproductive organs, tibia bone and hormonal profile in ovariectomised rats-animal model for menopause. *BMC Complement. Altern. Med.* **2011**, *10*, 82. [CrossRef] [PubMed]

34. Vijan, S.; Hayward, R.A. Pharmacologic lipid-lowering therapy in type 2 diabetes mellitus: Background paper for the American college of physicians. *Ann. Intern. Med.* **2004**, *140*, 650–658. [CrossRef] [PubMed]

35. Ahmadvand, H.; Noori, A.; Dehnoo, M.G.; Bagheri, S.; Cheraghi, R.A. Hypoglycemic, hypolipidemic and antiatherogenic effects of oleuropein in alloxan-induced type 1 diabetic rats. *Asian Pac. J. Trop. Dis.* **2014**, *4*, S421–S425. [CrossRef]

36. Ikewuchi, C.C. Effect of aqueous extract of sansevieria senegambica baker on plasma chemistry, lipid profile and atherogenic indices of alloxan-treated rats: Implications for the management of cardiovascular complications in diabetes mellitus. *Pac. J. Sci. Technol.* **2010**, *11*, 524–531.

37. Szkudelski, T. The mechanism of alloxan and streptozotocin action in beta cells of the rat pancreas. *Physiol. Res.* **2001**, *50*, 537–546. [PubMed]

38. Zheng, C.; Furtado, J.; Khoo, C. Apolipoprotein C-III and the metabolic basis for hypertriglyceridemia and the dense low-density lipoprotein phenotype. *Circulation* **2010**, *121*, 1722–1734. [CrossRef] [PubMed]

39. Klop, B.; Elte, J.W.F.; Cabezas, C.M. Dyslipidemia in obesity: Mechanisms and potential targets. *Nutrients* **2013**, *5*, 1218–1240. [CrossRef] [PubMed]

40. Winocour, P.H.; Durrington, P.N.; Bhatnagar, D.; Ishola, M.; Arrol, S.; Mackness, M. Abnormalities of VLDL, IDL, and LDL characterize insulin-dependent diabetes mellitus. *Arterioscler. Thromb.* **1992**, *12*, 920–928. [CrossRef] [PubMed]

41. Keevil, J.G.; Cullen, M.W.; Gangnon, R.; McBride, P.E.; Stein, J.H. Implications of cardiac risk and low-density lipoprotein cholesterol distributions in the United States for the diagnosis and treatment of dyslipidemia: Data from national health and nutrition examination survey 1999 to 2002. *Circulation* **2007**, *115*, 1363–1370. [CrossRef] [PubMed]

42. Katsilambros, N.L.; Philippides, P.; Touliatou, A. Metabolic effects of honey (alone or combined with other foods) in type II diabetics. *Acta Diabetol. Lat.* **1988**, *25*, 197–203. [CrossRef] [PubMed]

43. Bos, G.; Dekker, J.M.; Nijpels, G.; de Vegt, F.; Diamant, M.; Stehouwer, C.D.; Bouter, L.M.; Heine, R.J.; Hoorn, S. A combination of high concentrations of serum triglyceride and non-high-density-lipoprotein-cholesterol is a risk factor for cardiovascular disease in subjects with abnormal glucose metabolism—The hoorn study. *Diabetologia* **2003**, *46*, 910–916. [CrossRef] [PubMed]

44. Gasevic, D.; Frohlich, J.; Mancini, G.B.; Lear, S.A. Clinical usefulness of lipid ratios to identify men and women with metabolic syndrome: A cross-sectional study. *Lipids Health Dis.* **2014**, *13*, 159. [CrossRef] [PubMed]

45. Ingelsson, E.; Schaefer, E.; Contois, J.H.; McNamara, J.R.; Sullivan, L.; Keyes, M.J.; Pencina, M.J.; Schoonmaker, C.; Wilson, P.W.F.; D'Agostino, R.B.; et al. Clinical utility of different lipid measures for prediction of coronary heart disease in men and women. *JAMA* **2007**, *298*, 776–785. [CrossRef] [PubMed]

46. Salazar, M.R.; Carbajal, H.A.; Espeche, W.G.; Aizpurua, M.; Sisnieguez, C.E.; March, C.E.; Balbin, E.; Stavile, R.N.; Reaven, G.M. Identifying cardiovascular disease risk and outcome: Use of the plasma triglyceride/high-density lipoprotein cholesterol concentration ratio *versus* metabolic syndrome criteria. *J. Intern. Med.* **2013**, *273*, 595–601. [CrossRef] [PubMed]

47. Vega, G.L.; Barlow, C.E.; Grundy, S.M.; Leonard, D.; DeFina, L.F. Triglyceride-to high-density-lipoprotein-cholesterol ratio is an index of heart disease mortality and of incidence of type 2 diabetes mellitus in men. *J. Investig. Med.* **2014**, *62*, 345–349. [PubMed]

48. Azmi, M.B.; Qureshi, S.A. Methanolic root extract of rauwolfia serpentina benth improves the glycemic, antiatherogenic, and cardioprotective indices in alloxan-induced diabetic mice. *Adv. Pharm. Sci.* **2012**, 376429. [CrossRef] [PubMed]

49. Rizzo, M.; Berneis, K. Low-density lipoprotein size and cardiovascular risk assessment. *QJM* **2006**, *99*, 1–14. [CrossRef] [PubMed]

50. Brahm, A.; Hegele, R.A. Hypertriglyceridemia. *Nutrients* **2013**, *5*, 981–1001. [CrossRef] [PubMed]

51. Al-Waili, N.S. Natural honey lowers plasma glucose, C-reactive protein, homocysteine, and blood lipids in healthy, diabetic, and hyperlipidemic subjects: Comparison with dextrose and sucrose. *J. Med. Food* **2004**, *7*, 100–107. [CrossRef] [PubMed]

52. Erejuwa, O.O.; Sulaiman, S.A.; Wahab, M.S.; Salam, S.K.; Salleh, M.S.; Gurtu, S. Comparison of antioxidant effects of honey, glibenclamide, metformin, and their combinations in the kidneys of streptozotocin-induced diabetic rats. *Int. J. Mol. Sci.* **2011**, *12*, 829–843. [CrossRef] [PubMed]

53. Erejuwa, O.O.; Sulaiman, S.A.; Wahab, M.S.; Sirajudeen, K.N.; Salleh, M.S.; Gurtu, S. Antioxidant protection of Malaysian tualang honey in pancreas of normal and streptozotocin-induced diabetic rats. *Ann. Endocrinol.* **2010**, *71*, 291–296. [CrossRef] [PubMed]

54. Ihara, Y.; Toyokuni, S.; Uchida, K.; Odaka, H.; Tanaka, T.; Ikeda, H.; Hiai, H.; Seino, Y.; Yamada, Y. Hyperglycemia causes oxidative stress in pancreatic-cells of GK rats, a model of type 2 diabetes. *Diabetes* **1999**, *48*, 927–932. [CrossRef] [PubMed]

55. Ebbert, J.O.; Jensen, M.D. Fat depots, free fatty acids, and dyslipidemia. *Nutrients* **2013**, *5*, 498–508. [CrossRef] [PubMed]

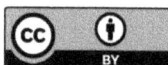

nutrients

MDPI

Article

Suppression of Endogenous Glucose Production by Isoleucine and Valine and Impact of Diet Composition

Isabel Arrieta-Cruz [1,†], Ya Su [2,†] and Roger Gutiérrez-Juárez [2,*]

[1]   National Institute of Geriatrics, Ministry of Health, Periférico Sur No. 2767,
     Col. San Jerónimo Lídice. Del. Magdalena Contreras, Mexico City 10200, Mexico; arrieta777@mail.com
[2]   Department of Medicine, Albert Einstein College of Medicine, Yeshiva University,
     1300 Morris Park Ave, Bronx, NY 10461, USA; ya.su@einstein.yu.edu
*   Correspondence: roger.gutierrez@einstein.yu.edu; Tel.: +718-430-3312; Fax: +718-430-8557
†   These authors contributed equally to this work.

Received: 14 November 2015; Accepted: 1 February 2016; Published: 15 February 2016

Abstract: Leucine has been shown to acutely inhibit hepatic glucose production in rodents by a mechanism requiring its metabolism to acetyl-CoA in the mediobasal hypothalamus (MBH). In the early stages, all branched-chain amino acids (BCAA) are metabolized by a shared set of enzymes to produce a ketoacid, which is later metabolized to acetyl-CoA. Consequently, isoleucine and valine may also modulate glucose metabolism. To examine this possibility we performed intrahypothalamic infusions of isoleucine or valine in rats and assessed whole body glucose kinetics under basal conditions and during euglycemic pancreatic clamps. Furthermore, because high fat diet (HFD) consumption is known to interfere with central glucoregulation, we also asked whether the action of BCAAs was affected by HFD. We fed rats a lard-rich diet for a short interval and examined their response to central leucine. The results showed that both isoleucine and valine individually lowered blood glucose by decreasing liver glucose production. Furthermore, the action of the BCAA leucine was markedly attenuated by HFD feeding. We conclude that all three BCAAs centrally modulate glucose metabolism in the liver and that their action is disrupted by HFD-induced insulin resistance.

Keywords: branched-chain amino acids; leucine; isoleucine; valine; glucose metabolism; nutrient sensing; hypothalamus; liver

1. Introduction

Excessive calorie intake resulting from the consumption of fat-rich diets is the most important environmental factor contributing to the emergence and worsening of the current world pandemic of diabetes and obesity [1,2]. Mammals have developed complex mechanisms for detecting changes in the availability of nutrients and responding to them with metabolic adaptations to maintain homeostasis. Multiple organs and tissues are involved in these physiological adaptive mechanisms of nutrient sensing, but the mediobasal hypothalamus (MBH) of the central nervous system (CNS) has been identified as a key integration center for these nutritional cues [3–6]. Dietary protein and amino acids (AA) exert a powerful influence on insulin action and glucose metabolism. The mechanisms underlying this effect are generally attributed to the metabolic actions of AAs in the liver and skeletal muscle [7–13]. Recently however, a number of metabolic actions of AAs have been localized to the MBH of rodents [14–17]. In particular, we have shown that the metabolism of leucine to acetyl-CoA in the MBH is coupled to the inhibition of endogenous glucose production (EGP) and a consequent decrease of circulating glucose levels [16]. In the brain, leucine is initially metabolized through the consecutive action of five enzymes [18,19]. First, leucine is transaminated to α-KIC by the branched-chain amino transferase (BCAT). Next, α-KIC is oxidatively decarboxylated by the action of the branched-chain α-ketoacid dehyrogenase (BCKDH) to form isovaleryl-CoA, which, after three more reactions, is converted to acetyl-CoA. In our studies [16], interventions that antagonized the activity of the enzyme BCKDH or otherwise prevented the formation of acetyl-CoA in the MBH markedly attenuated the glucoregulatory action of leucine. Thus, the conversion of leucine to acetyl-CoA was required to bring about the glucoregulatory effect. Further experiments also revealed that acetyl-CoA had to be converted to malonyl-CoA. More importantly, we showed that the incapacitation of leucine sensing in the MBH contributes to the development of hyperglycemia [16]. Interestingly, the first two enzymes, BCAT and BCKDH, also catalyze the metabolism of the other two members of the branched-chain amino acids (BCAA) family, isoleucine and valine, to form their respective ketoacid products. Successive enzymatic reactions give rise to various metabolites, including acetyl-CoA, a key intermediate for glucoregulation.

Several studies have shown that acute diet-induced insulin resistance partially obliterates the hypothalamic glucoregulatory response to fatty acids [20–22]. This acquired defect is induced by the consumption of a diet enriched in saturated fat. Furthermore, previous studies indicated that the hypothalamic sensing of glucose and lactate, both of which need to be converted to pyruvate, are attenuated by high-fat diet (HFD) feeding [23]. Importantly, studies in rats revealed that HFD feeding caused a marked decrease in the levels of hypothalamic long-chain fatty acyl CoAs (LCFA-CoA) and that their restoration normalized nutrient-dependent glucoregulation [22]. Based on these findings, we hypothesized that HFD feeding may also perturb the glucoregulatory response to BCAA.

Currently it is not known whether or not isoleucine and valine modulate glucose metabolism; furthermore, the effect of HFD on the central metabolic actions of BCAA has not yet been examined. Here we investigated the possibility that the central metabolism of isoleucine and valine may also be coupled to the regulation of glucose metabolism in the liver. Additionally, to determine whether HFD feeding has an impact on the glucoregulatory action of BCAAs, we infused leucine in the MBH of rats previously fed with a lard-enriched diet. In both cases we assessed glucose metabolism *in vivo* through a combination of pancreatic insulin clamps and measurements of whole body glucose kinetics.

2. Experimental Section

2.1. Animal Studies

The animal studies were approved by the Institutional Animal Care and Use Committee (IACUC) of the Albert Einstein College of Medicine. Ten-week-old Sprague-Dawley male rats (Charles River Laboratories, Wilmington, MA, USA) were used for the studies. The animals were individually housed and subjected to a light–dark cycle (0600–1800/1800–0600) with free access to water and food.

2.1.1. Animal Surgeries

Rats were subjected to stereotaxic surgery for implantation of a stainless steel bilateral cannula in the MBH as previously described [16]. The stereotaxic coordinates for cannula placement were (from bregma): −3.3 mm anterior–posterior axis; 0.4 mm lateral axis; and 9.6 mm vertical axis (depth) [24]. On recovery, the animals underwent a second surgery for the placement of indwelling vascular catheters that were used for infusions and blood sampling during the pancreatic clamp studies [16]. Postoperative recovery was monitored by measuring daily food intake and body weight. Only fully recovered animals were used for the experiments. Proper placement of the cannulas was confirmed histologically in brain slices prepared postmortem.

2.1.2. Diets

In the experiments where we compared leucine, isoleucine, and valine, the rats were fed with a regular chow diet (Cat#5001, Lab Diet, Richmond, IN, USA). In separate experiments designed to test the effect of saturated fat on leucine sensing, the animals were subjected to a 3-day regime of a HFD consisting of regular chow enriched with 10% of lard (Cat#01P5704C-K, Test Diet, Richmond, IN, USA) prior to the clamps.

2.1.3. Intrahypothalamic Infusions

Rats were randomized into three groups and received 6 hr intrahypothalamic (MBH) infusions of the following solutions: (1) Vehicle (artificial cerebrospinal fluid); (2) isoleucine; and (3) valine. For the glucose kinetics experiments, an additional group of animals received leucine at an equimolar dose for comparative purposes. Each AA was dissolved in vehicle and delivered at a total dose of 12 *n*moles over the course of 6 h (0.33 µL/h per side). The protocol and dose was based on our previous *in vivo* studies with leucine [16]. A separate group of rats were subjected to HFD feeding and then similarly infused with leucine during pancreatic clamps.

2.1.4. Pancreatic Clamp Studies and Glucose Kinetics Measurements

All rats on regular chow consumed 60 kcal of food the night prior to the study to ensure comparable nutritional status. Plasma levels of circulating glucose were monitored from the start (t = 0 min) of the central infusion (Figure 1A,B). A primed, continuous infusion of $[3\text{-}^3\text{H}]$ glucose (Perkin Elmer, San Jose, CA, USA; 40 µCi bolus; 0.4 µCi/min) was initiated at t = 120 min and maintained throughout the study to assess glucose kinetics by tracer dilution methodology [25], then a pancreatic clamp with insulin replaced at basal levels was performed (t = 240–360 min). At the end of the study, the animals were euthanized and tissue samples were freeze-clamped *in situ* and stored for subsequent analysis.

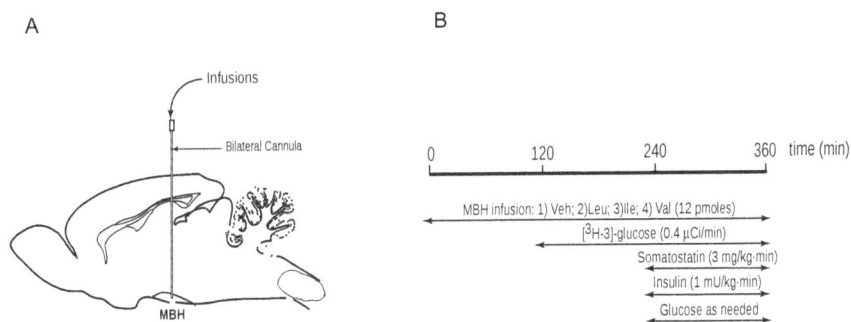

Figure 1. Experimental procedures. (**A**) Schematic of rat brain (sagittal view) with bilateral cannula implanted stereotactically for infusions into the mediobasal hypothalamus (MBH); (**B**) Time-line for *in vivo* central infusions of branched-chain amino acids (BCAAs) during euglycemic pancreatic clamp protocol with isotopic glucose tracer.

2.2. Analytical Procedures and Calculations

Plasma glucose was measured using an Analox instrument (Analox Instruments USA Inc., Lunenburg, MA, USA). The radioactivity of $[3\text{-}^3\text{H}]$ glucose in plasma was measured from supernatants of $Ba(OH)_2$ and from $ZnSO_4$ precipitates (Somogyi procedure) of plasma samples after each was evaporated to dryness to remove tritiated water. The rate of glucose uptake and endogenous glucose production were calculated as previously described [26].

2.3. Statistical Analysis

All data values are expressed as mean $\pm$ S.E.M. of the indicated number of experiments. Statistical comparisons were assessed by unpaired Student's *t* test or analysis of variance (ANOVA) followed by the Tukey HSD test. We used the customary threshold of $p < 0.05$ to declare statistical significance.

3. Results

We first asked if increasing the local levels of isoleucine or valine in the MBH of rats modifies circulating glucose levels. To answer this question we performed intrahypothalamic infusions of these BCAAs under basal conditions and measured blood glucose during the course of the infusion. As predicted, both isoleucine and valine individually decreased the plasma levels of glucose compared to vehicle-infused control animals (Figure 2). Thus isoleucine and valine replicated the glucose-lowering action of leucine.

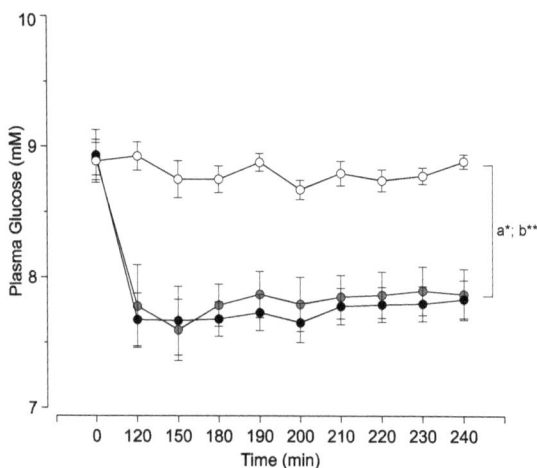

Figure 2. Effect of central isoleucine and valine on circulating glucose levels. Symbols (circles): white, vehicle; black, isoleucine; gray, valine. Each point represents the mean ± s.e.m for 6–8 individual experiments. * a, $p < 0.05$ Isoleucine *vs.* control; ** b, $p < 0.05$ Valine *vs.* control.

To determine if central isoleucine or valine modulates hepatic glucose metabolism, we performed pancreatic insulin clamps and glucose kinetics analysis in the same animals. During the clamps, when glucose and insulin levels in circulation are kept constant, both isoleucine and valine individually produced a marked increase in the glucose infusion rate (GIR) required to maintain euglycemia compared to vehicle (Figure 3A). Kinetic analysis revealed that the increase of GIR was the result of a marked inhibition of EGP (Figure 3B,C), since peripheral glucose utilization (GU) did not change (Figure 3D). The individual effect of isoleucine and valine on all these kinetic parameters was comparable in magnitude to that reported for leucine [16] at the equimolar dose (12 *p*moles) used here. Taken together these results indicate that isoleucine and valine fully replicated the effect of leucine on liver glucose metabolism. On close examination, the individual potency of isoleucine to inhibit EGP was approximately the same as for leucine but somewhat lower than for valine.

Short-term (3-day) feeding of rodents with a diet enriched in saturated fat (HFD) induces insulin resistance in the absence of changes in body weight compared to regular chow (RC) fed animals [27,28]. To examine the consequences of acutely-induced insulin resistance on the ability of BCAAs to inhibit EGP, we subjected rats to three days of HFD feeding and repeated our measurements during central infusions of leucine. We used leucine because its effects on glucose metabolism have been previously characterized in detail by our group [16]. During pancreatic clamps, acute insulin resistance was manifested by decreased GIR (RC = 2.3 ± 0.6 *vs.* HFD = 0.7 ± 0.2 mg/kg·min; $p < 0.05$) due to an increase of EGP (RC = 9.9 ± 0.4 *vs.* HFD = 11.6 ± 0.6 mg/kg·min; $p < 0.05$) without change in GU (RC = 12.3 ± 0.7 *vs.* HFD = 11.9 ± 0.5 mg/kg·min). Next, as shown in Figure 4A, animals treated with HFD required remarkably less glucose infusion to maintain appropriate plasma glucose levels than animals treated with regular chow (not insulin resistant) when infused centrally with leucine.

Analysis of the clamp tracer data revealed that the ability of leucine to reduce EGP was markedly attenuated in these HFD treated animals (Figure 4B,C). Importantly, there was no change in GU (Figure 4D), indicating that all the effect was essentially hepatic. In summary, these results indicate that the short-term consumption of HFD markedly blunts the glucoregulatory action of leucine.

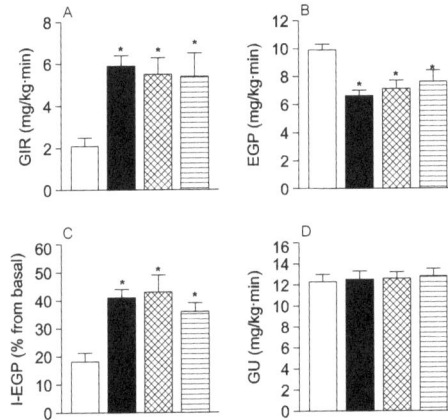

Figure 3. *In vivo* comparison of the central action of isoleucine, valine, and leucine on glucose kinetics during pancreatic insulin clamps. (**A**) Glucose infusion rate (GIR) to maintain euglycemia; (**B**) Endogenous glucose production (EGP); (**C**) Inhibition of EGP by insulin (I-EGP); (**D**) Peripheral glucose utilization (GU). White bars, vehicle; black bars, leucine; check-filled bars, isoleucine; striped bars, valine. Each bar represents the mean ± s.e.m for 6–8 individual experiments. * $p < 0.05$ *vs.* control.

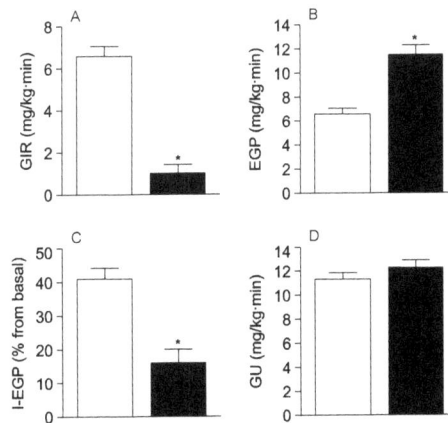

Figure 4. Impact of high-fat diet (HFD) feeding on the central glucoregulatory action of leucine. (**A**) Glucose infusion rate (GIR) to maintain euglycemia; (**B**) Endogenous glucose production (EGP); (**C**) Inhibition of EGP by insulin (I-EGP); (**D**) Peripheral glucose utilization (GU). White bars, regular chow-fed (control) animals; black bars, HFD-fed animals. Each bar represents the mean ± s.e.m for 6 individual experiments. * $p < 0.05$ *vs.* control.

4. Discussion

In the current studies, our measurements of whole body glucose kinetics during pancreatic clamps showed that isoleucine and valine each individually modified the main parameters in a very similar way: increased GIR, decreased EGP, and no change in peripheral GU. At an equimolar dose, the magnitude of their effects were comparable to those of leucine. These findings strongly support our hypothesis that all BCAAs are capable of signalling in the MBH through a common upstream metabolic mechanism. Although the goal of our work was to determine whether or not isoleucine and valine had central glucoregulatory activity rather than studying the mechanisms, it would be appropriate to discuss the possibilities. We think that it is the metabolic fate of these BCAAs that allows them to signal in the MBH. In the case of isoleucine, the explanation seems straightforward because this amino acid is directly converted to acetyl-CoA, which can then be used to generate malonyl-CoA. More intriguing, though, is the effect of valine, since this amino acid is not directly metabolized to acetyl-CoA but rather to propionyl-CoA. This metabolite is converted to succinyl-CoA, which then enters the tricarboxylic acid (TCA) cycle, a feature that makes it a glucogenic amino acid. As a glucogenic AA, valine is the second example of its kind, after proline [17], found to modulate glucose metabolism by acting in the hypothalamus. Interestingly, the glucogenic AA histidine was recently shown to inhibit liver glucose production when delivered in the third ventricle of rats, suggesting that it acts in the hypothalamus [29]. However, in contrast with proline, histidine requires binding to histamine receptors rather than its metabolism in the brain to modify liver glucose fluxes. More importantly, we have shown that physiologically relevant elevations of the circulating levels of leucine or proline modulate hepatic glucose metabolism *in vivo* [16,17]. Similarly, it is possible that physiological elevations of isoleucine and valine also regulate circulating glucose levels, but further studies are required to confirm (or rule out) this idea. Several studies in rodents appear to support a role for BCAAs in the improvement of glucose metabolism reported here. For example, dietary leucine supplementation improves glucose metabolism and prevents obesity in various mouse models [30,31]. Furthermore, mice lacking BCAT in the brain display high circulating levels of leucine in association with a lean phenotype and enhanced insulin sensitivity [32]. Interestingly, recent reports of studies in humans have identified a link between elevated levels of circulating BCAAs and the development of insulin resistance or diabetes [33,34]. However, the details of such an association are not clear, and therefore it is currently unknown how the elevated levels of BCAAs are connected to the development of these disorders of glucose metabolism. Interestingly, in one of these studies [33], the administration of BCAA to HFD-fed rodents induced insulin resistance while the administration of BCAA alone did not. These results not only indicate that BCAAs are not directly involved in the development of insulin resistance, but they also coincide with our report in that HFD feeding modifies the metabolic actions of BCAAs in a detrimental fashion. Thus, our current studies showing a blunting of central glucoregulation by leucine after short-term HFD feeding allows us to add amino acids, or leucine at least, to the list of nutrients whose hypothalamic sensing is nutritionally regulated. In this regard, our previous studies showing that molecular disruption of leucine sensing in the MBH precipitates the development of hyperglycemia in rats fed with a high-protein diet [16] further supports the idea that the faltering of central leucine sensing may contribute to disease development.

5. Conclusions

The MBH responded to a local increase of isoleucine or valine with an inhibition of EGP, which mainly reflects glucose production by the liver. At an equimolar dose, the magnitude of the individual glucoregulatory effect of either isoleucine or valine was similar to that of leucine. Importantly, insulin resistance induced by short-term high fat feeding markedly attenuated the central glucoregulatory effect of leucine. In summary, we conclude that not only leucine but also circulating isoleucine and valine may participate in the acute postprandial regulation of glycemia. Furthermore, consumption of diets rich in saturated fat incapacitates this centrally-mediated glucoregulation.

Acknowledgments: This work was supported by a grant from the National Institutes of Health (DK45024) and an Ajinomoto Amino Acid Research Program grant to R.G.-J. We thank Bing Liu for performing the animal vascular surgeries.

Author Contributions: I.A.-C. performed the experiments, analyzed the data and wrote the manuscript; Y.S. performed the experiments and analyzed the data; R.G.-J. conceived and designed the experiments, analyzed the data and wrote the manuscript.

Conflicts of Interest: The authors declare no conflict of interest.

References

1. Eaton, S.B.; Konner, M. Paleolithic nutrition. A consideration of its nature and current implications. *N. Engl. J. Med.* **1985**, *312*, 283–289.
2. Hill, J.O.; Peters, J.C. Environmental contributions to the obesity epidemic. *Science* **1998**, *280*, 1371–1374.
3. Ukropec, J.; Sebokova, E.; Klimes, I. Nutrient sensing, leptin and insulin action. *Arch. Physiol. Biochem.* **2001**, *109*, 38–51.
4. Obici, S.; Rossetti, L. Minireview: Nutrient sensing and the regulation of insulin action and energy balance. *Endocrinology* **2003**, *144*, 5172–5178.
5. Lindsley, J.E.; Rutter, J. Nutrient sensing and metabolic decisions. *Comp. Biochem. Physiol. B Biochem. Mol. Biol.* **2004**, *139*, 543–559.
6. Schwartz, G.J. Biology of eating behavior in obesity. *Obes. Res.* **2004**, *12* (Suppl. 2), 102S–106S.
7. Rossetti, L.; Rothman, D.L.; DeFronzo, R.A.; Shulman, G.I. Effect of dietary protein on *in vivo* insulin action and liver glycogen repletion. *Am. J. Physiol.* **1989**, *257*, E212–E219.
8. Patti, M.E.; Brambilla, E.; Luzi, L.; Landaker, E.J.; Kahn, C.R. Bidirectional modulation of insulin action by amino acids. *J. Clin. Investig.* **1998**, *101*, 1519–1529.
9. Gannon, M.C.; Nuttall, F.Q.; Saeed, A.; Jordan, K.; Hoover, H. An increase in dietary protein improves the blood glucose response in persons with type 2 diabetes. *Am. J. Clin. Nutr.* **2003**, *78*, 734–741.
10. Nuttall, F.Q.; Gannon, M.C.; Saeed, A.; Jordan, K.; Hoover, H. The metabolic response of subjects with type 2 diabetes to a high-protein, weight-maintenance diet. *J. Clin. Endocrinol. Metab.* **2003**, *88*, 3577–3583.
11. Tremblay, F.; Krebs, M.; Dombrowski, L.; Brehm, A.; Bernroider, E.; Roth, E.; Nowotny, P.; Waldhausl, W.; Marette, A.; Roden, M. Overactivation of S6 kinase 1 as a cause of human insulin resistance during increased amino acid availability. *Diabetes* **2005**, *54*, 2674–2684.
12. Promintzer, M.; Krebs, M. Effects of dietary protein on glucose homeostasis. *Curr. Opin. Clin. Nutr. Metab. Care* **2006**, *9*, 463–468.
13. Tremblay, F.; Lavigne, C.; Jacques, H.; Marette, A. Role of dietary proteins and amino acids in the pathogenesis of insulin resistance. *Annu. Rev. Nutr.* **2007**, *27*, 293–310.
14. Cota, D.; Proulx, K.; Smith, K.A.; Kozma, S.C.; Thomas, G.; Woods, S.C.; Seeley, R.J. Hypothalamic mTOR signaling regulates food intake. *Science* **2006**, *312*, 927–930.
15. Blouet, C.; Jo, Y.H.; Li, X.; Schwartz, G.J. Mediobasal hypothalamic leucine sensing regulates food intake through activation of a hypothalamus-brainstem circuit. *J. Neurosci.* **2009**, *29*, 8302–8311.
16. Su, Y.; Lam, T.K.; He, W.; Pocai, A.; Bryan, J.; Aguilar-Bryan, L.; Gutierrez-Juarez, R. Hypothalamic leucine metabolism regulates liver glucose production. *Diabetes* **2012**, *61*, 85–93.
17. Arrieta-Cruz, I.; Su, Y.; Knight, C.M.; Lam, T.K.T.; Gutiérrez-Juárez, R. Evidence for a role of proline and hypothalamic astrocytes in the regulation of glucose metabolism in rats. *Diabetes* **2013**, *62*, 1152–1158.
18. Suryawan, A.; Hawes, J.W.; Harris, R.A.; Shimomura, Y.; Jenkins, A.E.; Hutson, S.M. A molecular model of human branched-chain amino acid metabolism. *Am. J. Clin. Nutr.* **1998**, *68*, 72–81.
19. Brosnan, J.T.; Brosnan, M.E. Branched-chain amino acids: Enzyme and substrate regulation. *J. Nutr.* **2006**, *136*, 207S–211S.
20. Morgan, K.; Obici, S.; Rossetti, L. Hypothalamic responses to long-chain fatty acids are nutritionally regulated. *J. Biol. Chem.* **2004**, *279*, 31139–31148.
21. Lam, T.K.; Gutierrez-Juarez, R.; Pocai, A.; Rossetti, L. Regulation of blood glucose by hypothalamic pyruvate metabolism. *Science* **2005**, *309*, 943–947.
22. Pocai, A.; Lam, T.K.; Obici, S.; Gutierrez-Juarez, R.; Muse, E.D.; Arduini, A.; Rossetti, L. Restoration of hypothalamic lipid sensing normalizes energy and glucose homeostasis in overfed rats. *J. Clin. Investig.* **2006**, *116*, 1081–1091.
23. Lam, T.K.; Gutierrez-Juarez, R.; Pocai, A.; Bhanot, S.; Tso, P.; Schwartz, G.J.; Rossetti, L. Brain glucose metabolism controls the hepatic secretion of triglyceride-rich lipoproteins. *Nat. Med.* **2007**, *13*, 171–180.

24. Paxinos, G.; Watson, C. *The Rat Brain in Stereotaxic Coordinates*; Elsevier: Amsterdam, The Netherlands, 2007.

25. Gutierrez-Juarez, R.; Obici, S.; Rossetti, L. Melanocortin-independent effects of leptin on hepatic glucose fluxes. *J. Biol. Chem.* **2004**, *279*, 49704–49715.

26. Liu, L.; Karkanias, G.B.; Morales, J.C.; Hawkins, M.; Barzilai, N.; Wang, J.; Rossetti, L. Intracerebroventricular leptin regulates hepatic but not peripheral glucose fluxes. *J. Biol. Chem.* **1998**, *273*, 31160–31167.

27. Kraegen, E.W.; Clark, P.W.; Jenkins, A.B.; Daley, E.A.; Chisholm, D.J.; Storlien, L.H. Development of muscle insulin resistance after liver insulin resistance in high-fat-fed rats. *Diabetes* **1991**, *40*, 1397–1403.

28. Wang, J.; Obici, S.; Morgan, K.; Barzilai, N.; Feng, Z.; Rossetti, L. Overfeeding rapidly induces leptin and insulin resistance. *Diabetes* **2001**, *50*, 2786–2791.

29. Kimura, K.; Nakamura, Y.; Inaba, Y.; Matsumoto, M.; Kido, Y.; Asahara, S.I.; Matsuda, T.; Watanabe, H.; Maeda, A.; Inagaki, F.; *et al.* Histidine augments the suppression of hepatic glucose production by central insulin action. *Diabetes* **2013**, *62*, 2266–2277.

30. Zhang, Y.; Guo, K.; LeBlanc, R.E.; Loh, D.; Schwartz, G.J.; Yu, Y.H. Increasing dietary leucine intake reduces diet-induced obesity and improves glucose and cholesterol metabolism in mice via multimechanisms. *Diabetes* **2007**, *56*, 1647–1654.

31. Guo, K.; Yu, Y.H.; Hou, J.; Zhang, Y. Chronic leucine supplementation improves glycemic control in etiologically distinct mouse models of obesity and diabetes mellitus. *Nutr. Metab. (Lond.)* **2010**, *7*, 57.

32. She, P.; Reid, T.M.; Bronson, S.K.; Vary, T.C.; Hajnal, A.; Lynch, C.J.; Hutson, S.M. Disruption of BCATm in mice leads to increased energy expenditure associated with the activation of a futile protein turnover cycle. *Cell Metab.* **2007**, *6*, 181–194.

33. Newgard, C.B.; An, J.; Bain, J.R.; Muehlbauer, M.J.; Stevens, R.D.; Lien, L.F.; Haqq, A.M.; Shah, S.H.; Arlotto, M.; Slentz, C.A.; *et al.* A branched-chain amino acid-related metabolic signature that differentiates obese and lean humans and contributes to insulin resistance. *Cell Metab.* **2009**, *9*, 311–326.

34. Wang, T.J.; Larson, M.G.; Vasan, R.S.; Cheng, S.; Rhee, E.P.; McCabe, E.; Lewis, G.D.; Fox, C.S.; Jacques, P.F.; Fernandez, C.; *et al.* Metabolite profiles and the risk of developing diabetes. *Nat. Med.* **2011**, *17*, 448–453.

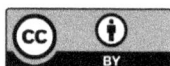

Article

Fermented Red Ginseng Potentiates Improvement of Metabolic Dysfunction in Metabolic Syndrome Rat Models

Min Chul Kho [1,2], Yun Jung Lee [1,2], Ji Hun Park [2], Hye Yoom Kim [1,2], Jung Joo Yoon [1,2], You Mee Ahn [1,2], Rui Tan [1,2], Min Cheol Park [3], Jeong Dan Cha [4], Kyung Min Choi [5], Dae Gill Kang [1,2,*] and Ho Sub Lee [1,2,*]

[1] College of Oriental Medicine and Professional Graduate School of Oriental Medicine, Wonkwang University, 460 Iksandae-ro, Iksan, Jeonbuk 54538, Korea; shadowzetx@hanmail.net (M.C.K.); shrons@wku.ac.kr (Y.J.L.); hyeyoomc@naver.com (H.Y.K.); morality16@hanmail.net (J.J.Y.); aum2668@naver.com (Y.M.A.); tanrui@hanmail.net (R.T.)

[2] Hanbang Body-Fluid Research Center, Wonkwang University, 460 Iksandae-ro, Iksan, Jeonbuk 54538, Korea; jihuncjstk@naver.com

[3] Department of Oriental Medical Ophthalmology & Otolaryngology & Dermatology, College of Oriental Medicine, Wonkwang University, 460 Iksandae-ro, Iksan, Jeonbuk 54538, Korea; shadowzetx@hanmail.net

[4] Department of Oral Microbiology and Institute of Oral Bioscience, Chonbuk National University, Jeonju, Jeonbuk 54896, Korea; joungdan@ijrg.re.kr

[5] Department of Research Development, Institute of Jinan Red Ginseng, Jinan, Jeonbuk 55442, Korea; kyungmc@ijrg.re.kr

* Correspondence: dgkang@wku.ac.kr (D.G.K.); host@wku.ac.kr (H.S.L.); Tel.: +82-63-850-6447 (D.G.K. & H.S.L.); Fax: +82-63-850-7260 (D.G.K. & H.S.L.)

Received: 10 March 2016; Accepted: 2 June 2016; Published: 16 June 2016

Abstract: Metabolic syndrome including obesity, dyslipidemia and hypertension is a cluster of risk factors of cardiovascular disease. Fermentation of medicinal herbs improves their pharmacological efficacy. Red ginseng (RG), a widely used traditional herbal medicine, was reported with anti-inflammatory and anti-oxidant activity. Aim in the present study was to investigate that the effects of fermented red ginseng (FRG) on a high-fructose (HF) diet induced metabolic disorders, and those effects were compared to RG and losartan. Animals were divided into four groups: a control group fed a regular diet and tap water, and fructose groups that were fed a 60% high-fructose (HF) diet with/without RG 250 mg/kg/day or FRG 250 mg/kg/day for eight weeks, respectively. Treatment with FRG significantly suppressed the increments of body weight, liver weight, epididymal fat weight and adipocyte size. Moreover, FRG significantly prevented the development of metabolic disturbances such as hyperlipidemia and hypertension. Staining with Oil-red-o demonstrated a marked increase of hepatic accumulation of triglycerides, and this increase was prevented by FRG. FRG ameliorated endothelial dysfunction by downregulation of endothelin-1 (ET-1) and adhesion molecules in the aorta. In addition, FRG induced markedly upregulation of Insulin receptor substrate 1 (IRS-1) and glucose transporter type 4 (Glut4) in the muscle. These results indicate that FRG ameliorates obesity, dyslipidemia, hypertension and fatty liver in HF diet rats. More favorable pharmacological effects on HF diet induced metabolic disorders were observed with FRG, compared to an equal dose of RG. These results showed that the pharmacological activity of RG was enhanced by fermentation. Taken together, fermentated red ginseng might be a beneficial therapeutic approach for metabolic syndrome.

Keywords: fermented red ginseng; metabolic syndrome; obesity; hyperlipidemia; hypertension

1. Introduction

Obesity, hyperinsulinemia, hyperlipidemia, and hypertension, *etc.*, such as variable coexistence diseases are characterized by metabolic syndrome [1]. Patients with various diseases have increased. There are several reasons for that is obesity population by western food, cardiovascular disease by hypertension, atherosclerosis, diabetes from insulin resistance, and so on. Patients with metabolic syndrome, as defined by the NCEP-ATP III (National Cholesterol Education Program Adult Treatment Panel III), simultaneously exhibit three or more of the following characteristics: increased blood pressure, increased waist circumference, decreased high-density lipoprotein (HDL) level, increased triglyceride level and hyperglycemia [2]. In metabolic syndrome, the liver is highly affected by excess dietary nutrients from the intestines and inflammatory adipocytokines from enlarged visceral adipose tissues. Thus, fatty liver is considered as a representative of metabolic syndrome [3–5].

Fructose is an isomer of glucose with a hydroxyl group on carbon-4 reversed in position. It is promptly absorbed and rapidly metabolized by the liver. Increased consumption of fructose commonly leads to rapid stimulation of lipogenesis and Triglyceride (TG) accumulation, which, in turn, leads to reduced insulin sensitivity and hepatic insulin resistance/glucose intolerance [6,7]. Thus, a high-fructose diet induces a well-characterized metabolic syndrome, generally resulting in hypertension, dyslipidaemia and low levels of HDL-cholesterol [8]. In addition, many recent studies suggest that consumption high fructose may be an important risk factor for the development of fatty liver [9]. Rodents, especially rats, are commonly used as a model to mimic human disease, including metabolic syndrome [10]. Similarly, lots of data suggests that experiments of fructose-diet rats tend to produce some of the changes associated with metabolic syndrome, such as altered lipid metabolism, fatty liver, hypertension, obesity and dyslipidemia [11].

Currently, available pharmacological agents for metabolic disorder have a number of limitations, such as various side effects and high rates of secondary failure. Therefore, the demand has increased from those interested in complementary and alternative approaches, including the use of natural herbs. Especially, natural substances and materials based on traditional medicines are of interest for the prevention or obstruction of diseases related to fatty liver, hypertension, high cholesterol and diabetes [12–14].

Red ginseng (RG), which is a famous herb of Korean origin,is produced by steaming and drying fresh and raw ginseng. During the steaming process, red ginseng formation allows for numerous chemical changes such as saponin deformation, amino acid changes, and browning reactions, in order to concentrate the activity principles [15,16]. The pharmacological components of red ginseng include various saponins (such as ginsenoside), non-saponins and amino acids. These components are known to have beneficial anti-inflammatory, anti-oxidant, anti-diabetic and anti-aging effects [17–19]. Recently, according to lots of literature, fermentation using microorganisms for the production of more effective compounds has been extensively studied. In particular, the pharmacological effects of new saponin generated by red ginseng fermentation have been reported, and this saponin can be mass produced. Fermented red ginseng (FRG) has displayed 30 types of metabolic factors, including Rb1, Rb2, Rc and Rd. Moreover, several studies have already reported that compound K exhibits anti-cancer, anti-diabetic and elevating immune system effects [20]. In addition, many studies have already reported that fermentation can also increase the effectiveness of pharmacological factors in red ginseng through easier and more effective endogenous absorption via degradation into small molecules, as well as disintegration of their toxicity [21]. In addition, several studies have recently reported that FRG elevates hyperlipidemia and protects pancreatic β-cells from streptozotocin toxicity [22,23]. However, the effect of fermented red ginseng on high fructose (HF) diet animal models has not been yet reported. Therefore, the aim of this study was to investigate and compare the effects of dietary supplied FRG and RG on high fructose diet-induced metabolic syndrome.

2. Materials and Methods

2.1. Preparation of Fermented Red Ginseng, Red Ginseng and Losartan

The fermented *Red ginseng* and *Red ginseng* extracts were provided from the Institute of JinAn Red Ginseng, Jinan, Jeonbuk Province, Korea. The losartan was purchased from Sigma-Aldrich (Yongin, Korea). For the fermentation of RG (FRG), a microbial strain, *Lactobacillus plantarum* A KFCC11611P, provided from the Korean Culture Center of Microorganisms (KCCM, Seodaemun-gun, Seoul, South Korea) was used for RG and *Rubuscoreanus* Miq. (RC) fermentation. The microbes were precultured in De Man–Rogosa–Sharpe (MRS) (BD biosciences, Sparks, MD, USA) broth medium for Lactobacillus at 30 °C for 24 h before being used for fermentation. For fermentation, 1 L of 0.05 g/m red ginseng (RG) and 1 L of 0.025 g/mL RG with RC mixture in distilled water was prepared and sterilized. After inoculation with 100 mL of precultured *L. plantarum* A, the RG and mixture solution containing the fermentation microbes was incubated at 35 °C for 10 and 5 days, respectively.

2.2. Animal Experiments and Diet

All experimental procedures and animal care were conducted in accordance with the National Institute of Health Guide for the Care and Use of Laboratory Animals and were published by the Institutional Animal Care and Utilization Committee for Medical Science of Wonkwang University (approve code WKU14-105). Seven-week-old male Sprague–Dawley (SD) rats were obtained from Samtako (Osan, Korea). All rats were housed in a room automatically maintained under a controlled 12 h light/dark cycle at 23 ± 2 °C with 45%–55% relative humidity. After acclimatization, animals were divided into 5 groups: a control group fed a regular diet, and fructose groups fed the 60% high-fructose (HF) diet with/without RG 250 mg/kg/day or FRG 250 mg/kg/day or losartan 30 mg/kg/day for 8 weeks, respectively. Both diets were purchased from Research Diet, Inc. (New Brunswick, NJ, USA). All groups received a regular diet and the HF diet, respectively, for 8 weeks. The composition of both diets is listed in Table S1.

2.3. Estimation of Blood Pressure

Systolic blood pressure (SBP) of rats in all groups were measured at 1, 2, 5 and 8 weeks of period, respectively. SBP was determined by using non-invasive tail-cuff plethysmogrphy method and recorded with an automatic sphygmotonography (MK2000, Muromachi Kikai, Tokyo, Japan).

2.4. Estimation of Oral Glucose Tolerance Tests

The oral glucose tolerance tests (OGTT) were performed 2 days apart at 7 weeks. For the OGTT, rats were deprived of food for 12 h. After the food deprivation period, the basalblood samples were obtained from the tail veins of fully conscious rats and were analyzed using a glucometer (Onetouch® UltraTM, Boston, MA, USA) and Test Strip (Life Scan, Chesterbrook, CA, USA), respectively. Rats were then given 2 g/kg body weight as glucose solution by oral gavage. The tail blood samples were taken at 30, 60, 90 and 120 min after glucose administration.

2.5. Estimation of Biochemical Analysis of Plasma

The levels of triglyceride (TG), blood urea nitrogen (BUN), total billiubin (T-bill), glutamic-oxaloacetic transaminase (GOT) and glutamic-pyruvic transaminase (GPT) in plasma were enzymatically measured using commercially available kits (ARKRAY, Inc., Minami-ku, Kyoto, Japan). Plasma total cholesterol, low density lipoprotein (LDL)-cholesterol and HDL-cholesterol were determined using HDL and LDL/very low density lipoprotein (VLDL) Assay kit (E2HL-100, BioAssay Systems, Hayward, CA, USA). The plasma concentration ofleptin and insulin were measured based on the ELISA method using commercial rat leptin and insulin ELISA kit (Leptin Rat ELISA ab100773, Abcam, Cambridge, MA, USA; Insulin, 80-INSRT-E01, ALPCO, Cambridge, MA, USA).

2.6. Protein Preparation and Immunoblotting in the Rat Aorta and Muscle

Thoracic aorta and muscle were homogenized in a buffer consisting of 250 mM sucrose, 1 mM EDTA, 0.1 mM phenyl methylsulfonyl fluoride, and 20 mM potassium phosphate buffer (pH 7.6). Large tissue debris and nuclear fragments were removed by two successive low-speed spins (3500 rpm, 5 min; 8000 rpm, 10 min, 4 °C). Quantity of protein was measured by the Bradford method. An equal amount (35 μg) of protein was separated by 10% Sodium Dodecyl Sulfate (SDS)-PAGE. After electrophosis, protein was transferred electrophoretically to nitrocellulose membranes using a Mini-Protean II apparatus (Bio-Rad, Hercules, CA, USA). The membranes were then blocked by 5% bovine serum albumin (BSA) powder in 0.05% Tween 20-Tris-bufferd saline (TBS-T) for 1 h, and subsequently washed and incubated with primary antibodies to VCAM-1, ICAM-1, E-selectin and ET-1 (in aorta) and Insulin receptor substrate-1 (IRS-1) and glucose transporter type 4 (Glut4) (in muscle) (Santa Cruz Biotechnology, Santa Cruz, CA, USA) at a final dilution of 1:1000 overnight at 4 °C. After washing with TBS-T, membranes were incubated with the appropriate horseradish peroxidase-conjugated secondary antibody for 1 h. Signals were detected by a chemiluminescence (ECL) using detection system (Amersham, Buchinghamshire, UK). The bands were analyzed densitometrically by using a Chemi-doc image analyzer (Bio-Rad, Hercules, CA, USA).

2.7. Histopathological and Oil Red OStaining of Aortic Tissues, Epididymal Fat and Liver Tissues

For histopathological staining, aortic tissues were fixed in 10% (*v/v*) formalin in 0.01 M phosphate buffered saline (PBS) for 2 days with a change of formalin solution every day to remove traces of blood from tissue. The tissue samples were embedded in paraffin, and then thin sections (6 μm) of the aortic arch in each group were cut and stained with hematoxylin and eosin (H & E) stain for histopathological comparisons.

Epididymal fat and liver tissues were fixed by immersion in 4% paraformaldehyde for 2 days at 4 °C, and incubated with 30% sucrose for 2 days. Each fat and liver was embedded in an optimum cutting temperature (OCT) compound (Tissue-Tek, Sakura Finetek, Torrance, CA, USA), frozen in liquid nitrogen, and stored at −80 °C. Frozen sections were cut with a Shandon Cryotome Special Motorized Electronic (SME) (Thermo Electron Corporation, Pittsburg, PA, USA) and placed on poly-L-lysine-coated slide. Epididymal fat sections were stained with H & E. For quantitative histopathological comparisons, each section was determined by Axiovision 4 Imaging/Archiving software (Axiovision 4, Carl Zeiss, Oberkochen, Germany). Liver sections were assessed by using Oil red o staining. Each section was stained with Oil red O for 20 min at room temperature after rinsing with 60% isopropyl alcohol and distilled water. Images of Oil red O stained liver were taken with Axiovision 4 Imaging/Archiving software. For quantitative analysis, the average scores of 10–20 randomly selected areas were calculated by using National institutes of health (NIH) Image analysis software, Image J (NIH, Bethesda, MD, USA).

2.8. Immunihistochemical Staining of Aortic Tissues

Parraffin sections for immunohistochemical staining were placed on poly-L-lysine-coated slides (Fisher Scientific, Pittsburgh, PA, USA). Slides were immunostained by Invitrogen's HISOTO-STAIN®-SP kits (Carlsbad, CA, USA) using the Labeled-[strept] Avidin-Biotin (LAB-SA) method. After antigen retrieval, slides were immersed in 3% hydrogen peroxide for 10 min to block endogenous peroxidase activity. After being rinsed with PBS, slides were incubated with 10% non-immune goat serum for 10 min and incubated with primary antibodies of ICAM-1, VCAM-1 and ET-1 (1:200; Santa Cruz, CA, USA) in humidified chambers overnight at 4 °C. All slides were then incubated with biotinylated secondary antibody for 20 min, and then incubated with horseradish peroxidase-conjugated streptavidin for 20 min. Peroxidase activity was visualized by 3,3'-Diaminobenzidine (DAB; Novex®, Los Angeles, CA, USA) substrate-chromogen system, and counterstaining with hematoxylin (Zymed, Carlsbad, CA, USA). For quantitative analysis, the average scores of 10–20 randomly selected areas were calculated by using NIH Image analysis software, Image J (NIH, Bethesda, MD, USA).

2.9. Statistical Analysis

All the experiments were repeated at least three times. The results were expressed as a mean $\pm$ S.E., and the data were analyzed using one-way ANOVA followed by a Dunnett's test or Student's *t*-test to determine any significant differences. $p < 0.05$ was considered as statistically significant.

3. Results

3.1. Effects of FRG on Changes in Body Weight, Liver Weight and Epididymal Fat Pad Weight

Rats from all five groups showed significant increases in body weight gain during the experimental period. There was no significant change in body weight after eight weeks of high-fructose feeding in HF diet groups compared with the control group. However, treatment of FRG and losartan (Los.) groups showed significant decreases in body weight (Table 1). There was no significant change in food intake in all groups. Although there were no significant changes in body weight between HF groups and RG groups, there were decrease those levels. Moreover, HF diet resulted in a significant increase in liver weight and epididymal fat pad weight. Liver weight and epididymal fat pad weight were 34.81% and 40.92% higher than that of the HF diet group compared with the control group, respectively. However, treatment of the FRG group significantly reduced the liver weight and epididymal fat pad weight (23.44%, 38.26%) compared with HF diet groups, respectively. Similarly, treatment of losartan showed similar results to the FRG group. Although there was no significant change in liver weight between HF groups and RG groups, they decrease at those levels (Table 1).

Table 1. Effect of fermented red ginseng FRG on body weight, liver weight and epididymal fat pads.

Groups	Control	HF	HF		
			Los.	RG	FRG
Initial BW (g)	270.5 $\pm$ 3.3	270.0 $\pm$ 3.1	275.8 $\pm$ 3.6	272.6 $\pm$ 1.8	275.5 $\pm$ 4.3
Terminal BW (g)	399.6 $\pm$ 7.4	421.2 $\pm$ 6.0	384.1 $\pm$ 9.8 [#]	405.8 $\pm$ 10.5	393.9 $\pm$ 6.4 [#]
Food intake (g/day)	18.5 $\pm$ 0.3	18.4 $\pm$ 0.4	18.2 $\pm$ 0.5	18.8 $\pm$ 0.4	18.4 $\pm$ 0.5
Liver weight (g)	9.0 $\pm$ 1.3	12.3 $\pm$ 0.4 [*]	9.2 $\pm$ 0.4 [##]	10.5 $\pm$ 0.7	9.9 $\pm$ 0.3 [#]
Epididymal fat pads weight (g)	6.4 $\pm$ 0.9	9.0 $\pm$ 0.4 [*]	5.5 $\pm$ 0.4 [##]	7.6 $\pm$ 0.7 [#]	6.6 $\pm$ 0.7 [#]

Values were expressed as mean $\pm$ S.E. ($n = 10$). [*] $p < 0.05$ *versus* Cont.; [#] $p < 0.05$, [##] $p < 0.01$ *versus* HF. Abbreviations: HF, high fructose; HF + Los., high fructose diet with losartan; HF + RG, high fructose diet with red ginseng; HF + FRG, high fructose diet with fermented red ginseng; BW, body weight.

3.2. Effect of FRG on the Morphology of Epididymal Fat Pads

Because FRG effectively reduced the epididymal fat pad weight, we prepared frozen sections of epididymal fat pads and stained them with H & E. Histological findings, as shown in Figure 1, revealed hypertrophy of adipocytes in HF diet groups compared with the control group (+34.86%, $p < 0.01$). However, treatment of FRG, Los. and RG groups showed significantly decreases in the hypertrophy of adipocytes (-23.81%, -29.62% and -21.44% respectively, $p < 0.01$) (Figure 1).

3.3. Effect of FRG on Plasma Lipid Levels

After eight weeks of fructose feeding, rats of HF diet groups showed a significant increase in plasma triglycerides, total cholesterol, and LDL-cholesterol levels compared with the control group. However, biochemical analysis of blood samples of the FRG groups showed significant decreases of T-Cho (104.2 $\pm$ 11.5 *versus* 70.3 $\pm$ 7.1 mg/dL, $p < 0.05$) and LDL-c (30.0 $\pm$ 2.6 *versus* 22.2 $\pm$ 1.7 mg/dL, $p < 0.05$) when compared with HF diet groups (Table 2), respectively.Although there was no significant change in triglyceride levels between HF group and FRG groups, there tended to decrease at those levels. Similarly, Los. group, TG, T-Cho and LDL-c were significantly lower than those levels of the HF diet group. Moreover, FRG was found to be more effective in reducing the elevated plasma triglycerides, total cholesterol, and LDL-cholesterol levels compared with RG groups. Besides the plasma levels of HDL-c levels in administration of Los., RG and FRG groups increased compared with HF diet groups (45.2 ± 4.1 *versus* 56.4 ± 1.6, 56.0 ± 3.1 and 60.5 ± 4.4 mg/dL, respectively, *p* < 0.05) (Table 2).

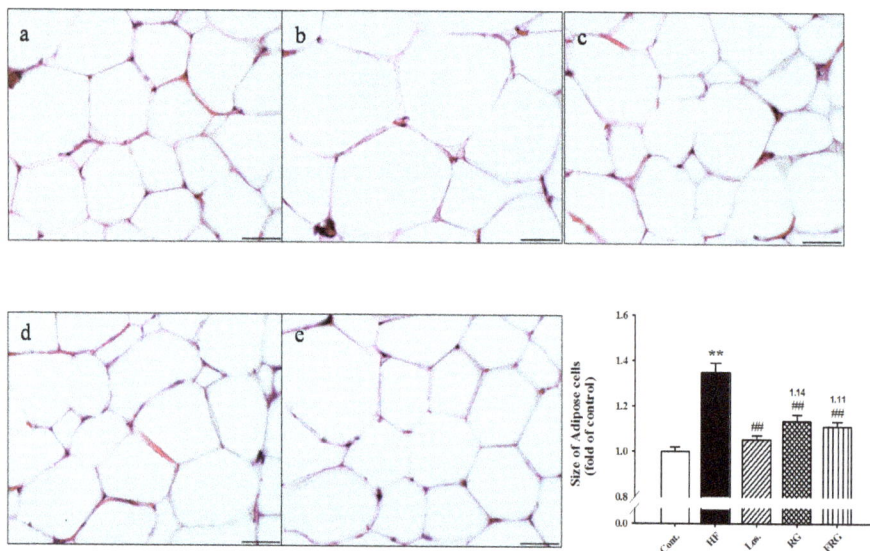

Figure 1. Effects of fermented red ginseng (FRG) on adipocytes on high fructose (HF) diet rats. Representative microscopic photographs of hematoxylin and eosin (H & E) stained sections of epididymal fat pads in HF diet rats. The lower panels indicated the size of adipose cells (magnification ×400). Scale bar shows 50 μm. (**a**) control; (**b**) HF; (**c**) HF + Losartan (Los.); (**d**) HF + RG (red ginseng); (**e**) HF + FRG (fermented red ginseng). Values were expressed as mean ± S.E. (*n* = 3). ** *p* < 0.01 *versus* Cont.; ## *p* < 0.01 *versus* HF.

Table 2. Effect of FRG on plasma lipids.

Groups	Control	HF	HF		
			Los.	RG	FRG
T-Cho (mg/dL)	69.1 ± 7.2	104.2 ± 11.5 *	72.5 ± 5.5 #	80.0 ± 4.1 #	70.3 ± 7.1 #
TG (mg/dL)	155.0 ± 12.8	243.6 ± 27.5 *	117.8 ± 17.1 ##	180.3 ± 32.6	169.0 ± 25.1
HDL-c (mg/dL)	57.7 ± 5.5	45.2 ± 4.1	56.4 ± 1.6 #	56.0 ± 3.1 #	60.5 ± 4.4 #
LDL-c (mg/dL)	22.2 ± 2.1	30.0 ± 2.6*	20.2 ± 1.8 #	26.0 ± 1.6	22.2 ± 1.7 #

Values were expressed as mean ± S.E. (*n* = 10). * *p* < 0.05 *versus* Cont.; # *p* < 0.05 *versus* HF. Abbreviations: HF, high fructose; HF + Los., high fructose diet with losartan; HF + RG, high fructose diet with red ginseng; HF + FRG, high fructose diet with fermented red ginseng; T-Cho, total cholesterol; TG, triglyceride; HDL-c, high-density lipoprotein cholesterol; LDL-c, low-density lipoprotein cholesterol.

3.4. Effect of FRG on Plasma Parameters

Although there was no significant change of glutamic oxaloacetic transaminase (GOT), glutamic pyruvic transaminase (GPT), T-bills and non-fasting blood glucose levels in HF groups and administration drug groups, they decrease at those levels (Table 3). Similar to the plasma lipid levels, the plasma levels of leptin and insulin were significantly increased in HF diet groups compared with the control group. However, treatment of drug groups, especially FRG and Los. Groups, showed a significantly decreased in those levels compared with HF diet groups (Table 2). Moreover, FRG was found to be more effective in reducing the elevated plasma insulin level compared with RG groups.

Table 3. Effect of FRG treatment on plasma parameters.

Groups	Control	HF	HF		
			Los.	RG	FRG
GOT (IU/L)	137.9 ± 10.5	164.3 ± 15.0	155.1 ± 9.8	161.8 ± 28.6	137.00 ± 16.4
GPT (IU/L)	22.2 ± 3.8	29.3 ± 6.7	30.3 ± 4.5	26.8 ± 1.8	28.1 ± 6.5
T-bill (mg/mL)	0.49 ± 0.04	0.48 ± 0.04	0.48 ± 0.03	0.49 ± 0.02	0.38 ± 0.03
Leptin (ng/mL)	5.76 ± 1.0	10.93 ± 2.0 *	3.80 ± 0.7 ##	6.32 ± 1.1	5.41 ± 1.3 #
Insulin (ng/mL)	2.1 ± 0.5	4.1 ± 0.6 *	2.0 ± 0.5 #	2.4 ± 0.6	2.2 ± 0.3 #
Blood glucose (mg/dL)	129.4 ± 5.6	136.9 ± 3.2	128.1 ± 4.6	129.4 ± 7.1	130.3 ± 2.9

Values were expressed as mean ± S.E. (n = 10). * $p < 0.05$ *versus* Cont.; # $p < 0.05$ *versus* HF. Abbreviations: HF, high fructose; HF + Los., high fructose diet with losartan; HF + RG, high fructose diet with red ginseng; HF + FRG, high fructose diet with fermented red ginseng; GOT, glutamic-oxaloacetic transaminase; GPT, glutamic-pyruvic transaminase; T-bill, total billiubin.

3.5. Effect of FRG on Oral Glucose Tolerance Tests

Oral glucose tolerance tests were carried out to check insulin resistance in high-fructose diet rats after eight weeks. The results showed that HF diet groups maintained a significant increase in blood glucose levels at 30 ($p < 0.01$), 60 and 90 min ($p < 0.05$), respectively. However, the plasma glucose levels in treatment of FRG and RG groups were significantly decreased at 30 min as compared with HF diet groups ($p < 0.05$) (Figure 2A). Similarly, treatment of Los. groups was significantly decreased at 30 and 60 min as compared with HF diet groups. Moreover, area analysis (AUC) showed that HF diet groups significantly increased compared with the control group. However, FRG and Los. groups was significantly decreased compared to that of the HF groups (Figure 2B). Moreover, FRG was found to be more effective in reducing the elevated plasma glucose level compared with RG group.

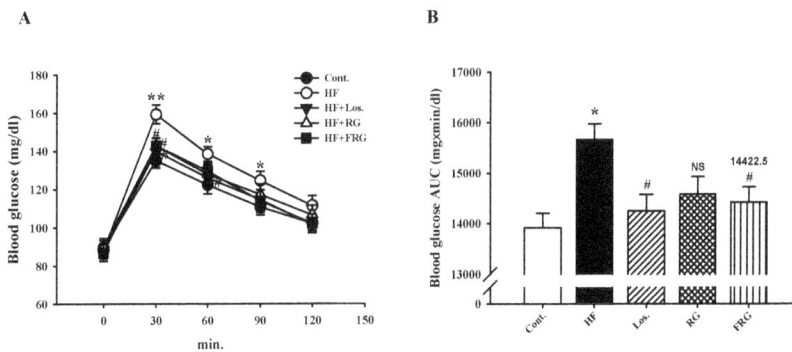

Figure 2. Effect of an FRG on oral glucose tolerance tests (**A**) and the blood glucose area under curve (AUC) (**B**). Values were expressed as mean ± S.E. (n = 10). * $p < 0.05$, ** $p < 0.01$ *versus* Cont.; # $p < 0.05$ *versus* HF. Abbreviations: HF, high fructose; HF + Los., high fructose diet with losartan; HF + RG, high fructose diet with red ginseng; HF + FRG, high fructose diet with fermented red ginseng.

3.6. Effect of FRG on Blood Pressure

At the beginning of the experimental feeding period, the levels of systolic blood pressure in all groups were approximately 106–108 mmHg as investigated by the tail-cuff technique. After eight weeks, systolic blood pressure of HF groups were significantly increased compared to that of the control groups ($p < 0.01$). However, treatment of FRG and RG groups was significantly decreased compared to that of the HF groups during all experimental period (135.7 ± 1.3 *versus* 120.7 ± 1.1 and 122.0 ± 1.1, respectively, $p < 0.01$) (Figure 3A). Similarly, treatment of losartan showed similar results to FRG and RG groups. In addition, the protein expression of ET-1 level was increased in the HF diet group compared with the control group. However, administration drug groups showed significantly decreased expression levels of protein compared with HF diet groups (Figures 3B and 4).

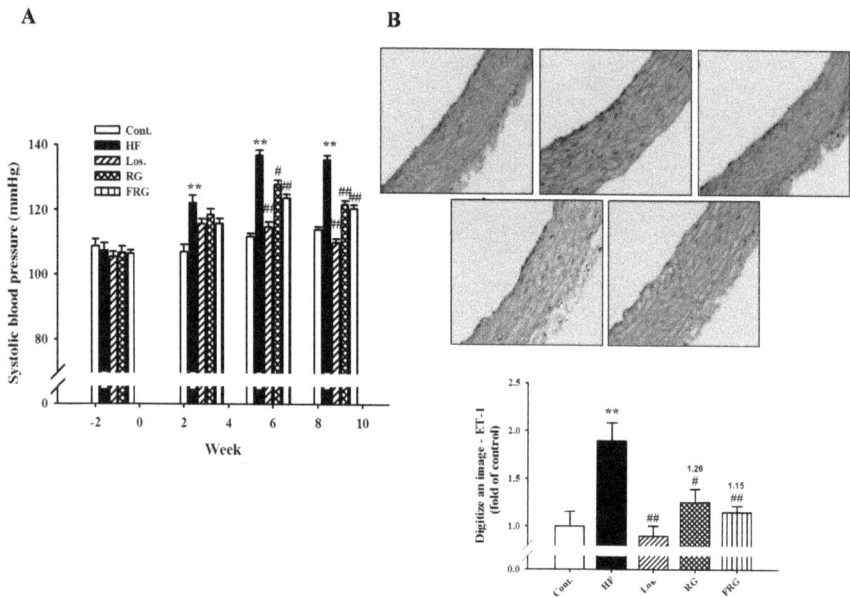

Figure 3. Effects of FRG on systolic blood pressure (**A**) and expression of ET-1 immunoreactivity (**B**) in aortic tissues of HF diet rats. Representative immunohistochemistry and quantifications are shown. Values were expressed as mean $\pm$ S.E. $n = 10$ (**A**) and $n = 3$ (**B**). ** $p < 0.01$ *versus* Cont.; # $p < 0.05$, ## $p < 0.01$ *versus* HF.

3.7. Effect of FRG on the Morphology of Aortas

FRG effectively decreased blood pressure. Thus, we examined staining with hematoxilin-eosin in thoracic aortas. Figure 5 showed that thoracic aortas of HF diet groups revealed roughened endothelial layers and increased tunica intima-media of layers compared with the control group. However, treatment of FRG and RG groups significantly maintained the smooth character of the intima endothelial layers and decreased tunica intima-media thickness in aortic sections. Similarly, treatment of losartan showed similar results to FRG and RG groups. Moreover, FRG was found to be more effective in maintaining the smooth character of the intima endothelial layers and decreased tunica intima-media thickness compared with RG groups.

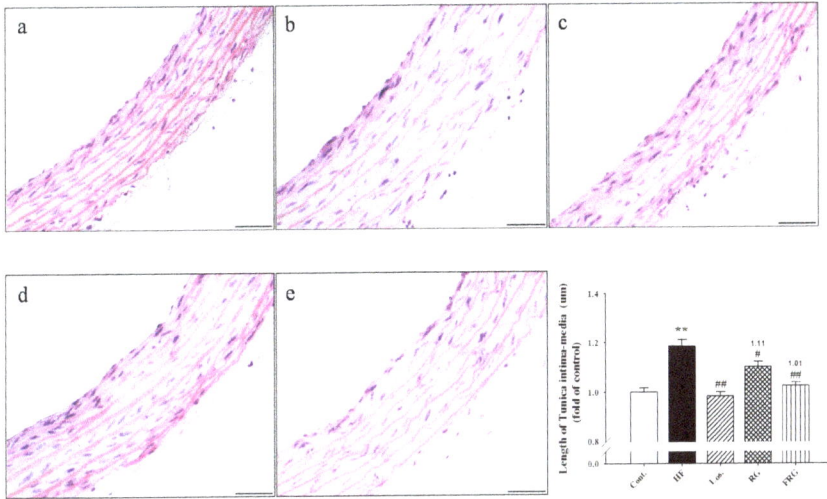

Figure 4. Representative microscopic photographs of H & E stained section of the thoracic aorta in HF diet rats. Lower panel indicated length of intima-media. Lower panel indicated the size of adipose cells (magnification ×400). (**a**) control; (**b**) HF; (**c**) HF + Los.; (**d**) HF + RG; (**e**) HF + FRG. Values were expressed as mean ± S.E. (*n* = 3). ** $p < 0.01$ *versus* Cont.; ## $p < 0.01$ *versus* HF.

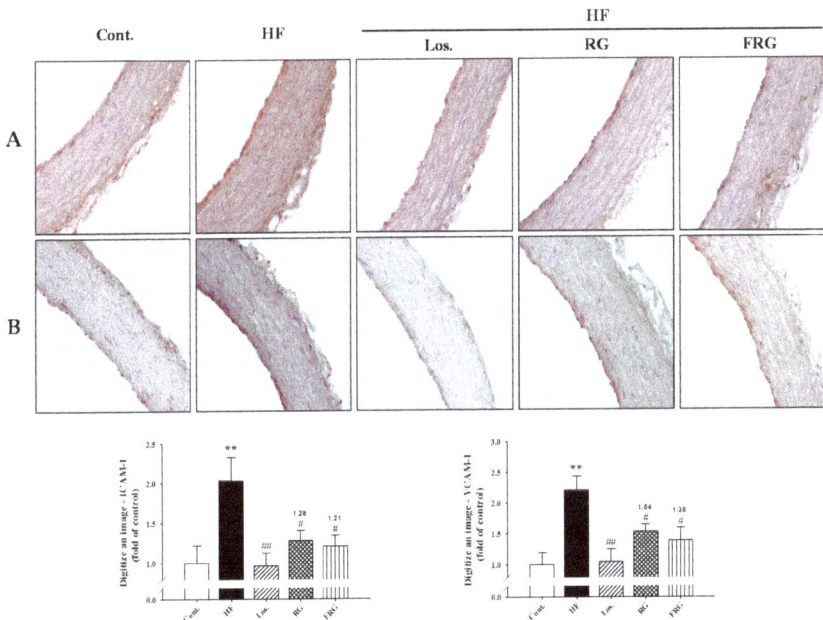

Figure 5. Effects of FRG on ICAM-1 (**A**) and VCAM-1 (**B**) immunoreactivity in aortic tissues of HF diet rats. Representative immunohistochemistry and quantifications are shown (magnification ×400. Values were expressed as mean ± S.E. (*n* = 3). ** $p < 0.01$ *versus* Cont.; # $p < 0.05$, ## $p < 0.01$ *versus* HF. Abbreviations: HF, high fructose; HF + Los., high fructose diet with losartan; HF + RG, high fructose diet with Red ginseng; HF + FRG, high fructose diet with fermented Red ginseng.

3.8. Effect of FRG on the Expressions Levels of Adhesion Molecules and ET-1 in Aortas

The protein expression of VCAM-1, ICAM-1, E-selectin and ET-1 in the descending aortas of all groups of rats was examined by Western blot analysis. Expression of adhesion molecules (VCAM-1, ICAM-1 and E-selectin) and ET-1 levels were increased in the HF diet groups compared with the control group. However, treatment of FRG and RG groups showed significantly decreased expression levels of protein compared with HF diet groups (Figure 6). Similarly, treatment of losartan groups showed similar results to FRG and RG groups.

Immunohistochemistry was performed to determine the direct expression of adhesion molecules in the aortic wall. Adhesion molecule expressions such as ICAM-1 and VCAM-1 were increased in the HF diet groups ($p < 0.01$). However, treatment of FRG and RG groups was significantly decreased expression levels of protein (ICAM-1 and VCAM-1, $p < 0.05$) (Figure 4). Similarly, treatment of losartan groups showed similar results to FRG and RG groups. Moreover, FRG was found to be more effective in decreased expression levels of protein levels compared with RG groups.

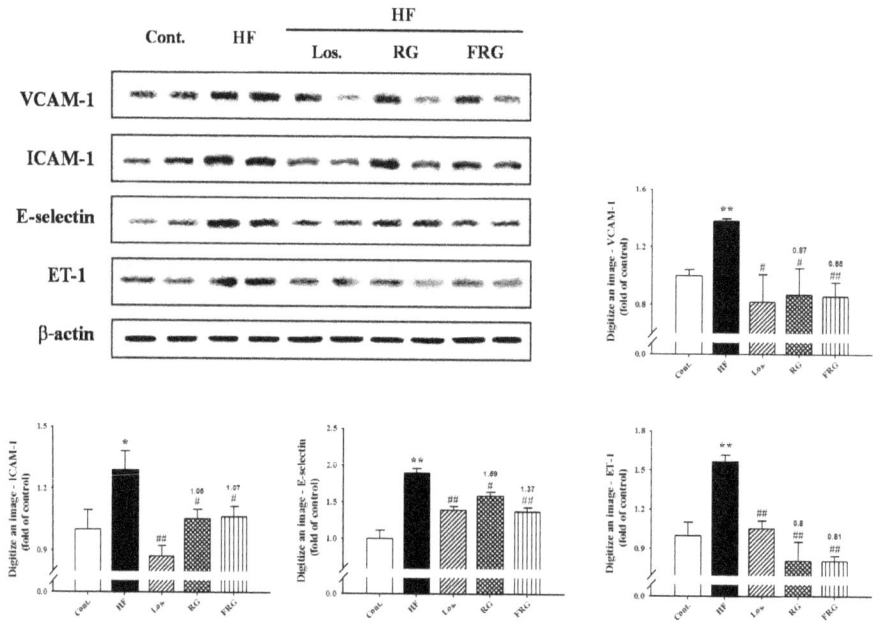

Figure 6. Effects of FRG on VCAM-1, ICAM-1, E-selectinm and ET-1 immunoreactivity in aortic tissues. Representative western blots of VCAM-1, ICAM-1, E-selectinm and ET-1 protein levels are quantifications are shown. Values were expressed as mean ± S.E. ($n = 3$). ** $p < 0.01$ *versus* Cont.; # $p < 0.05$, ## $p < 0.01$ *versus* HF.

3.9. Effect of FRG on Hepatic Lipids

To investigate the existence of fat accumulation in the livers in all experimental groups, we prepared frozen sections of livers and stained them with Oil red O. Lipid droplets were detected in HF diet groups. However, treatment of FRG groups showed that the number of lipid droplets significantly decreased compared with HF diet groups (Figure 7). Similarly, treatment of losartan group showed similar results to the FRG groups. However, RG groups was no significant in RG groups compared with HF group. These results also showed that FRG was found to be more effective in decreased lipid droplets compared with RG groups.

3.10. Effect of FRG on the Expressions Levels of IRS-1 and Glut4 in Muscle Tissue

To investigate the signals in insulin signaling, we examined the expression of IRS-1 and Glut4 in muscle tissue. The expression of IRS-1 and Glut4 were significantly decreased in HF diet groups. However, treatment of FRG groups increased expression levels of protein compared with HF diet groups (Figure 8). Similarly, treatment of losartan groups showed similar results to FRG groups.

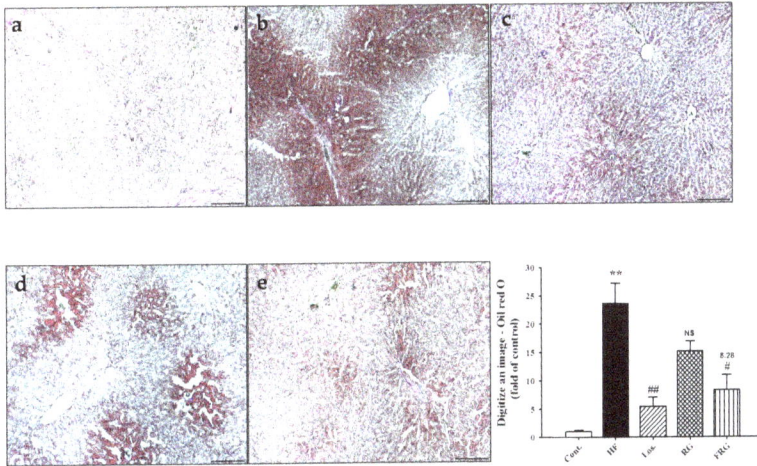

Figure 7. Representative microscopic photographs of Oil red O stained sections of the livers in HF diet rats. Representative Oil red O staining and quantifications are shown (magnification ×100). Values were expressed as mean ± S.E. (n = 3). ** $p < 0.01$ *versus* Cont.; [#] $p < 0.05$, [##] $p < 0.01$ *versus* HF. (**a**) control; (**b**) HF; (**c**) HF + Los.; (**d**) HF + RG (red ginseng); (**e**) HF + FRG (fermented red ginseng).

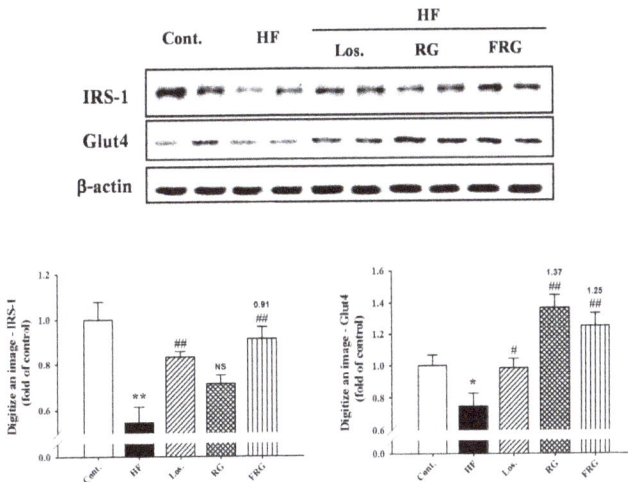

Figure 8. Effect of FRG on the expression of IRS-1 and Glut4 in the muscle of HF diet rats. Each electrophoretogram is representative of the results from three individual experiments. Values were expressed as mean ± S.E. (n = 3). ** $p < 0.01$ *versus* Cont.; [##] $p < 0.01$ *versus* HF. Abbreviations: HF, high fructose; HF + Los., high fructose diet with losartan; HF + RG, high fructose diet with red ginseng; HF + FRG, high fructose diet with fermented red ginseng.

4. Discussion

Past several years, many various plant extracts have been clinically evaluated for the treatment of metabolic disorder disease, such as diabetes, hypertension, dyslipidemia and atherosclerosis [24]. RG has been shown to possess beneficial clinical activity *in vivo* and *in vitro* studies [25,26]. Interestingly, the pharmacological effects of RG were further increased by fermentation. It has been reported that during the fermentation, the chemical composition of ginsenosides are transformed into their readily absorbable and more potent deglycosylated forms. In addition, FRG contains a much higher concentration of total ginsenosides and metabolites [27]. Therefore, future study will be required to clarify the active compounds of FRG and their pharmacological relevance for treatment of metabolic syndrome.

In the present study, we investigated anti-obesity, hypotension, hypolipidemia improved glucose tolerance and ameliorated fatty liver effects of FRG in HF diet rats for eight weeks, and the efficacies were compared to those of RG and losartan. The HF diet induced rodent model is a well-established model of induced hypertension, hypertriglyceridemia, obesity, impaired glucose tolerance, fatty liver and vascular remodeling [28,29]. As expected, the present study showed that the results marked hypertension (increased systolic blood pressure and protein levels of ET-1), obese states (increased body weight, fat weight, adipocyte size and plasma levels of leptin), hyperlipidemia (increased plasma total cholesterol, triglycerides and LDL-cholesterol), impaired glucose tolerance (decreased protein levels of IRS-1 and Glut4), fatty liver (increased liver weight and fat accumulation) and vascular remodeling (increased endothelial dysfunction and adhesion molecules) through eight weeks of an HF diet.

It is reported that a high fructose diet induced high blood pressure, intima-media thickness of the aorta and progress of blood vessel inflammation, which is correlated with prognosis and extension of the initial stage of atherosclerosis and initial stage of cardiovascular disease [30,31]. In addition, endothelial dysfunction was also related with lipid metabolism disorders [32]. The present results showed that an HF diet induced hypertension, dyslipidemia and endothelial dysfunction. However, administering FRG improved endothelial dysfunction with the amelioration of hypertension and dyslipidemia. In addition, interestingly, more favorable anti-hypertension, anti-vascular, inflammatory and regulating lipid homeostasis effects were observed with FRG as compared with an equal dose of RG.

The accumulation of fat deposition and increase in adipocyte size in the body is a major characteristic of obesity, as well as an increase of leptin level processes of leptin resistance, which classically has been characterized by expansion of intra-adipose tissue [33]. Although some studies have reported that losartan has no anti-obesity effects [34], the present results shows losartan has anti-obesity effects that decreased body weight, epididymal fat pad weight, adipocyte size and induced development of leptin resistance [35,36]. Further study is required to clarify the regulatory mechanisms of obesity and leptin levels in metabolic syndrome models. In addition, FRG effectively inhibited the leptin resistance with the amelioration of downregulation of body weight, epididymal fat pad weight and adipocyte size. These results suggest that FRG may be useful for inhibiting the development of leptin resistance and obesity. In addition, FRG was observed to homeostasis about anti-obesity and regulating leptin.

Recently, report has been found a low activation state of AMP-activated protein kinase (AMPK) with metabolic disorder associated with impaired insulin sensitivity, fat accumulation and dyslipidemia [37,38]. It is suggested that fructose-driven leptin resistance in the present study may be associated with impaired leptin-mediated decrease in AMPK phosphorylation. Although we did not examine specific research related to energy metabolism in the AMPK pathway, we speculate that treatment of FRG could be related to the improvements of metabolic disorders by activation of AMPK-related signal pathways.

It is reported that a high fructose diet induced impaired glucose tolerance via the elevation of plasma triglyceride levels, which plays an important role in the development of such abnormalities as insulin resistance, type 2 diabetes, dyslipidemia and fatty liver [39,40]. In addition, there are two signal transduction pathways for glucose/insulin transport in skeletal muscles. IRS-1 is an important tool for stimulating glucose transport induced by insulin [41]. The magnitude of a dense membrane compartment of Glut4 is related to the degree of insulin stimulated and thereby improves glucose uptake in skeletal muscles [42]. Thus, these factors are important key elements in insulin-dependent signal transduction pathways [43]. The present results showed that an HF diet impaired glucose tolerance, which is downregulation of IRS-1 and Glut4 expression. Moreover, an HF diet produced increased liver weight and accumulation of fat deposition in the liver, whereas, FRG improved impaired glucose tolerance with upregulation of IRS-1 and Glut4 protein level expression and decreased liver weight and accumulation of fat deposition in the liver. Hepatic steatosis is associated with metabolic syndrome and is a risk factor for the development of chronic hepatitis. Hyperinsulinemia and hyperglycemia associated with various metabolic disorders may act directly to promote hepatic injury including inflammation and fatty liver. In addition to investigating damage of the liver with aggravation of inflammation, the present study measured plasma levels of GPT, GOT and T-bill. Although all groups did not observe significant changes in plasma levels of GPT, GOT and T-bill, FRG tended to ameliorate those levels. Taken together, the present results showed direct/indirect evidence that FRG has regulated insulin signals and hepatoprotective effects. Moreover, FRG was observed to have more favorable regulating insulin signals and hepatoprotective effects compared with equal doses of RG.

In the future, we plan for more studies that clarify specific mechanism research in relation to other energy metabolic controls in an intestinal body and what ingredients or compounds are most effective in fermented red ginseng in HF diet induced metabolic syndrome.

5. Conclusions

Oral treatment of fermented red ginseng (FRG) effectively ameliorated HF diet induced metabolic disorders such as obesity, dyslipidemia, hypertension and fatty liver. Moreover, treatment of FRG had more favorable pharmacological effects on HF diet induced metabolic disorders compared with an equal dose of red ginseng. Taken together, fermented red ginseng might be a beneficial therapeutic approach for metabolic syndrome.

Supplementary Materials: The following are available online at http://www.mdpi.com/2072-6643/8/6/369/s1, Table S1: Composition of diet obtained from Research diet.

Acknowledgments: This work was supported by the National Research Foundation of Korea (NRF) grant funded by the Korea government (MSIP) (2008-0062484) (2015M3A9E3051054).

Author Contributions: M.C.K., Y.J.L. conceived and designed the experiment; J.H.P., H.Y.K., J.J.Y., Y.M.A., and R.T. performed the experimentalwork and data analyses; J.D.C. and K.M.C. provided the RG and FRG; M.C.P., D.G.K., and H.S.L. supervised the experimental work. All authors read and approved the final manuscript.

Conflicts of Interest: The authors declare no conflict of interest.

References

1. El-Bassossy, H.M.; Shaltout, H.A. Allopurinol alleviateshypertension and proteinuria in high fructose, high salt and high fat induced model of metabolic syndrome. *Transl. Res.* **2015**, *165*, 621–630. [CrossRef] [PubMed]
2. Journal of the American Medical Association (JAMA). National cholesterol education program: Executive summary of the third report of the national cholesterol education program (NCEP) expert panel on detection, evaluation and treatment of high blood cholesterol in adults (adults treatment panel III). *Circulation* **2001**, *285*, 2487–2497.
3. Tilg, H.; Hotamisligil, G.S. Nonalcoholic fatty liver disease: Cytokine-adipokine interplay and regulation of insulin resistance. *Gastroenterology* **2006**, *131*, 934–945. [CrossRef] [PubMed]
4. Shoelson, S.E.; Herrero, L.; Naaz, A. Obesity, inflammation, and insulin resistance. *Gastroenterology* **2007**, *132*, 2169–2180. [CrossRef] [PubMed]

5. Stanhope, K.L.; Havel, P.J. Endocrine and metabolic effects of consuming beverages sweetened with fructose, glucose, sucrose or high-fructose corn syrup. *Am. J. Clin. Nutr.* **2008**, *88*, 1733S–1737S. [CrossRef] [PubMed]
6. Stanhope, K.L.; Havel, P.J. Fructose consumption: Recentresults and their potential implications. *Ann. N. Y. Acad. Sci.* **2010**, *1190*, 15–24. [CrossRef] [PubMed]
7. Basciano, H.; Federico, L.; Adeli, K. Fructose, insulin resistance,and metabolic dyslipidemia. *Nutr. Metab.* **2005**, *2*, 5. [CrossRef] [PubMed]
8. Kim, H.Y.; Okubo, T.; Juneja, L.R.; Yokozawa, T. Theprotective role of amla (*Emblica officinalis* Gaertn.) againstfructose-induced metabolic syndrome in a rat model. *Br. J. Nutr.* **2010**, *103*, 502–512. [CrossRef] [PubMed]
9. Ouyang, X.; Cirillo, P.; Sautin, Y.; McCall, S.; Bruchette, J.L.; Diehl, A.M.; Johnson, R.J.; Abdelmalek, M.F. Fructose consumptionas a risk factor for non-alcoholic fatty liver disease. *J. Hepatol.* **2008**, *48*, 993–999. [CrossRef] [PubMed]
10. Panchal, S.K.; Brown, L. Rodent models for metabolicsyndrome research. *J. Biomed. Biotechnol.* **2011**, *2011*, 351982. [CrossRef] [PubMed]
11. Ferder, L.; Ferder, M.D.; Inserra, F. The role of high-fructosecorn syrup in metabolic syndrome and hypertension. *Curr. Hypertens. Rep.* **2010**, *12*, 105–112. [CrossRef] [PubMed]
12. Yotsumoto, H.; Yanagita, T.; Yamamoto, K.; Ogawa, Y.; Cha, J.Y.; Mori, Y. Inhibitory effect of Oren-Gedoku-to and its components on cholesterol ester synthesis in cultured human hepatocyte HepG2 cells: Evidence from the cultured HepG2 cells and *in vitro* assay of ACAT. *Planta Med.* **1997**, *63*, 141–145. [CrossRef] [PubMed]
13. Miettinen, T.A. Cholesterol absorption inhibition: A strategy for cholesterol-lowering therapy. *Int. J. Clin. Pract.* **2001**, *55*, 710–716. [PubMed]
14. Shin, M.K.; Han, S.H. Effects of methanol extracts from bamboo (*Pseudosasa japonica* Makino) leaves extracts on lipid metabolism in rats fed high fat and high cholesterol diet. *Korean J. Food Cult.* **2002**, *17*, 30–36.
15. Ko, S.K.; Lee, C.R.; Choi, Y.E.; Im, B.O.; Sung, J.H.; Yoon, K.R. Analysis of ginsenosides of white and red ginseng concentrates. *Korean J. Food Sci. Technol.* **2003**, *35*, 536–539.
16. Kim, N.D. Pharmacological effects of red ginseng. *J. Ginseng Res.* **2001**, *25*, 2–10.
17. Ramesh, T.; Kin, S.W.; Hwang, S.Y.; Sohn, S.H.; Yoo, S.K.; Kim, S.K. Panax ginseng reduces oxidative stress and restores antioxidant capacity in aged rats. *Nutr. Res.* **2012**, *32*, 718–726. [CrossRef] [PubMed]
18. Lee, B.; Heo, H.; Oh, S.; Lew, J. Comparison study of Korean and Chinese ginsengs on the regulation of lymphocyte proliferation and cytokine production. *J. Ginseng Res.* **2008**, *32*, 250–256.
19. Lee, H.; Park, D.; Yoon, M. Korean red ginseng (*Panax ginseng*) prevents obesity by inhibiting angiogenesis in high fat diet induced obes C57BL/6J mice. *Food Chem. Toxicol.* **2013**, *53*, 402–408. [CrossRef] [PubMed]
20. Kim, DH. Metabolism of ginsenosides to bioactive compounds by intestinal microfloraand its industrial application. *J. Ginseng Res.* **2009**, *33*, 165–176.
21. Bae, E.A.; Han, M.J.; Kim, E.J.; Kim, D.H. Transformation of ginseng saponins to ginsenoside Rh2 by acids and human intestinal bacteria and biological activities of their transformants. *Arch. Pharm. Res.* **2004**, *27*, 61–67. [CrossRef] [PubMed]
22. Yasuda, M.; Tachibana, S.; Kuba-Miyara, M. Biochemical aspects of red koji and tofuyo preparedusing Monascus fungi. *Appl. Microbiol. Biotechnol.* **2012**, *96*, 49–60. [CrossRef] [PubMed]
23. Trinh, H.T.; Han, S.J.; Kim, S.W.; Lee, Y.C.; Kim, D.H. Bifidus fermentation increaseshypolipidemic and hypoglycemic effects of red ginseng. *J. Microbiol. Biotechnol.* **2007**, *17*, 1127–1133. [PubMed]
24. Kim, H.Y.; Kim, K. Regulation of signaling molecules associated with insulin action, insulin secretion and pancreatic beta-cell mass in the hypoglycemic effect of Korean red ginseng in Goto-Kakizaki rat. *J. Ethnopharmacol.* **2012**, *142*, 53–58. [CrossRef] [PubMed]
25. Ha, K.S.; Jo, S.H.; Kang, B.H.; Apostolidis, E.; Lee, M.S.; Jang, H.D.; Kwon, Y.I. *In vitro* and *in vivo* antihyperglycemic effect of 2 amadori rearrangement compounds, arginyl-fructose and arginyl-fructose-glucose. *J. Food Sci.* **2011**, *76*, H188–H193. [CrossRef] [PubMed]
26. Vuksan, V.; Sung, M.K.; Sievenpiper, J.L.; Stavro, P.M.; Jenkins, A.L.; Buono, M.D.; Lee, K.S.; Leiter, L.A.; Nam, K.Y.; Arnason, J.T.; *et al.* Korean red ginseng (*Panax ginseng*) improves glucose and insulin regulation in well-controlled, type 2 diabetes: results of a randomized, double-blind, placebo-controlled study of efficacy and safety. *Nutr. Metab. Cardiovasc. Dis.* **2008**, *18*, 46–56. [PubMed]
27. Kim, B.G.; Choi, S.Y.; Kim, M.R.; Suhd, H.J.; Park, H.J. Changes of ginsenosides in Korean red ginseng (*Panax ginseng*) fermented by *Lactobacillus plantarum* M1. *Process. Biochem.* **2010**, *45*, 1319–1324. [CrossRef]

28. Miatello, R.; Vázquez, M.; Renna, N.; Cruzado, M.; Zumino, A.P.; Risler, N. Chronic administration of resveratrol prevents biochemical cardiovascular changes in fructose-fed rats. *Am. J. Hypertens.* **2005**, *18*, 864–870. [CrossRef] [PubMed]

29. Renna, N.F.; Vazquez, M.A.; Lama, M.C.; González, E.S.; Miatello, R.M. Effect of chronic aspirin administration on an experimental model of metabolic syndrome. *Clin. Exp. Pharmacol. Physiol.* **2009**, *36*, 162–168. [CrossRef] [PubMed]

30. Johnson, J.L. Matrix metalloproteinases:influence on smooth muscle cells and atherosclerotic plaque stability. *Expert. Rev. Cardiovasc. Ther.* **2007**, *5*, 265–282. [CrossRef] [PubMed]

31. Li, G.; Sanders, J.M.; Phan, E.T.; Ley, K.; Sarembock, I.J. Arterial macrophages and regenerating endothelial cells express P-selectin in atherosclerosis-prone apolipoprotein E-deficient mice. *Am. J. Pathol.* **2005**, *167*, 1511–1518. [CrossRef]

32. Endemann, D.H.; Schiffrin, E.L. Nitric oxide, oxidative excess, and vascular complications of diabetes mellitus. *Curr. Hypertens. Rep.* **2004**, *6*, 85–89. [CrossRef] [PubMed]

33. Friedman, J.M.; Halass, J.L. Leptin and the regulation of body weight in mammals. *Nature* **1998**, *1*, 1155–1161.

34. Carter, C.S.; Giovannini, S.; Seo, D.O.; DuPree, J.; Morgan, D.; Chung, H.Y.; Lees, H.; Daniels, M.; Hubbard, G.B.; Lee, S.; *et al.* Differential effects of enalapril and losartan on body composition and indices of muscle quality in aged male Fischer 344 × Brown Norway rats. *Age* **2011**, *33*, 167–183. [CrossRef] [PubMed]

35. Brink, M.; Wellen, J.; Delafontaine, P. Angiotensin II causes weight loss and decreases circulating insulin-like growth factor I in rats through a pressor-independent mechanism. *J. Clin. Invest.* **1996**, *97*, 2509–2516. [CrossRef] [PubMed]

36. Guo, Q.; Mori, T.; Jiang, Y.; Hu, C.; Ohsaki, Y.; Yoneki, Y.; Nakamichi, T.; Ogawa, S.; Sato, H.; Ito, S. Losartan modulates muscular capillary density and reverses thiazide diuretic-exacerbated insulin resistance in fructose-fed rats. *Hypertens. Res.* **2012**, *35*, 48–54. [CrossRef] [PubMed]

37. Luo, Z.; Saha, A.K.; Xiang, X.; Ruderman, N.B. AMPK, the metabolic syndrome and cancer. *Trends Pharmacol. Sci.* **2005**, *26*, 69–76. [CrossRef] [PubMed]

38. Majithiya, J.B.; Balaraman, R. Metformin reduces blood pressure and restores endothelial function in aorta of streptozotocin-induced diabetic rats. *Life Sci.* **2006**, *78*, 2615–2624. [CrossRef] [PubMed]

39. Miller, A.; Adeli, K. Dietary fructose and the metabolic syndrome. *Curr. Opin. Gastroenterol.* **2008**, *24*, 204–209. [CrossRef] [PubMed]

40. Tran, L.T.; Yuen, V.G.; McNeill, J.H. The fructose-fed rat: A review on the mechanisms of fructose-induced insulin resistance and hypertension. *Mol. Cell. Biochem.* **2009**, *332*, 145–159. [CrossRef] [PubMed]

41. Thong, F.S.L.; Bilan, P.J.; Klip, A. The RabGTPase-activating protein AS160 integrates Akt, protein kinase C, and AMP-activated protein kinase signals regulating GLUT4 traffic. *Diabetes* **2007**, *56*, 414–423. [CrossRef] [PubMed]

42. Garvey, W.T.; Maianu, L.; Zhu, J.H.; Brechtel-Hook, G.; Wallace, P.; Baron, A.D. Evidence for defects in the trafficking and translocation of GLUT4 glucose transporters in skeletal muscle as a cause of human insulin resistance. *J. Clin. Invest.* **1998**, *101*, 2377–2386. [CrossRef] [PubMed]

43. Mackenzie, R.W.; Elloitt, B.T. Akt/PKB activation and insulin signaling: A novel insulin signaling pathway in the treatment of type 2 diabets. *Diabetes Metab. Syndr. Obes.* **2014**, *7*, 55–64. [CrossRef] [PubMed]

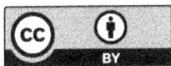

![nutrients logo] *nutrients*

MDPI

Article

Glutamine Modulates Macrophage Lipotoxicity

Li He [1,2], Kassandra J. Weber [1,2] and Joel D. Schilling [1,2,3,*]

[1] Diabetic Cardiovascular Disease Center, Washington University School of Medicine, St. Louis, MO 63110, USA; Lhe@dom.wustl.edu (L.H.); kweber@wayne.med.edu (K.J.W.)
[2] Department of Medicine, Washington University School of Medicine, St. Louis, MO 63110, USA
[3] Department of Pathology and Immunology, Washington University School of Medicine, St. Louis, MO 63110, USA
[*] Correspondence: schillij@wustl.edu; Tel.: +1-314-747-8499

Received: 17 February 2016; Accepted: 6 April 2016; Published: 12 April 2016

Abstract: Obesity and diabetes are associated with excessive inflammation and impaired wound healing. Increasing evidence suggests that macrophage dysfunction is responsible for these inflammatory defects. In the setting of excess nutrients, particularly dietary saturated fatty acids (SFAs), activated macrophages develop lysosome dysfunction, which triggers activation of the NLRP3 inflammasome and cell death. The molecular pathways that connect lipid stress to lysosome pathology are not well understood, but may represent a viable target for therapy. Glutamine uptake is increased in activated macrophages leading us to hypothesize that in the context of excess lipids glutamine metabolism could overwhelm the mitochondria and promote the accumulation of toxic metabolites. To investigate this question we assessed macrophage lipotoxicity in the absence of glutamine using LPS-activated peritoneal macrophages exposed to the SFA palmitate. We found that glutamine deficiency reduced lipid induced lysosome dysfunction, inflammasome activation, and cell death. Under glutamine deficient conditions mTOR activation was decreased and autophagy was enhanced; however, autophagy was dispensable for the rescue phenotype. Rather, glutamine deficiency prevented the suppressive effect of the SFA palmitate on mitochondrial respiration and this phenotype was associated with protection from macrophage cell death. Together, these findings reveal that crosstalk between activation-induced metabolic reprogramming and the nutrient microenvironment can dramatically alter macrophage responses to inflammatory stimuli.

Keywords: lysosome; cell death; metabolism; inflammasome

1. Introduction

Diabetes and obesity are common metabolic disorders that are associated with macrophage dysfunction. Moreover, pathologic inflammation driven by macrophages is recognized as a contributing factor to the impaired tissue repair responses observed in obese and diabetic patients [1–4]. Therefore, understanding the mechanisms by which the nutrient microenvironment alters macrophage inflammatory responses is highly relevant to human disease. Individuals with obesity and diabetes have excess circulating triglycerides and free fatty acids (FFAs) leading to ectopic lipid deposition in non-adipose tissues including macrophages [5,6]. Toll-like receptor 4 (TLR4) is an inflammatory receptor expressed at high levels on macrophages, which is activated in response to bacterial infection and/or sterile tissue damage [7,8]. Recently, we demonstrated that activation of macrophage TLR4 in a lipid rich environment triggers lysosome damage, which contributes to NLRP3 inflammasome activation and macrophage cell death [9–11]. However, the molecular pathways that precede lysosome pathology are not well understood.

Macrophage activation leads to dramatic reprogramming of cellular metabolism to facilitate ATP generation and the production of macromolecules such as proteins, nucleotides, and lipids [12]. Activation of TLR4 on macrophages triggers an increase in glycolysis with variable effects on fatty acid oxidation (FAO) [13,14]. Glutamine uptake and metabolism is also enhanced in response to TLR4 activation [15]. Although metabolic reprogramming is important for macrophage activation, it remains unclear how changes in the nutrient microenvironment interface with these changes in cellular metabolism to influence cell phenotype. This is particularly relevant in situations of nutrient excess where mitochondria can be presented with energetic substrates in excess of what is needed for ATP generation. In this context, oversupply of substrates and reducing equivalents to the mitochondria has the potential to lead to accumulation of metabolites and reactive oxygen species [16].

Glutamine is a non-essential amino acid that is consumed by growing or activated cells. Following uptake, glutamine can be broken down to produce glutamate and α-ketoglutarate (α-KG), the latter of which enters into the TCA cycle. In addition to feeding energetic pathways glutamine also facilitates the uptake of other amino acids, such as leucine via SLC7A5, and promotes activation of growth kinases such as mTOR [17,18]. In line with these observations, when glutamine concentrations are low, mTOR activation is suppressed, and catabolic processes such as autophagy are enhanced [19]. Therefore, glutamine and its metabolites significantly alter cell stress responses, making this a relevant nutrient to consider in the context of lipid-induced macrophage dysfunction. To date, the role of glutamine in macrophage responses to excess FAs has not been explored.

In light of previous data that TLR4 activation in primary macrophages triggers enhanced glucose and glutamine metabolism in macrophages we hypothesized that excess SFA could lead to metabolic gridlock from nutrient overload. This scenario would be expected to result in the accumulation of toxic metabolites that could mediate lysosome damage. Based on prior evidence that lipid-induced cell death is independent of glucose concentration we focused our analysis on how glutamine influences macrophage lipotoxicity [9]. In the absence of glutamine, macrophage cell death and inflammasome activation in response to excess dietary SFAs was attenuated. We provide evidence that glutamine deficiency attenuates the toxic effects of lipid overload likely through its impact on mitochondrial metabolism.

2. Experimental Section

2.1. Reagents

Bafilomycin A was from Enzo life sciences (Farmingdale, NY, USA). The α-tubulin antibody, α-actin antibody, α-ketoglutarate, and BPTES were from Sigma Chemical (St. Louis, MO, USA). C968 was from Millipore-EMD-Calbiochem (Bellerica, MA, USA). Phospho- and total S6Kinase and AKT S473 antibodies were from Cell Signaling (Danvers, MA, USA). L-glutamine was from Corning (Manassas, VA, USA). The α-LC3 antibody was from Novus Biologicals (NB100-2220; Littleton, CO, USA). The α-p62 antibody was from Abcam (ab56416; Cambridge, MA USA). Lysotracker red was from Life Technologies (Carlsbad, CA, USA). Ultrapure *E. coli* LPS was from Invivogen (San Diego, CA, USA). Thioglycollate was from Difco-BD (Franklin Lakes, NJ, USA). Fatty acids were from Nu-Chek Prep (Waterville, MN, USA). Ultrapure-bovine serum albumin (BSA) was from Lampire (Ottsville, PA, USA) and was tested for TLR ligand contamination prior to use by treating primary macrophages and assaying for TNFα release.

2.2. Cell Culture

Peritoneal macrophages were isolated from C57BL/6, or the indicated knockout mice 4 days after intraperitoneal injection of 1 mL, 3.85% thioglycollate and plated at a density of 1×10^6 cells/mL in DMEM containing 10% inactivated fetal serum (IFS), 50 U/mL penicillin G sodium, and 50U/mL streptomycin sulfate (pen-strep). For glutamine free experiments media was prepared with dialyzed serum (Gibco-ThermoFisher, Waltham, MA, USA) to remove all sources of glutamine. Stimulations were performed on the day after harvest. For flow cytometry experiments, peritoneal cells were cultured on low adherence plates (Greiner Bio-One) to facilitate cell harvest. Cells were removed from low adherence plates by washing with PBS followed by 10 min with Cell Stripper (Gibco) and then

10 min with EDTA/trypsin (Sigma). Growth medium was supplemented with palmitate or stearate complexed to BSA at a 2:1 molar ratio, as described previously [9], and BSA-supplemented media was used as control. For cell stimulations, PBS or LPS (100 ng/mL) were added to BSA or free fatty acid containing media.

2.3. Mice

Wild type (WT) C57BL/6 mice were bred in our mouse facility; ATG5flox X LysM-Cre, were from Skip Virgin (Washington University). All lines were in the C57BL/6 background. Mice were maintained in a pathogen free facility on a standard chow diet ad libitum (6% fat). All animal experiments were conducted in strict accordance with NIH guidelines for humane treatment of animals and were reviewed by the Animal Studies Committee of Washington University School of Medicine.

2.4. RNA Isolation and Quantitative RT-PCR

Total cellular RNA was isolated using Qiagen RNeasy columns and reverse transcribed using a high capacity cDNA reverse transcription kit (Applied Biosystems, Thermo-Fisher Scientific, Waltham, MA, USA). Real-time qRT-PCR was performed using SYBR green reagent (Applied Biosystems) on an ABI 7500 fast thermocycler. Relative gene expression was determined using the delta-delta CT method normalized to 36B4 expression. Mouse primers sequences were as follows (all $5'$-$3'$): *36B4* (forward- ATC CCT GAC GCA CCG CCG TGA, reverse-TGC ATC TGC TTG GAG CCC ACG TT); *LC3* (forward-CGT CCT GGA CAA GAC CAA GT, reverse-ATT GCT GTC CCG AAT GTC TC); *p62* (forward-GCT GCC CTA TAC CCA CAT CT, reverse-CGC CTT CAT CCG AGA AAC).

2.5. Western Blotting

Total cellular protein was isolated by lysing cells in 150 mM NaCl, 10 mM Tris (pH 8), triton X-100 1% and 1X Protease Complete and phosphatase inhibitors (Thermo-Fisher Scientific). Subsequently, 25 µg of protein from each sample was separated on a TGX gradient gel (4%–20%; Biorad) and transferred to a nitrocellulose membrane. For blots of Phospho-S6, S6K, and AKT transfer was for 1 h on ice. For LC3 blots, proteins were transferred overnight in the cold room at 140 mAmp constant current.

2.6. Lysosome Imaging

After the indicated stimulations, cells were stained with 500 nM lysotracker red in tissue culture media for 15 min at 37 °C. After staining, cells were washed three times with PBS, harvested as described above, and analyzed by flow cytometry.

2.7. Metabolism Assays

Cells were plated into 96 well Seahorse plates at density of 75,000 cells/well and stimulated as indicated in the text. After stimulation the cells were washed and placed in XF media (non-buffered RPMI 1640 containing, 25 mM glucose, 2 mM L-glutamine and 1 mM sodium pyruvate) with 10% FCS. Oxygen consumption rates (OCR) and extracellular acidification rates (ECAR) were measured under basal conditions and following the addition the following drugs: 1.5 µM flurorcarbonyl cynade phenylhydrazon (FCCP), and 100 nM rotenone + 1 µM antimycin A (all Sigma). Measurements were taken using a 96 well Extracellular Flux Analyzer (Seahorse Bioscience; North Bellerica, MA, USA).

2.8. Ammonia Quantification

After stimulation, supernatants were collected from 0.5×10^6 pMACs macrophages grown in a 24 well plate. The ammonia concentration was determined using an ammonia assay kit (BioVision, Milpitas, CA, USA) as per the manufacturer's instructions.

2.9. Intracellular Glutamine Quantification

Two million pMACs were grown in 6 well plates. After stimulation the cells were washed 3 times with PBS and then were snap frozen and scraped in liquid nitrogen. Intracellular metabolites were quantified by LC-MS/MS at Sanford Burnham Metabolomics Core, Medical Discovery Institute (Lake Nona, FL, USA).

3. Results

3.1. Glutamine Deficiency Attenuates Macrophage Lipotoxic Responses

We have previously shown that resting macrophages are largely resistant to the effects of SFA excess; however, upon activation exposure to SFAs leads to lysosome damage, cell death, and inflammasome activation [9,11]. An important consequence of macrophage activation is dramatic reprogramming of cellular metabolism, raising the intriguing possibility that interplay between the internal and external metabolic milieu might be relevant to the toxic effects of lipids. Glutamine metabolism is modulated by TLR4-activation, but the influence of this nutrient pathway on lipid stress responses has not been explored. Consistent with increased uptake of glutamine, we observed that macrophages treated with LPS or LPS with palmitate had increased intracellular glutamine levels (Figure 1A). To further investigate glutamine handling in activated macrophages we quantified ammonia release, a byproduct of glutamine catabolism. Treatment with LPS increased release of ammonia from macrophages under control and lipid stress conditions. In contrast, baseline and LPS-induced ammonia release were significantly decreased when cells were activated in glutamine free conditions (Figure 1B,C).

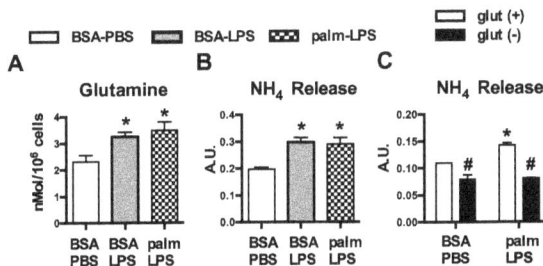

Figure 1. Glutamine metabolism is increased in activated macrophages. (**A**) Peritoneal macrophages (pMACs) were treated with control (BSA-PBS), BSA-LPS (100 ng), or palm (250 μM)-LPS (100 ng) for 16 h; and intracellular glutamine levels were quantified by mass spectroscopy; (**B**) After the indicated stimulations for 16 h, NH_4 release was quantified in the supernatant; (**C**) pMACs were stimulated in glutamine sufficient (open bars) or glutamine deficient (filled bars) media and NH_4 release into the media was quantified at 16 h. Bar graphs report the mean $\pm$ standard error (SE) for a minimum of 3 experiments, each performed in triplicate. *, $p < 0.05$ for PBS *vs.* LPS; #, $p < 0.05$ glutamine *vs.* no glutamine.

To elucidate the impact of glutamine on lipid-induced macrophage lysosome damage we activated pMACs with palmitate and LPS in control media or media deficient in glutamine. In the absence of glutamine, macrophage cell death and lysosome damage in response to palmitate and LPS were significantly decreased (Figure 2A,B). In addition, release of the inflammasome regulated cytokine IL-1β was also diminished when glutamine was absent. TNFα secretion, which is not regulated by the inflammasome or lysosome damage, was not reduced with glutamine deficiency indicating that macrophage inflammatory function was not globally suppressed (Figure 2C,D). Thus, alterations in TLR4 activation-induced glutamine metabolism are required for FAs in the nutrient microenvironment to produce toxicity in macrophages.

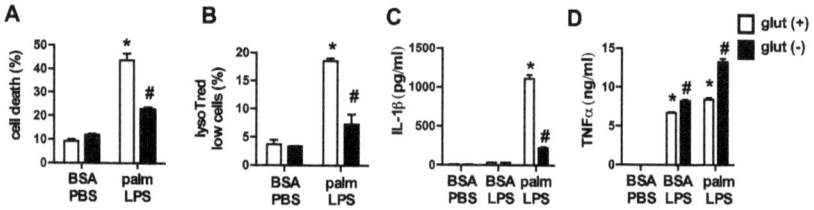

Figure 2. Glutamine deficiency protects against lipotoxicity in macrophages. (**A,B**) pMACs were stimulated with BSA-PBS or palm-LPS in glutamine sufficient (open bars) or glutamine deficient (black bars) media and cell death was assessed at 30 h by annexin-PI (**A**), or lysosome damage was determined at 24 h by lysotracker red staining (**B**), both coupled with flow cytometry; (**C,D**) After the indicated stimulations IL-1β (**C**) or TNFα (**D**) release was quantified in the supernatant using ELISA. Bar graphs report the mean ± SE for a minimum of 3 experiments, each performed in triplicate. *, $p < 0.05$ for PBS *vs.* LPS; #, $p < 0.05$ glutamine *vs.* no glutamine.

3.2. Oxidative Glutamine Metabolism Is Partially Responsible for the Protection from Lipid Toxicity

Upon entering the cell, glutamine can be broken down by glutaminase to glutamate, which is then converted to α-ketoglutarate (α-KG) for oxidation in the TCA cycle. To determine whether depletion of α-KG was the cause of reduced macrophage lipotoxicity we added a membrane permeable form of α-KG to glutamine deficient or sufficient media and assessed the lipotoxic phenotypes. Restoration of α-KG significantly increased cell death and lysosome damage in macrophages stimulated in glutamine deficient media (Figure 3A,B). In contrast, the addition of α-KG to macrophages cultured in glutamine sufficient media did not increase macrophage cell death. Similar findings were observed for IL-1β release (Figure 3C,D). However, the lysosome damage and cell death observed with α-KG supplementation was still less severe compared to glutamine sufficient media, arguing that some of the effects of glutamine are independent of glutamine breakdown. To further address this issue we used two chemically distinct inhibitors of glutaminase, Bis-2-(5-phenylacetamido-1,3,4-thiadiazol-2-yl)ethyl sulfide (BPTES) or compound 968. With both agents cell death and IL-1β release were attenuated, although the compounds were significantly less effective than glutamine deprivation (Figure 4A–C). These findings are consistent with the α-KG add-back experiments, and suggest that glutamine deprivation protects through pathways that are both dependent and independent of its catabolism.

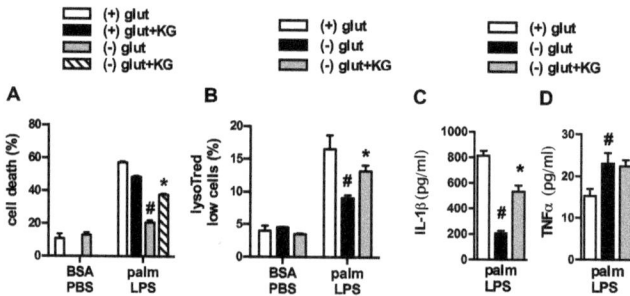

Figure 3. α-ketoglutarate partially restores macrophage lipotoxic phenotypes under glutamine deficient conditions. (**A**) Macrophages were treated as indicated in glutamine sufficient and deficient media ± 440 nM α-ketoglutarate (α-KG) and cell death (**A**) or lysotracker low cells (**B**) were quantified by flow cytometry; (**C,D**) pMACs were stimulated with palm-LPS in glutamine sufficient and deficient media ± α-KG and IL-1β (**C**) or TNF α (**D**) release was quantified by ELISA. Bar graphs report the mean ± SE for a minimum of 3 experiments, each performed in triplicate. *, $p < 0.05$ for veh *vs.* α-KG; #, $p < 0.05$ glutamine *vs.* no glutamine.

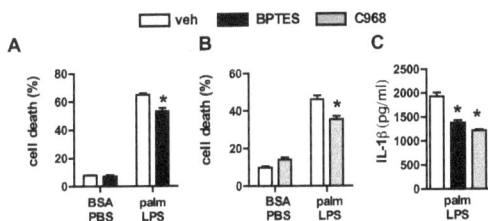

Figure 4. Inhibition of glutaminolysis partially mimics glutamine deficiency. (**A,B**) Primary macrophages were stimulated with BSA-PBS in the presece of the glutaminolysis inhibitors BPTES ((**A**) 10 µM) or C698 ((**B**) 10 µM); (**C**) IL-1β release was quantified from pMACs treated with palm-LPS in the presence of BTPES of C968. Bar graphs report the mean ± SE for a minimum of 3 experiments, each performed in triplicate. *, $p < 0.05$ for veh *vs.* inhibitor.

3.3. Glutamine Deficiency Is Protective Independent of Leucine

Glutamine is required for the cellular import of branched chain amino acids such as leucine [20]. Thus, a possible catabolism-independent function of glutamine deprivation could be explained by reduced leucine uptake. To investigate whether leucine deprivation could mimic the effects of glutamine removal we used media deficient in glutamine or leucine and analyzed macrophage cell death. Removal of leucine from glutamine containing media did not protect the macrophages from cell death (Figure 5). Thus, the phenotype of glutamine deficiency cannot be explained by reduced uptake and metabolism of leucine.

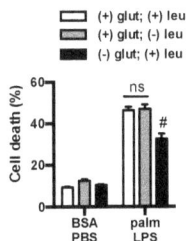

Figure 5. Leucine deficiency does not protect macrophage from lipotoxicity. Macrophages were incubated in complete RPMI media (open bars) or RPMI lacking leucine (gray filled bars) or glutamine (black filled bars), and after the indicated stimulation cell death was determined by annexin-PI flow cytometry. Bar graphs report the mean ± SE for a minimum of 3 experiments, each performed in triplicate. #, $p < 0.05$ glutamine *vs.* no glutamine.

3.4. mTOR Signaling Is Reduced in the Absence of Glutamine

mTOR is a nutrient responsive kinase that is activated by growth factors and/or amino acids, including glutamine. mTOR exists as two complexes known as mTORC1 and mTORC2 in which mTOR pairs with the adaptor proteins raptor or rictor, respectively (Figure 6A) [21]. To assess activation of these mTOR complexes in the presence and absence of glutamine we analyzed phosphorylation of the mTORC1 substrate S6kinase (S6K) and the mTORC2 substrate AKT. Consistent with prior reports, LPS led to increased phosphorylation of both S6K and AKT. In the absence of glutamine S6K phosphorylation was impaired, but no effect was observed on AKT phosphorylation. In contrast, the SFA palmitate reduced AKT phosphorylation, but did not significantly affect S6K phosphorylation (Figure 6B). We next determined whether the addition of α-KG could restore activation of S6K. As can be seen in Figure 6C, α-KG add-back did not increase S6K phosphorylation in the absence of glutamine, suggesting this was a direct effect of glutamine on mTORC1 activation and less likely to be involved in the protection from lipotoxicity.

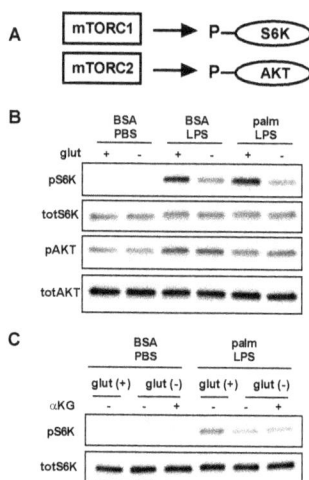

Figure 6. Glutamine deficiency impairs activation of mTORC1. (**A**) mTORC can assemble in two distinct complexes known as mTORC1 and mTORC2 which lead to the phosphorylation of S6K and AKT, respectively; (**B**) pMACs were stimulated with BSA-PBS, BSA-LPS, or palm-LPS for 16 h in the presence or absence of glutamine and phosphorlyation of S6K and AKT were assessed by Western blotting. Total S6K and total AKT are shown as control; (**C**) Macrophages were treated as indicated for 16 h in glutamine sufficient or deficient media ± α-KG (440 nM) and S6K phosphorylation was determined by Western blotting.

3.5. Glutamine Deficiency Modulates Macrophage Autophagy

One important function of mTORC1 is to regulate autophagy, a fundamental process involved the starvation response and in cell quality control. Glutamine availability has also been implicated as a regulator of autophagy. Thus, to monitor autophagic flux in our system we performed western blots of the autophagy proteins LC3 and p62 with or without bafilomycin present for the last 2 h of the stimulation to block lysosomal flux. Under control conditions with BSA-PBS there were no differences in LC3II or p62 protein levels whether or not glutamine was present. Treatment with bafilomycin to block lysosomal degradation of autophagosomes increased both LC3II and p62 consistent with active autophagic flux in these macrophages. Again, glutamine deficiency did not alter autophagic flux under control conditions. In contrast, the absence of glutamine in cell treated with palm-LPS led to decreased protein levels of LC3II and p62 and this response was partially restored by α-KG. In bafilomycin treated samples LC3II levels increased in all of the treatment groups, although the greatest increase was observed for BSA-PBS treated samples (Figure 7A). These findings are consistent with reduced flux through the lysosome under lipid stress conditions. Even in the presence of bafilomycin, LC3II levels were still reduced in palm-LPS samples from glutamine free conditions. As LC3 and p62 are also regulated at the transcriptional level we assessed whether the observed differences between glutamine sufficient or deficient conditions were driven by transcriptional changes using qRT-PCR. Treatment with palm-LPS decreased LC3 and increased p62 mRNA levels compared to control, but glutamine status did not alter this profile (Figure 7B). Together this data reveals that under lipid stress conditions the absence of glutamine results in reduced LC3II protein likely through a combination of increased autophagic degradation together with another post-translational regulatory pathway, perhaps autophagolysosomal exocytosis [22].

To determine whether augmentation of macrophage autophagy under glutamine free conditions was required for the protection against lipid stress, we turned to a model of autophagy deficiency. ATG5 is absolutely required for classical autophagy. Therefore, we utilized macrophages in which

ATG5 had been knocked out using a myeloid specific Cre driver (lysM-Cre). In ATG5 knockout (KO) macrophages we observed that LC3 was predominantly in the non-lipidated form known as LC3I and p62 levels were increased at baseline (Figure 8A). These observations indicate a block at the initiation step of autophagy. Wild type (WT) and ATG5KO macrophages were then activated in the presence or absence of the FA palmitate ± glutamine. As we had shown previously, palm-LPS induced macrophage cell death was not affected by ATG5 deficiency [9]. Importantly, the protection afforded by glutamine deficiency occurred in both WT and ATG5KO macrophages, demonstrating that this rescue phenomenon is independent of autophagy (Figure 8B).

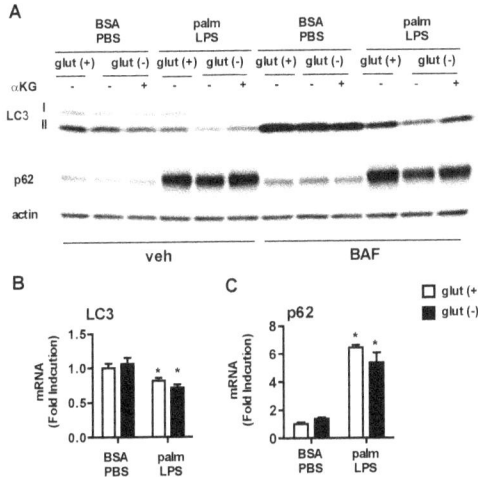

Figure 7. Autophagy is modulated by glutamine deficiency. (**A**) pMACs were treated with BSA-PBS or palm-LPS in glutamine sufficient or glutamine deficient media ± α-KG (440 nM). The cells were incubated for 16 h followed by 2 h of veh or bafilomycin (BAF; 50 nM). Protein lysates were analyzed for expression of LC3 or p62. Actin is shown as a loading control; (**B**) Cells were stimulated as indicated for 16 h in media with or without glutamine followed by qRT-PCR assessment of LC3 and p62 mRNA expression. Bar graphs report the mean ± SE for a minimum of 3 experiments, each performed in triplicate. *, $p < 0.05$ for PBS *vs.* LPS; #, $p < 0.05$ glutamine *vs.* no glutamine.

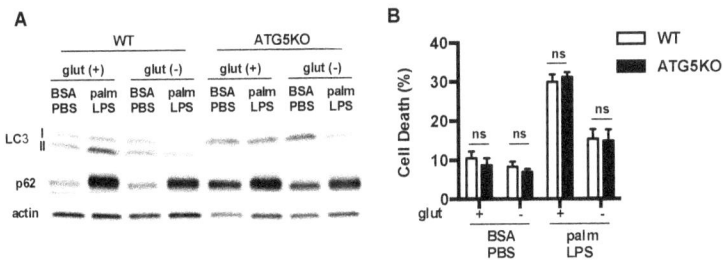

Figure 8. Autophagy is dispensable for protective effects of glutamine deficiency. (**A**) Primary macrophages were isolated from WT (ATG5 flx/flx) or ATG5KO (ATG5 flx/flx-LysM-Cre) followed by stimulation with BSA-PBS or palm-PLS in the presense or absence of glutamine. The levels of LC3 and p62 protein protein expression were assessed by western blotting. Actin is shown as a protein loading control; (**B**) pMACs from WT and ATG5KO mice were stimulated as indicated and cell death was determinded at 30 h using annexin-PI flow cytometry. The bar graph reports the mean ± SE for a minimum of 3 experiments, each performed in triplicate. *, $p < 0.05$ for WT *vs.* ATG5KO.

3.6. Glutamine Deficiency Prevents the Suppression of Mitochondrial Function by Palmitate

Glutamine is a critical substrate for mitochondrial metabolism and TCA function and can directly or indirectly impact mitochondrial metabolism. To investigate the affects of glutamine deficiency on cellular metabolism we employed a Seahorse flux analyzer to measure mitochondrial oxygen consumption rate (OCR) and extracellular acidification rate (ECAR), a marker of glycolytic flux. In response to LPS, macrophage OCR at baseline dramatically increased and this response was suppressed by the presence of palmitate. Maximal OCR, assessed after injection of the uncoupling agent FCCP, was also increased with LPS (Figure 9A). In the absence of glutamine, macrophages had similar baseline OCR under control conditions compared to glutamine sufficient conditions; however, upon activation with LPS the increase in mitochondrial OCR was significantly less than that seen in glutamine sufficient conditions. In addition, palmitate no longer suppressed LPS-induced mitochondrial respiration as it did when glutamine was present. The addition of α-KG to glutamine deficient media yielded only a small increase in LPS-induced OCR, but the suppression of mitochondrial respiration in response to palmitate returned (Figure 9A–D). Glycolytic flux as estimated by ECAR was also reduced in the absence of glutamine, but unlike OCR this response was unaffected by the presence of palmitate. The addition of α-KG to glutamine deficient media led to a very small increase in ECAR (Figure 9E). These results indicate that the toxicity of excess SFA appears to track with mitochondrial respiration dynamics as opposed to changes in ECAR/glycolysis.

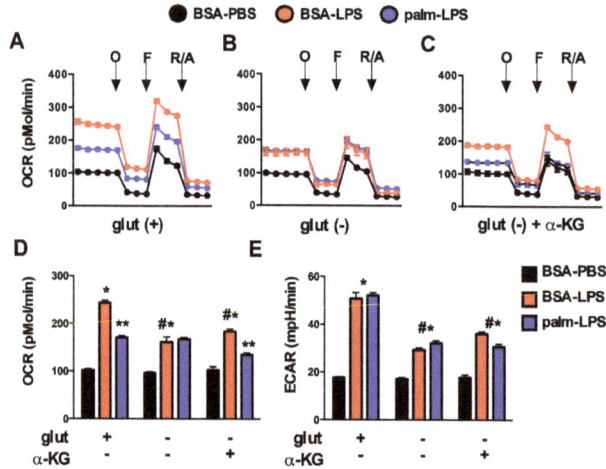

Figure 9. Glutamine deficiency alters mitochondrial metabolism. (**A–C**) pMACs were stimulated for 16 h with BSA-PBS (black), BSA-LPS (red), or palm-LPS (blue) in glutamine sufficient media (**A**) or glutamine deficient media $\pm$ α-KG (**B,C**) and mitochondrial metabolism was assessed using a Seahorse flux analyzer. Mitochondrial oxygen consumption rate (OCR) was assessed at baseline and after the injection of oligomycin (**O**), FCCF (**F**) and rotenone/antamycin (R/A); (**D,E**) Baesline OCR (**D**) or extracellular acidification rate (ECAR; (**E**)) are reported from cells stimulated as in (**A–C**). Bar graphs report the mean $\pm$ SE for a minimum of 3 experiments, each performed in triplicate. *, $p < 0.05$ for BSA-PBS *vs.* BSA-LPS; **, $p < 0.05$ BSA-LPS *vs.* palm-LPS; #, $p < 0.05$ glutamine *vs.* no glutamine.

4. Discussion

It is increasingly being recognized that the nutrient composition present in tissues can influence the phenotypes and inflammatory functions of macrophages [23]. The central finding of this study is that the removal of glutamine from the nutrient microenvironment renders activated macrophages resistant to the toxic effects of dietary SFAs. Consistent with a role for glutaminolysis in this process, the sensitivity to lipid stress is partially restored by the addition of α-KG, an important metabolite of glutamine breakdown. Although mTOR activation and autophagic flux are altered by glutamine deficiency, the mechanism of protection appears to be independent of these pathways. Instead alterations in mitochondrial oxidative metabolism that occur in the absence of glutamine are associated with macrophage sensitivity to cell death. These findings add to a growing body of literature arguing that the interplay between lipid and amino acid metabolism in the mitochondria is relevant to cell dysfunction in metabolic disease [24,25].

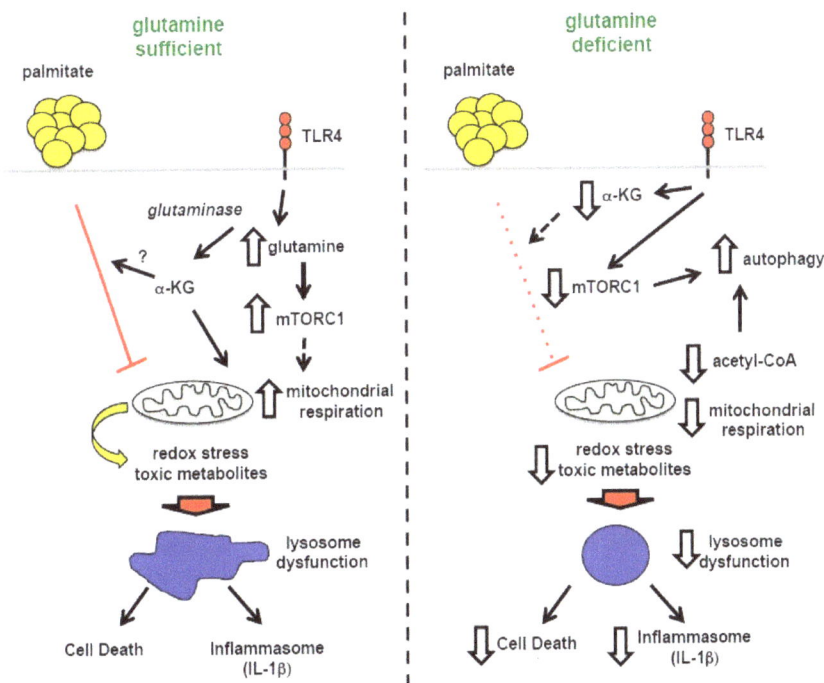

Figure 10. Model of macrophage lipotoxicity under glutamine sufficient and deficient conditions. When glutamine is available, TLR4 activation stimulates glutamine uptake, mTORC1 activation, enhanced formation of TCA intermediates, such as α-KG, and increased mitochondrial respiration. The presence of excess fatty acids like palmitate leads to suppression of mitochondrial respiration, which in the setting of LPS activation likely promotes accumulation of toxic metabolites, lipids and/or redox stress. Lysosome dysfunction ensues leading to macrophage cell death and inflammasome activation. In the absence of glutamine, mTORC1 activation and mitochondrial respiration are diminished leading to enhanced rates of autophagy. In this scenario palmitate no longer suppresses mitochondrial function, which appears to protect against lysosome dysfunction, perhaps by decreasing the formation of damaging metabolites and lipids.

Glutamine is the most abundant amino acid in the body and its uptake and utilization are significantly increased in macrophages following activation signals, such as LPS [15]. Once inside the cell glutamine has several potential fates; however, the best-described metabolic pathway is its break down to glutamate and α-KG by the enzymes glutaminase and glutamate dehydrogenase, respectively. The activity of both of these enzymes is enhanced in LPS-activated macrophages [26]. The α-KG generated by these reactions is critical for TCA cycle anapleurosis, particularly since oxidation of citrate is reduced by LPS activation [27]. However, the majority of glutamine does not undergo complete oxidation and instead is converted to ammonia, aspartate, or pyruvate/lactate [28].

To determine the importance of glutaminolysis in cell death we used two approaches. First, we added back the glutaminolysis product α-KG to cells lacking glutamine and discovered a partial restoration of lipotoxicity. We also inhibited glutaminolysis using two chemically distinct inhibitors of glutaminase. Both of these approaches suggested that glutamine catabolic pathways were partially responsible for the observed effects on lipotoxicity. We also considered that an important non-catabolic function of glutamine might be related to its role in the import of leucine via SLC7A5 [18]. However, cell death was not affected under leucine free conditions arguing that impaired uptake of this branched chain amino acid did not contribute to the protection afforded by glutamine deficiency.

Glutamine directly and indirectly modulates pathways related to the kinase mTOR and autophagy [17,20]. In this study we showed that removal of glutamine from the nutrient microenvironment during LPS activation modestly decreased the activity of mTORC1 as assessed by the phosphorylation status of S6K. This phenotype was specific to mTORC1 as the mTORC2 substrate AKT was unaffected under these conditions. However, the addition of α-KG to glutamine deficient media did not restore mTOR activation, suggesting that suppression of mTORC1 was not the primary mechanism accounting for reduced lipotoxicity. Autophagy is also regulated by glutamine, where glutamine deficiency increases flux through this pathway [29]. Reduced mTORC1 activity is at part of this response; however, decreased levels of other metabolites, such as cytosolic acetyl-CoA, may also play a role in increasing autophagy [17,30]. In other systems autophagy has been shown to protect against cell death related to accumulation of damaged organelles and proteins [31,32]. We show that in macrophages the absence of glutamine did not change autophagic flux at baseline; however, after LPS activation autophagy rates were increased in glutamine deficient macrophages. However, genetic disruption of autophagy using ATG5KO macrophages did not reverse the protection afforded by lack of glutamine. Thus, although mTORC1 activity is reduced and autophagy is enhanced in a glutamine-free nutrient microenvironment, the protection from lipotoxicity occurs independent of these events.

As discussed above, glutamine is an important contributor to mitochondrial metabolism in part through the replenishment of TCA cycle intermediates. Using functional metabolism studies we discovered an interesting mitochondrial phenotype in LPS activated cells lacking glutamine. As expected, the increase in mitochondrial OCR induced by LPS activation was substantially attenuated in the absence of glutamine. Interestingly, addition of α-KG to glutamine deficient media did not reverse this OCR phenotype indicating that the mitochondrial reprograming is more than just a loss of TCA cycle flux. The most striking difference was that the suppressive effect of palmitate on LPS-induced OCR was reversed in glutamine free media and partially restored with addition of α-KG. Although glycolytic flux, as estimated by ECAR, was also suppressed by ~50% in glutamine deficient media neither palmitate nor α-KG significantly changed this phenotype.

It is now appreciated that obesity and diabetes impose a multifaceted nutrient stress on the mitochondria. Specifically, the excess delivery of an uptake of FAs and amino acid metabolites to the mitochondria can produce metabolic gridlock, especially when energy stores are replete [16]. In this context, a "back pressure" develops on the mitochondrial electron transport chain due to lower activity of ATP synthase. The consequence of this backlog can be the generation of reactive oxygen species and/or accumulation of other metabolites, which have the potential to damage proteins and organelles. Our data suggest that glutamine deficiency reduces the mitochondrial substrate burden, which may be protective against cell damage in the setting of lipid overload. As we have previously shown that scavenging of ROS does not reduce lysosome damage or cell death in our system, we expect other pathways connecting mitochondrial metabolites (acetyl-CoA, acylcarnitines, etc.) with lysosome damage exist [9] (Figure 10). This is an area of active exploration.

Our findings may be relevant to several physiologic situations in obese and diabetic hosts. In the context of acute infection or tissue injury glutamine is released from skeletal muscle and its uptake by macrophages is enhanced [33]. When excess lipids are present, as in diabetes, macrophage inflammasome activation and cell death are anticipated to increase, contributing to the persistent inflammatory response seen in diabetics. The potential relevance of this pathway is supported by recent data revealing that the inflammasome is a major contributor to diabetic inflammation *in vivo*, including in humans [34–36]. In addition to acute inflammation, diabetes is associated with a chronic inflammatory response [37]. Macrophages are recruited to adipose tissue during obesity and are thought to contribute to the development of systemic insulin resistance [38,39]. It is well established that macrophages accumulate lipid in obese adipose tissue suggesting that interaction between FAs and glutamine metabolism would be of interest to explore in this situation [40]. Such studies could be performed using macrophage specific knockout of glutamine transporters. Further investigation into the role of glutamine in other inflammatory conditions that often co-exist with diabetes such as vascular and rheumatologic disease could also be of interest.

There are several limitations of the current study that must be acknowledged. In order to perturb the nutrient microenvironment, we used an *in vitro* system with thioglycollate-elicited peritoneal cells as a model of monocyte-derived macrophages. Therefore, *in vivo* approaches will be necessary to determine the relevance of these findings to diabetic inflammation. Moreover, the studies were performed with murine macrophages and therefore additional studies with human monocyte-derived macrophages are warranted. It is also important to acknowledge that glutamine uptake by immune cells is important for full activation and therefore deprivation of this nutrient could lead to increased risk of infection [26]. The relative balance of risk and benefit in diabetic patients will require further investigation.

Macrophage dysfunction is a hallmark of lipid overload disorders such as obesity and diabetes. In response to excess dietary saturated FAs activated macrophages develop lysosome damage, inflammasome activation, and cell death and these events appear to be involved in clinical complications of these metabolic conditions [3,36,41–43]. However, the mechanisms that lead to these phenotypes are not well understood. Herein we describe an intriguing example whereby TLR4-induced metabolic reprogramming of glutamine metabolism can be maladaptive in the setting of lipid overload. These findings suggest that nutritional or pharmacologic interventions could potentially be used to modulate macrophage function for therapeutic benefit in metabolic disease.

Acknowledgments: We thank Skip Virgin for the generous provision of ATG5KO mice. This work was funded in part by NIH DRC P30 DK020579 (JDS).

Author Contributions: Li He conducted experiments; Kassandra J. Weber conducted experiments; Joel D. Schilling conceived experiments, interpreted experiments and wrote the manuscript.

Conflicts of Interest: The authors declare no conflict of interest.

References

1. Mirza, R.; Koh, T.J. Dysregulation of monocyte/macrophage phenotype in wounds of diabetic mice. *Cytokine* **2011**, *56*, 256–264. [CrossRef] [PubMed]
2. Aronson, D.; Rayfield, E.J.; Chesebro, J.H. Mechanisms determining course and outcome of diabetic patients who have had acute myocardial infarction. *Ann. Intern. Med.* **1997**, *126*, 296–306. [CrossRef] [PubMed]
3. Khanna, S.; Biswas, S.; Shang, Y.; Collard, E.; Azad, A.; Kauh, C.; Bhasker, V.; Gordillo, G.M.; Sen, C.K.; Roy, S. Macrophage dysfunction impairs resolution of inflammation in the wounds of diabetic mice. *PLoS ONE* **2010**, *5*, e9539. [CrossRef] [PubMed]
4. Wetzler, C.; Kampfer, H.; Stallmeyer, B.; Pfeilschifter, J.; Frank, S. Large and sustained induction of chemokines during impaired wound healing in the genetically diabetic mouse: Prolonged persistence of neutrophils and macrophages during the late phase of repair. *J. Investig. Dermatol.* **2000**, *115*, 245–253. [CrossRef] [PubMed]
5. Hallgren, B.; Stenhagen, S.; Svanborg, A.; Svennerholm, L. Gas chromatographic analysis of the fatty acid composition of the plasma lipids in normal and diabetic subjects. *J. Clin. Investig.* **1960**, *39*, 1424–1434. [CrossRef] [PubMed]
6. Schaffer, J.E. Lipotoxicity: When tissues overeat. *Curr. Opin. Lipidol.* **2003**, *14*, 281–287. [CrossRef] [PubMed]

7. Kaczorowski, D.J.; Tsung, A.; Billiar, T.R. Innate immune mechanisms in ischemia/reperfusion. *Front. Biosci. (Elite Ed.)* **2009**, *1*, 91–98. [PubMed]

8. Takeda, K.; Akira, S. Tlr signaling pathways. *Semin. Immunol.* **2004**, *16*, 3–9. [CrossRef] [PubMed]

9. Schilling, J.D.; Machkovech, H.M.; He, L.; Diwan, A.; Schaffer, J.E. Tlr4 activation under lipotoxic conditions leads to synergistic macrophage cell death through a trif-dependent pathway. *J. Immunol.* **2013**, *190*, 1285–1296. [CrossRef] [PubMed]

10. Schilling, J.D.; Machkovech, H.M.; He, L.; Sidhu, R.; Fujiwara, H.; Weber, K.; Ory, D.S.; Schaffer, J.E. Palmitate and lipopolysaccharide trigger synergistic ceramide production in primary macrophages. *J. Biol. Chem.* **2013**, *288*, 2923–2932. [CrossRef] [PubMed]

11. Weber, K.J.; Schilling, J.D. Lysosomes integrate metabolic-inflammatory crosstalk in primary macrophage inflammasome activation. *J. Biol. Chem.* **2014**, *289*, 9158–9171. [CrossRef] [PubMed]

12. Loftus, R.M.; Finlay, D.K. Immunometabolism: Cellular metabolism turns immune regulator. *J. Biol. Chem.* **2016**, *291*, 1–10. [CrossRef] [PubMed]

13. Liu, T.F.; Vachharajani, V.T.; Yoza, B.K.; McCall, C.E. Nad+-dependent sirtuin 1 and 6 proteins coordinate a switch from glucose to fatty acid oxidation during the acute inflammatory response. *J. Biol. Chem.* **2012**, *287*, 25758–25769. [CrossRef] [PubMed]

14. Rodriguez-Prados, J.C.; Traves, P.G.; Cuenca, J.; Rico, D.; Aragones, J.; Martin-Sanz, P.; Cascante, M.; Bosca, L. Substrate fate in activated macrophages: A comparison between innate, classic, and alternative activation. *J. Immunol.* **2010**, *185*, 605–614. [CrossRef] [PubMed]

15. Newsholme, P.; Curi, R.; Pithon Curi, T.C.; Murphy, C.J.; Garcia, C.; Pires de Melo, M. Glutamine metabolism by lymphocytes, macrophages, and neutrophils: Its importance in health and disease. *J. Nutr. Biochem.* **1999**, *10*, 316–324. [CrossRef]

16. Muoio, D.M. Metabolic inflexibility: When mitochondrial indecision leads to metabolic gridlock. *Cell* **2014**, *159*, 1253–1262. [CrossRef] [PubMed]

17. Jewell, J.L.; Kim, Y.C.; Russell, R.C.; Yu, F.X.; Park, H.W.; Plouffe, S.W.; Tagliabracci, V.S.; Guan, K.L. Metabolism. Differential regulation of mtorc1 by leucine and glutamine. *Science* **2015**, *347*, 194–198. [CrossRef] [PubMed]

18. Meier, C.; Ristic, Z.; Klauser, S.; Verrey, F. Activation of system l heterodimeric amino acid exchangers by intracellular substrates. *EMBO J.* **2002**, *21*, 580–589. [CrossRef] [PubMed]

19. Meijer, A.J.; Lorin, S.; Blommaart, E.F.; Codogno, P. Regulation of autophagy by amino acids and mtor-dependent signal transduction. *Amino Acids* **2015**, *47*, 2037–2063. [CrossRef] [PubMed]

20. Nicklin, P.; Bergman, P.; Zhang, B.; Triantafellow, E.; Wang, H.; Nyfeler, B.; Yang, H.; Hild, M.; Kung, C.; Wilson, C.; et al. Bidirectional transport of amino acids regulates mtor and autophagy. *Cell* **2009**, *136*, 521–534. [CrossRef] [PubMed]

21. Laplante, M.; Sabatini, D.M. Mtor signaling in growth control and disease. *Cell* **2012**, *149*, 274–293. [CrossRef] [PubMed]

22. Takenouchi, T.; Nakai, M.; Iwamaru, Y.; Sugama, S.; Tsukimoto, M.; Fujita, M.; Wei, J.; Sekigawa, A.; Sato, M.; Kojima, S.; et al. The activation of p2x7 receptor impairs lysosomal functions and stimulates the release of autophagolysosomes in microglial cells. *J. Immunol.* **2009**, *182*, 2051–2062. [CrossRef] [PubMed]

23. El Kasmi, K.C.; Stenmark, K.R. Contribution of metabolic reprogramming to macrophage plasticity and function. *Semin. Immunol.* **2015**, *27*, 267–275. [CrossRef] [PubMed]

24. Huffman, K.M.; Shah, S.H.; Stevens, R.D.; Bain, J.R.; Muehlbauer, M.; Slentz, C.A.; Tanner, C.J.; Kuchibhatla, M.; Houmard, J.A.; Newgard, C.B.; et al. Relationships between circulating metabolic intermediates and insulin action in overweight to obese, inactive men and women. *Diabetes Care* **2009**, *32*, 1678–1683. [CrossRef] [PubMed]

25. Bhattacharya, S.; Granger, C.B.; Craig, D.; Haynes, C.; Bain, J.; Stevens, R.D.; Hauser, E.R.; Newgard, C.B.; Kraus, W.E.; Newby, L.K.; et al. Validation of the association between a branched chain amino acid metabolite profile and extremes of coronary artery disease in patients referred for cardiac catheterization. *Atherosclerosis* **2014**, *232*, 191–196. [CrossRef] [PubMed]

26. Murphy, C.; Newsholme, P. Importance of glutamine metabolism in murine macrophages and human monocytes to l-arginine biosynthesis and rates of nitrite or urea production. *Clin. Sci.* **1998**, *95*, 397–407. [CrossRef] [PubMed]

27. Jha, A.K.; Huang, S.C.; Sergushichev, A.; Lampropoulou, V.; Ivanova, Y.; Loginicheva, E.; Chmielewski, K.; Stewart, K.M.; Ashall, J.; Everts, B.; *et al.* Network integration of parallel metabolic and transcriptional data reveals metabolic modules that regulate macrophage polarization. *Immunity* **2015**, *42*, 419–430. [CrossRef] [PubMed]

28. Newsholme, P.; Newsholme, E.A. Rates of utilization of glucose, glutamine and oleate and formation of end-products by mouse peritoneal macrophages in culture. *Biochem. J.* **1989**, *261*, 211–218. [CrossRef] [PubMed]

29. van der Vos, K.E.; Eliasson, P.; Proikas-Cezanne, T.; Vervoort, S.J.; van Boxtel, R.; Putker, M.; van Zutphen, I.J.; Mauthe, M.; Zellmer, S.; Pals, C.; *et al.* Modulation of glutamine metabolism by the pi(3)k-pkb-foxo network regulates autophagy. *Nat. Cell Biol.* **2012**, *14*, 829–837. [CrossRef] [PubMed]

30. Eisenberg, T.; Schroeder, S.; Andryushkova, A.; Pendl, T.; Kuttner, V.; Bhukel, A.; Marino, G.; Pietrocola, F.; Harger, A.; Zimmermann, A.; *et al.* Nucleocytosolic depletion of the energy metabolite acetyl-coenzyme a stimulates autophagy and prolongs lifespan. *Cell Metab.* **2014**, *19*, 431–444. [CrossRef] [PubMed]

31. Mizushima, N.; Levine, B.; Cuervo, A.M.; Klionsky, D.J. Autophagy fights disease through cellular self-digestion. *Nature* **2008**, *451*, 1069–1075. [CrossRef] [PubMed]

32. Choi, A.M.; Ryter, S.W.; Levine, B. Autophagy in human health and disease. *N. Engl. J. Med.* **2013**, *368*, 651–662. [CrossRef] [PubMed]

33. Karinch, A.M.; Pan, M.; Lin, C.M.; Strange, R.; Souba, W.W. Glutamine metabolism in sepsis and infection. *J. Nutr.* **2001**, *131*, 2535S–2538S. [PubMed]

34. Lee, H.M.; Kim, J.J.; Kim, H.J.; Shong, M.; Ku, B.J.; Jo, E.K. Upregulated nlrp3 inflammasome activation in patients with type 2 diabetes. *Diabetes* **2013**, *62*, 194–204. [CrossRef] [PubMed]

35. Luo, B.; Li, B.; Wang, W.; Liu, X.; Xia, Y.; Zhang, C.; Zhang, M.; Zhang, Y.; An, F. Nlrp3 gene silencing ameliorates diabetic cardiomyopathy in a type 2 diabetes rat model. *PLoS ONE* **2014**, *9*, e104771. [CrossRef] [PubMed]

36. Mirza, R.E.; Fang, M.M.; Ennis, W.J.; Koh, T.J. Blocking il-1beta induces a healing-associated wound macrophage phenotype and improves healing in type-2 diabetes. *Diabetes* **2013**, *62*, 2579–2587. [CrossRef] [PubMed]

37. Hotamisligil, G.S.; Erbay, E. Nutrient sensing and inflammation in metabolic diseases. *Nat. Rev. Immunol.* **2008**, *8*, 923–934. [CrossRef] [PubMed]

38. Weisberg, S.P.; McCann, D.; Desai, M.; Rosenbaum, M.; Leibel, R.L.; Ferrante, A.W., Jr. Obesity is associated with macrophage accumulation in adipose tissue. *J. Clin. Investig.* **2003**, *112*, 1796–1808. [CrossRef] [PubMed]

39. Weisberg, S.P.; Hunter, D.; Huber, R.; Lemieux, J.; Slaymaker, S.; Vaddi, K.; Charo, I.; Leibel, R.L.; Ferrante, A.W., Jr. Ccr2 modulates inflammatory and metabolic effects of high-fat feeding. *J. Clin. Investig.* **2006**, *116*, 115–124. [CrossRef] [PubMed]

40. Xu, X.; Grijalva, A.; Skowronski, A.; van Eijk, M.; Serlie, M.J.; Ferrante, A.W., Jr. Obesity activates a program of lysosomal-dependent lipid metabolism in adipose tissue macrophages independently of classic activation. *Cell Metab.* **2013**, *18*, 816–830. [CrossRef] [PubMed]

41. Thakker, G.D.; Frangogiannis, N.G.; Bujak, M.; Zymek, P.; Gaubatz, J.W.; Reddy, A.K.; Taffet, G.; Michael, L.H.; Entman, M.L.; Ballantyne, C.M. Effects of diet-induced obesity on inflammation and remodeling after myocardial infarction. *Am. J. Physiol. Heart Circ. Physiol.* **2006**, *291*, H2504–H2514. [CrossRef] [PubMed]

42. Greer, J.J.; Ware, D.P.; Lefer, D.J. Myocardial infarction and heart failure in the db/db diabetic mouse. *Am. J. Physiol. Heart Circ. Physiol.* **2006**, *290*, H146–H153. [CrossRef] [PubMed]

43. Mirza, R.E.; Fang, M.M.; Novak, M.L.; Urao, N.; Sui, A.; Ennis, W.J.; Koh, T.J. Macrophage ppargamma and impaired wound healing in type 2 diabetes. *J. Pathol.* **2015**, *236*, 433–444. [CrossRef] [PubMed]

![nutrients logo]
nutrients

MDPI

Article

High Risk of Metabolic and Adipose Tissue Dysfunctions in Adult Male Progeny, Due to Prenatal and Adulthood Malnutrition Induced by Fructose Rich Diet

Ana Alzamendi [1], Guillermina Zubiría [1], Griselda Moreno [2], Andrea Portales [1], Eduardo Spinedi [3] and Andrés Giovambattista [1,*]

[1] IMBICE (CICPBA-CONICET La Plata-National University of La Plata (UNLP)), La Plata 1900, Argentina; aalzamendi@imbice.gov.ar (A.A.); gzubiria@imbice.gov.ar (G.Z.); andreaeportales@gmail.com (A.P.)
[2] IIFP (CONICET La Plata) School of Exact Sciences, National University of La Plata (UNLP), La Plata1900, Argentina; gmoreno@iifp.laplata-conicet.gov.ar
[3] CENEXA (CONICET La Plata-UNLP, a PAHO/WHO (Collaborating Centre for Diabetes)), School of Medicine, National University of La Plata (UNLP), La Plata1900, Argentina; spinedi@cenexa.org
* Correspondence: agiovamba@imbice.gov.ar; Tel.: +54-221-421-0112

Received: 29 December 2015; Accepted: 14 March 2016; Published: 22 March 2016

Abstract: The aim of this work was to determine the effect of a fructose rich diet (FRD) consumed by the pregnant mother on the endocrine-metabolic and *in vivo* and *in vitro* adipose tissue (AT) functions of the male offspring in adulthood. At 60 days of age, rats born to FRD-fed mothers (F) showed impaired glucose tolerance after glucose overload and high circulating levels of leptin (LEP). Despite the diminished mass of retroperitoneal AT, this tissue was characterized by enhanced LEP gene expression, and hypertrophic adipocytes secreting *in vitro* larger amounts of LEP. Analyses of stromal vascular fraction composition by flow cytometry revealed a reduced number of adipocyte precursor cells. Additionally, 60 day-old control (C) and F male rats were subjected to control diet (CC and FC animals) or FRD (CF and FF rats) for three weeks. FF animals were heavier and consumed more calories. Their metabolic-endocrine parameters were aggravated; they developed severe hyperglycemia, hypertriglyceridemia, hyperleptinemia and augmented AT mass with hypertrophic adipocytes. Our study highlights that manipulation of maternal diet induced an offspring phenotype mainly imprinted with a severely unhealthy adipogenic process with undesirable endocrine-metabolic consequences, putting them at high risk for developing a diabetic state.

Keywords: metabolic programming; adipocyte precursor cells; dysfunctional adipose tissue; altered glucose tolerance; insulin resistance; pre-diabetes; metabolic syndrome

1. Introduction

Metabolic Syndrome (MS), obesity and type 2 diabetes have drastically increased to epidemic levels worldwide in the last few decades. The World Health Organization has defined obesity as an increment in adipose tissue (AT) mass which may or may not be detrimental to health [1]. These illnesses have been attributed mainly to changes in lifestyle, including dietary habits. Fructose rich diet (FRD) consumption has been shown to be associated with insulin resistance [2], hyperadiposity, hypertriglyceridemia, hyperleptinemia [3], hyperglycemia, hyperinsulinemia, impaired glucose tolerance [4] and hepatic steatosis [5], in both animal models and humans.

Diseases in adulthood may originate during an individual's development, due to changes in the environment in which the individual is subjected to [6]. Factors that may alter the environment can include maternal nutrition, either during gestation and lactation [7,8]. Several studies highlighted the undesirable consequences of maternal unbalanced diet intake during gestation and/or lactation for the offspring's health in adult life [9,10]. Different works have focused on the effects of feeding mothers a FRD during gestation and lactation, showing that their offspring displayed an increased risk of developing obesity in adult life [11,12]. We previously reported deleterious metabolic-endocrine function of pups born to FRD-fed lactating mothers [13]. These pups developed changes in the hypothalamic circuitry controlling appetite, impaired peripheral insulin sensitivity, and both hyperleptinemia and visceral adipocyte hypertrophy [13].

Carbohydrates are major metabolites involved in fetal growth and metabolism, and it is accepted that fructose is present in fetal circulation [14]. The intake of refined sugar, particularly high-fructose corn syrup, has increased in the United States from a yearly estimate of 8.1 kg/individual at the beginning of the 19th century up to 65 kg/person in 2010 [15]. However, limited data exist on the consequences of FRD intake through the mother for the offspring's metabolic programming [16,17]. Indeed, most of the international literature showed studies wherein experimental designs were devoted to mothers consuming FRD throughout gestation and lactation or only while lactating [11,18–20].

It was reported recently that adult male offspring born to FRD-fed dams throughout gestation developed insulin resistance, dyslipidemia, a distorted pattern of peripheral adipokines and enhanced oxidative stress [21]. Interestingly, later in life, the offspring normalized leptinemia, but became hypoadiponectinemic [22]. Conversely, a recent study showed that FRD intake by gestating mothers resulted in pronounced maternal dysfunctions but no major undesirable metabolic effects on offspring, even after following their progress up to 6 months of age [23].

The current study was designed to test whether or not the feeding of mothers with a FRD throughout gestation modifies endocrine-metabolic biomarkers and *in vivo* and *in vitro* AT functions in adult male progeny. Moreover, we aimed to determine *in utero* fructose exposure impact on adult rats challenged or not with a FRD during adult lifetime.

2. Materials and Methods

2.1. Animals and Experimental Designs

Sprague-Dawley (S-D) rats were kept in controlled conditions of temperature (21 ± 2 °C) and lights (on between 07:00 a.m. and 7:00 p.m. with free access to standard commercial rat chow (Ganave Lab., Argentina) and tap water. Virgin females (3 per cage) were mated with a male in plastic cages until positive detection of sperm in their vaginal smears (daily examined at 08:00 a.m.). Sperm positive dams were then individually housed and provided with standard chow *ad libitum* and allocated into two groups: (a) drinking tap water only (control mothers, CM; $n = 19$); and (b) drinking a FRD (fructose 10% w/v in tap water, fructose mothers, FM; $n = 20$) throughout pregnancy [24]. Fresh fructose solution was provided every 2 days. Body weight (BW), food and fluid intakes were recorded daily during pregnancy. Immediately after delivery, and as previously validated by our laboratory [13], litter-size was adjusted to eight pups per dam (average male pups per litter ranged between 60% and 65%, approximately). Lactating mothers were provided with standard chow and water *ad libitum*. Weaned (21 days old) male pups (born to CM and FM, assigned as C and F rats, respectively) were individually housed and fed standard purina chow diet and tap water *ad libitum* until experimentation. These groups of male rats (C and F) were made by including one male rat from each litter (see Figure 1). Rats were euthanized following protocols in the National Institute of Health Guidelines for care and use of experimental animals. All experiments also received approval from our Institutional Committee on Animal Experimentation.

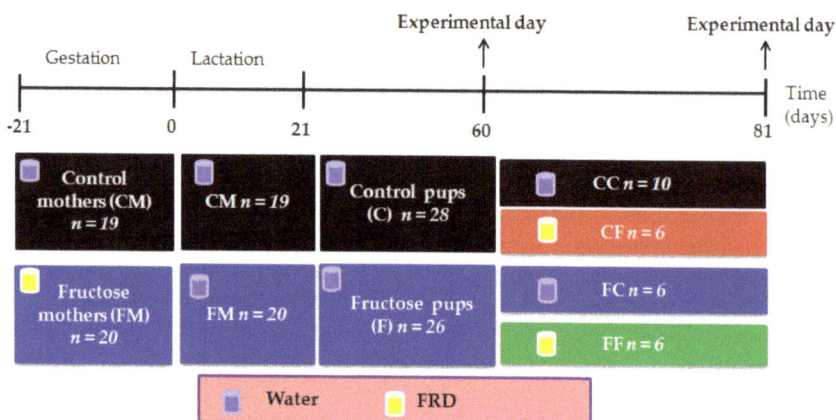

Figure 1. Experimental design. Sperm positive dams fed standard chow *ad libitum* were allocated in two groups: drinking water (control mothers, CM, *n* = 19) and drinking FRD (fructose mothers, FM, *n* = 20). This diet was maintained until delivery. During lactation, both mothers groups were fed standard chow *ad libitum* and drink tap water. The weaning day, male pups born to CM and FM, assigned as C and F rats, respectively, were fed standard purina chow diet and tap water *ad libitum*. At 60 days of age, 6 C and 7 F males were killed for basal determinations and AT studies. Others 6 C and 7 F rats were subjected to an i.v. GTT at 60 day-old. The remaining 16 C rats were divided in two sub-groups; 10 animals receive water (CC) and 6 receive FRD (CF). The remaining 12 F animals, they also were subdivided into two sub-groups; 6 animals receive water (FC) and 6 receive FRD (FF) from day 60 until 81 days of age. Groups were made by including one male rat from each litter, so as not to include pups from the same litter in the same experiment.

2.1.1. Sixty-Day-Old Rats

Six C and seven F rats were killed (08:00–09:00 a.m.) by decapitation in non-fasting conditions and trunk blood was collected into plastic tubes containing EDTA (10% w/v, in normal saline solution). Plasma samples were then stored frozen ($-20\ ^\circ$C) until determination of several metabolites. Immediately after euthanization, retroperitoneal adipose tissue (RPAT) pads were dissected and weighed. RPAT was used for histological, gene expression, stromal vascular fraction (SVF) cell composition and adipocyte functional studies (see below). Additionally, six C and seven F rats were subjected to an intravenous glucose tolerance test (i.v. GTT) (Figure 1).

2.1.2. Eighty-One Day-Old Rats

Sixteen C and 12 F 60-day-old male rats were allocated to four sub-groups according to the drinking solution provided, either tap water only CC (*n* = 10) and FC (*n* = 6) groups; or FRD CF (*n* = 6) and FF (*n* = 6) groups (Figure 1). All groups were fed standard purina chow *ad libitum* and treatments lasted for three weeks. Rat BW and food and fluid intakes were recorded daily. Rats were killed by decapitation (08:00 a.m.) in non-fasting conditions. Trunk blood was collected and plasma samples kept frozen ($-20\ ^\circ$C) until measurement of different metabolites. Additionally, RPAT pads were dissected, weighed, and used for histological studies.

2.2. RPAT Adipocyte Isolation and Incubation

Isolated adipocytes from RPAT pads were obtained as previously described [25]. Cells were diluted to a density of approximately 200,000 cells per 900 µL of DMEM-1% BSA medium and distributed into 5 mL plastic tubes. Substances tested (diluted in 100 µL) were either medium alone (basal) or contained insulin (INS) (final concentrations: 0.1, 1 or 10 nM; Novo Nordisk Pharma AG,

Switzerland) [26]. Adipocytes were then incubated for 45 min at 37 °C in a 95% air-5% CO_2 atmosphere. At the end of incubation, media were carefully aspirated and kept frozen (-20 °C) until measurement of LEP concentrations as described below.

2.3. RPAT Pad Histology

For histological studies, freshly dissected RPAT pads were fixed in 4% paraformaldehyde, then washed with tap water, immersed in a series of graded ethanol (70%, 96% and 100%), and clarified in xylene before being embedded in paraffin [13]. Four-micrometer sections were taken from different levels of the blocks and stained with hematoxylin-eosin. Quantitative morphometric analysis was performed using a RGB CCD Sony camera together with Image Pro-Plus 4.0 software (magnification, ×400). For each tissue sample, seven sections and three levels were selected ($n = 4$ animals per group). Systematic random sampling was used to select 15 fields for each section, and 2500 cells per group were examined. Adipocyte diameter was measured [24] and cell volume was later calculated ($4/3\pi r^3$).

2.4. RNA Isolation and Real-Time Quantitative PCR

Total RNA was isolated from RPAT pads by the single-step acid guanidinium isothiocyanate-phenol-chloroform extraction method (TRIzol; Invitrogen, LifeTech.). One µg of total RNA was reverse-transcribed using random primers (0.2 µg/µL) and RevertAid Reverse Transcriptase (200 U/µL Thermo Scientific). Primers applied were β-actin (ACTB; sense, 5′-GGTCCACACCCGCCACCAG-3′ and anti-sense, 5′-GGGCCTCGTCGCCCACGTA-3′; 200 bp; Gene Code: NM_031144.3), ADIPOQ (sense, 5′-AATCCTGCCCAGTCATGAAG-3′ and anti-sense, 5′-TCTCCAGGAGTGCCATCTCT-3′; 159 bp; Gene Code: NM_144744.3) and LEP (sense, 5′-GAGACCTCCTCCATCTGCTG-3′ and anti-sense, 5′-CTCAGCATTCAGGGCTAAGG-3′; 192 bp; Gene Code: NM_013076.3). One microliter of the RT mix was amplified with Hot FIREPol EvaGreen qPCR Mix Plus (Solis BioDyne) containing 0.5 µM of each specific primer and using the Light Cycler Detection System (MJMini Opticon, Bio-Rad). PCR efficiency was near 1. Threshold cycles (Ct) were measured in separate tubes by duplicate. Identity and purity of the amplified product were checked by electrophoresis on agarose mini-gels, and the melting curve was analyzed at the end of amplification. Relative changes in the expression levels of one specific gene were calculated by ΔCt analysis [13].

2.5. SVF Cell Composition Analysis by Flow Cytometry (FACS)

SVF cells from RPAT pads of C and F animals were isolated and at least 2×10^5 cells (in 100 µL PBS/0.5% BSA) incubated with fluorescent antibodies or respective isotype controls for 1 h at 4 °C. After washing steps, flow cytometry was analyzed using a FACS Calibur flow cytometer (Becton Dickinson Biosciences). A combination of surface cell markers were used to identify adipocyte precursor cells (APCs) as: $CD34^+/CD45^-/CD31^-$ [27]. Conjugated monoclonal antibodies used were: anti-rat CD34:PE (Santa Cruz Biotechnology Inc., Santa Cruz, CA, USA), anti-rat CD45:FITC (Santa Cruz Biotechnology Inc., Santa Cruz, CA, USA) and anti-rat CD31:FITC (Santa Cruz Biotechnology Inc., Santa Cruz, CA, USA). Samples were analyzed using CellQuest Pro (Becton-Dickinson, San Jose, CA, USA) and FlowJo softwares (TreeStar, San Carlo, CA, USA) [27].

2.6. Intravenous Glucose Tolerance Test (i.v. GTT)

This test has been widely validated in our laboratory [13]. Briefly, 60 day-old C and F rats ($n = 6$ C and $n = 7$ F rats) were subjected to an i.v. GTT. Rats were implanted (under light ketamine anesthesia) with an i.v. cannula (in the right jugular vein 48 h before experimentation) kept patent by administering heparin (10 U/mL in sterile saline solution: 100 µL). On the morning of the experimental day (08:00–09:00 a.m.) a small volume of blood was taken in non-fasting condition before (time 0) and 5, 15, 30, 60, and 90 min after i.v. glucose (GLU) (2 g/kg BW; dissolved in sterile saline solution) administration [28]; the blood withdrawn was immediately replaced by a similar volume of sterile artificial plasma. Plasma samples were kept frozen (-20 °C) until determination of GLU and INS concentrations. The area under the curve (AUC) was calculated with GraphPad Prism software using basal (time 0) plasma GLU and INS as baseline.

2.7. Peripheral Metabolite Measurements

Circulating levels of GLU, triglycerides (TG) and total cholesterol (TC) were measured by commercial kits (Wiener Lab., Rosario, Argentina). Plasma and medium LEP concentrations [25] and circulating levels of INS [26] and corticosterone (CORT) [29] were determined by specific radioimmunoassays (RIAs) previously validated. LEP (standard curve 0.05–25 ng/mL) coefficients of variation (CV) intra- and inter-assay were 4%–7% and 9%–11%, respectively. INS (standard curve 0.08–10 ng/mL) CV intra- and inter-assay were 3%–7% and 8%–11%, respectively. CORT (standard curve 0.05–50 μg/dL) CV intra- and inter-assay were 4%–6% and 8%–10%, respectively. Plasma levels of adiponectin (ADIPOQ) were measured by commercial ELISA kit following manufacturer's instructions (Linco Research, Cat. #EZRADP-62 K, standard curve: 3–100 ng/mL CV intra- and inter-assay were 0.43%–1.96% and 4.3%–8.44%, respectively).

2.8. Statistical Analysis

Results (expressed as means $\pm$ SEM) were analyzed by Student t-test when appropriate. One way ANOVA followed by post hoc comparisons of mean values with the Newman Keuls test, was used to compare different groups. ANOVA with repeated measures was used for analyses of i.v. GTT values. Two-way ANOVA followed by Tukey's multiple comparison test was used for analyses of the effect of INS on LEP release by adipocytes; and for analyses of male caloric intake from weaning until 60 day-old. The non-parametric Mann-Whitney test was employed to analyze data on tissue mRNA expression [13]. All data was analyzed using the software GraphPad Prism 6.0 on Windows (GraphPad Software Inc., San Diego, CA, USA). P values lower than 0.05 were considered statistically significant.

3. Results

3.1. Pregnant Rats' Body Weight and Food-Provided Energy Intake

The individual BW of pregnant rats were similar in both groups at the beginning (CM: 249.37 $\pm$ 9.83 g, and FM: 244.28 $\pm$ 6.16 g; $n = 19$ CM and $n = 20$ FM) and at the end (CM: 366.86 $\pm$ 19.04 g, and FM: 366.87 $\pm$ 10.11 g; $n = 19$ CM and $n = 20$ FM) of the gestational period. The 21-day average of individual daily energy intake through diet was significantly higher in FM than in CM (84.71 $\pm$ 3.41 *vs.* 68.17 $\pm$ 5.07 kCal/day/100 g BW, respectively; $p < 0.05$, $n = 19$ CM and $n = 20$ FM).

3.2. Body Weight and Caloric Intake in Adult Male Offspring Born to CM and FM

The first male offspring born to CM and FM mothers ($n = 12$ and $n = 14$ rats in group C and F, respectively) displayed similar BW between birth and 60 days of age (Figure 2A). No group-difference was observed in 48 h-caloric intake corrected per 100g of BW (Figure 2B). Nevertheless, when a two-way ANOVA analyses was performed, we observed that caloric intake is both influenced by time and FRD intake during gestation was ($p < 0.05$). Even the interaction between these two factors was statistically different ($p < 0.05$).

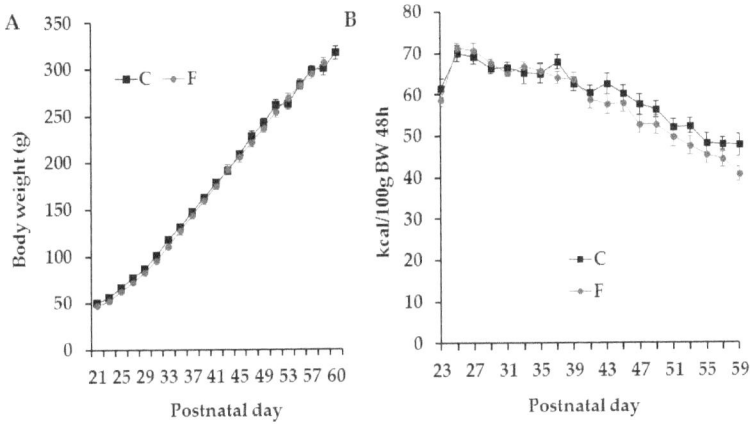

Figure 2. Body weight and caloric intake. (**A**) Body weight and (**B**) mean 48 h cumulative caloric intake corrected by 100 g of BW, between weaning and 60 days of age, in C and F rats. Values are means ± SEM (*n* = 12 and *n* = 14 rats in group C and F, respectively). FRD during gestation, time, and the interaction between them are considered significantly different between C and F rats, based on two-way ANOVA.

3.3. Peripheral Levels of Several Metabolites and i.v. GTT in Adult Male Offspring

In non-fasting conditions, adult (60 day-old; *n* = 6 C rats and *n* = 7 F rats per group) F rats displayed significantly ($p < 0.05$) higher circulating levels of LEP and lower levels of TG (Table 1). Circulating concentrations of GLU, TC, CORT, INS and ADIPOQ remained the same (Table 1).

Table 1. Metabolic markers in 60 day-old rats.

	C	F
GLU (mmol/L)	6.58 ± 0.18	6.08 ± 0.24
TG (mmol/L)	1.44 ± 0.14	1.12 ± 0.06 *
TC (mmol/L)	1.56 ± 0.07	1.88 ± 0.13
CORT (nmol/L)	4.67 ± 1.08	3.43 ± 1.02
INS (nmol/L)	0.31 ± 0.02	0.26 ± 0.05
LEP (ng/mL)	2.41 ± 0.35	4.10 ± 0.31 *
ADIPOQ (μg/mL)	5.87 ± 0.72	5.60 ± 0.44

Circulating levels (in non-fasting conditions) of several metabolic markers in 60 day-old male rats born to either normal diet (C)- or FRD (F)-fed mothers throughout pregnancy. Values are means ± SEM. *n* = 6 C rats and *n* = 7 F rats. * $p < 0.05$ *vs.* C values, based on Student's *t*-test.

Circulating GLU levels (Figure 3A) and the AUC of these peripheral GLU levels (Figure 3B) throughout the i.v. GTT were significantly ($p < 0.05$) higher in F than in C rats (*n* = 6 C and *n* = 7 F rats per group). Moreover, while C rats did recover initial plasma GLU values 60 min after GLU load, F rats failed to do so (Figure 3A). The altered tolerance to GLU overload observed in F rats was related to changes in INS secretion in plasma throughout the test. The profile of circulating levels of INS and the AUC of INS values in both groups are depicted in Figure 3 (C and D, respectively). As shown, plasma INS peak values (time 15 min) were significantly ($p < 0.05$) higher in F than in C rats (Figure 3C). Moreover, we found a significantly ($p < 0.05$) higher AUC for INS values in F than in C rats (Figure 3D).

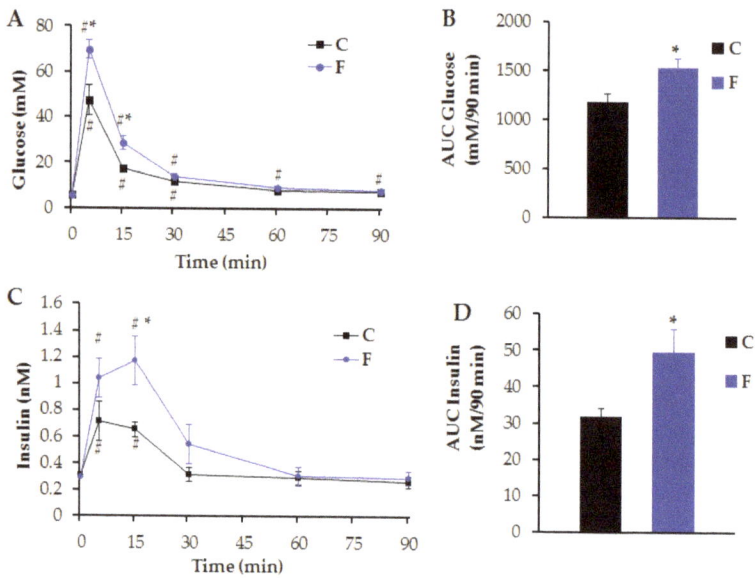

Figure 3. Glucose Tolerance Test. Circulating levels of GLU (**A**), INS (**C**) and the area under the curve (AUC) of GLU (**B**) and INS (**D**) during an i.v. GTT in C and F rats. Values are means ± SEM (n = 6 C rats, and n = 7 F rats; [#] $p < 0.05$ *vs.* time-zero values in the same group, * $p < 0.05$ *vs.* C values in similar conditions). One way ANOVA with repeated measures was used to compare different groups. Student's *t*-test was used for AUC differences.

3.4. Retroperitoneal Adipose Tissue Characteristics and Functionality in Adult Male Offspring

Whereas no difference was found in RPAT mass in 30 day-old C and F rats (data not shown), RPAT fat mass was significantly ($p < 0.05$ *vs.* C) lower in F rats at 60 days of age (Table 2). However, RPAT adipocyte diameter, area and volume were significantly ($p < 0.05$ *vs.* C) higher in F pads (Table 2 and Figure 4A,B, respectively).

Table 2. RPAT pad characteristics in 60 day-old rats.

	C	F
Pad mass (g per 100g BW)	0.71 ± 0.07	0.54 ± 0.03 *
Adipocyte diameter (μm)	37.21 ± 0.09	48.45 ± 0.28 *
Adipocyte area (μm^2)	1182.34 ± 10.64	2057.79 ± 23.57 *
Adipocyte volume (μm^3 × 10^3)	26.97 ± 1.84	59.97 ± 3.47 *
LEP mRNA (AU)	1.09 ± 0.19	2.99 ± 0.18 *
ADIPOQ mRNA (AU)	1.28 ± 0.40	1.94 ± 0.41

RPAT pad characteristics in 60 day-old male rats born to either control diet- (C) or FRD-fed (F) mothers throughout pregnancy. Values are means ± SEM. n = 6 C rats and n = 7 F rats. * $p < 0.05$ *vs.* C values; based on Student's *t*-test. mRNA expression levels were analyze by the non-parametric Mann-Whitney test.

Figure 4C shows the results of *in vitro* LEP release by isolated RPAT adipocytes incubated in the absence or presence of graded concentrations of INS. Spontaneous (INS 0 nM) LEP output was significantly ($p < 0.05$) higher in the F than in the C cell-group. While INS 0.1 nM failed to enhance LEP secretion over the baseline in both groups of cells, INS 1 and 10 nM were able to significantly ($p < 0.05$) increase LEP release over the baseline, regardless of the group examined. Interestingly, the amount of LEP released into the medium was significantly ($p < 0.05$) higher in F than in C cell-media, regardless of the condition examined (Figure 4C). These results tally with both circulating levels of LEP (Table 1) and the RPAT LEP mRNA expression levels in these rats (Table 2), although no significant group-difference was noticed in the RPAT mRNA levels of ADIPOQ (Table 2). The adipogenic cell population (CD34$^+$/CD31$^-$/CD45$^-$ cells) in the RPAT SVF from both groups was evaluated in order to assess a possible effect of maternal FRD intake on their APC number (Figure 4D,E). Interestingly, maternal high fructose exposure significantly ($p < 0.05$ *vs.* C) decreased APC number (Figure 4F). This result strongly suggests that the low APC number could be related to the finding of both RPAT adipocyte hypertrophy and decreased pad mass in the F male progeny.

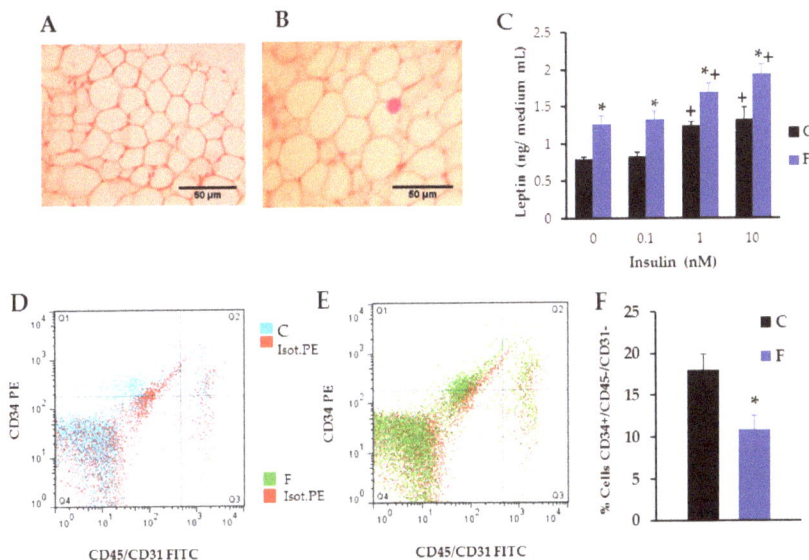

Figure 4. RPAT Characteristics. (**A** and **B**) Histological characteristics, representative fields, in C (**A**) and F (**B**) RPAT pads stained with hematoxylin eosin (scale bar: 50 µm; magnification: ×400); (**C**) Effects of INS on LEP release by adipocytes. Values are means ± SEM (n = 4–5 different experiments; * $p < 0.05$ *vs.* C values in similar conditions, $^+$ $p < 0.05$ *vs.* 0 nM INS values in the same group, based on two way ANOVA); (**D** and **E**) Representative dot plots showing the staining profile of RPAT SVF cells isolated from C (**D**) and F (**E**) male adult rats; (**F**) Percentage of CD34$^+$/CD45$^-$/CD31$^-$ cells, determined by flow citometry. * $p < 0.05$ *vs.* C values, based on Student's *t*-test.

3.5. Challenging Adult Male Offspring with a FRD

In these experiments, four groups of rats (CC, CF, FC and FF) were studied. The growth curves of rats (studied over a 21 day-period: between 60 and 81 days of age) are shown in Figure 5A. Rat BWs were similar in all groups on the initial day of diet administration. Throughout the indicated period, energy intake (expressed as a 21 day-average) was similar in CC and CF rats. Conversely, this parameter was significantly ($p < 0.05$) higher in FC than in CC rats. Notably, FF rats incorporated the highest ($p < 0.05$ *vs.* remaining group-values) amount of energy (Figure 5B) and, as a result, FF rats were heavier ($p < 0.05$ *vs.* CC rats) from day 68 until 81 days of age, although their final BWs were similar to those from CF and FC rats (Figure 5A). Furthermore, no significant differences were found in final BW values among CC, CF and FC rats (Figure 5A).

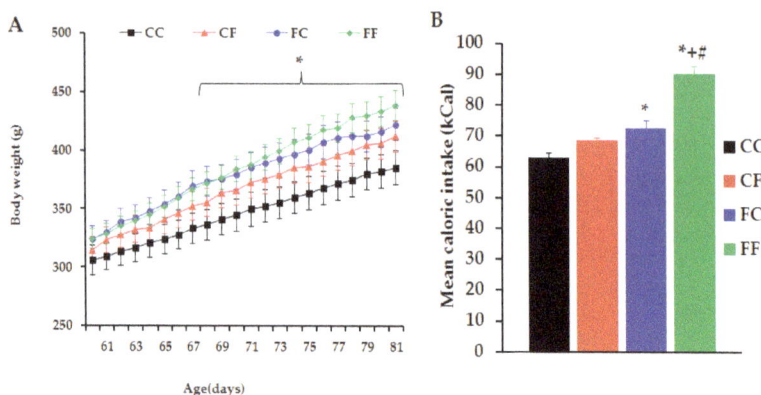

Figure 5. Body weight and mean caloric intake. (**A**) Body weight of male rats, born to CM or FM, fed with either control diet (CC and FC groups) or FRD (CF and FF groups), since postnatal day 60 until day 81; (**B**) Mean caloric intake of animals from four different groups. Values are means $\pm$ SEM. $n = 10$ CC rats, $n = 6$ CF rats, $n = 6$ FC rats and $n = 6$ FF rats. * $p < 0.05$ *vs.* CC values, $^{+}$ $p < 0.05$ *vs.* CF values, $^{\#}$ $p < 0.05$ *vs.* FC values, based on one way ANOVA.

When evaluated in basal conditions, CF animals displayed (Table 3) significantly ($p < 0.05$ *vs.* CC values) higher circulating levels of TG, LEP and ADIPOQ; conversely, no difference in plasma GLU and INS levels were noticed. FC rats displayed a severely distorted peripheral profile in several endocrine-metabolic parameters: hyperglycemia, hypertriglyceridemia and hyperleptinemia ($p < 0.05$ *vs.* CC values) although unchanged plasma for INS, TC and CORT (Table 3 data indicating a highly compromised basal metabolic state. Notably, both FC and FF rats showed similar (even *vs.* CC values) basal plasma adiponectinemia, and FF rats were unable (as CF rats did) to mount their adiponectinemia for protection against the FRD challenge applied; moreover, they displayed the highest peripheral levels of GLU, TG and LEP, although with normoinsulinemia (Table 3).

Table 3. Metabolic markers in 81 day-old rats.

	CC	CF	FC	FF
GLU (mmol/L)	4.96 ± 0.27	5.1 ± 0.33	5.88 ± 0.28 *	7.91 ± 0.56 *,+,#
TG (mmol/L)	1.19 ± 0.16	1.89 ± 0.17 *	1.7 ± 0.12 *	2.62 ± 0.11 *,+,#
TC (mmol/L)	0.26 ± 0.03	0.23 ± 0.01	0.23 ± 0.001	0.21 ± 0.02
CORT (nmol/L)	140.81 ± 37.41	87.45 ± 24.15	84.52 ± 12.99	190.98 ± 58.14
INS (nmol/L)	0.28 ± 0.04	0.31 ± 0.04	0.37 ± 0.06	0.34 ± 0.05
LEP (ng/mL)	2.87 ± 0.14	3.89 ± 0.38 *	3.89 ± 0.43 *	5.57 ± 1.4 *
ADIPOQ (µg/mL)	14.82 ± 0.94	20.08 ± 2.77 *	13.61 ± 1.95	14.89 ± 2.72

Circulating levels (in non-fasting conditions) of plasma metabolites in 81 day-old male rats from different groups. Values are means $\pm$ SEM. $n = 10$ CC rats, $n = 6$ CF rats, $n = 6$ FC rats and $n = 6$ FF rats.* $p < 0.05$ *vs.* CC values, $^{+}$ $p < 0.05$ *vs.* CF values, $^{\#}$ $p < 0.05$ *vs.* FC values, based on one-way ANOVA.

Regarding RPAT characteristics, we found that at 81 days-old, pad mass (in g per 100 g BW) was significantly ($p < 0.05$ *vs.* CC values) increased in CF rats and that, although no pad mass difference was observed in FC rats, FF rats also displayed an increased RPAT mass ($p < 0.05$ *vs.* CC values) (Figure 6E). Figure 6A–D displays the morphological characteristics of adipocytes isolated from RPAT pads of different groups. As expected [30], three-week-FRD administration to normal animals (CF group) resulted in enlarged ($p < 0.05$ *vs.* CC) RPAT adipocytes (Figure 6F). Moreover, RPAT pads from rats either challenged (FF) or not (FC) with a FRD at adult age displayed hypertrophic adipocytes ($p < 0.05$ *vs.* CC values), the first being the largest (Figure 6F).

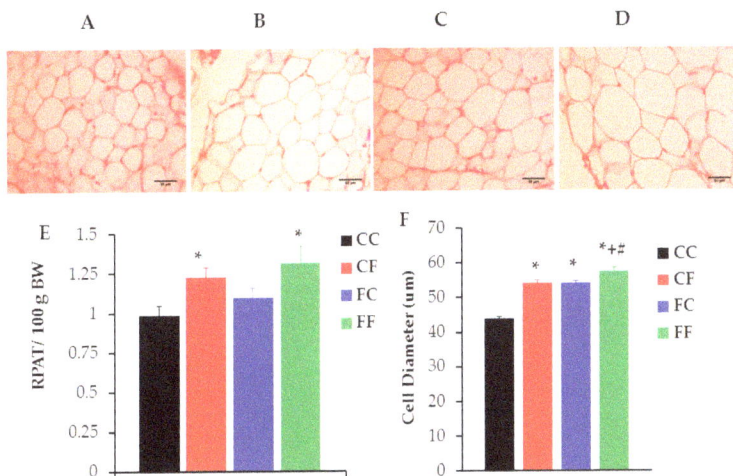

Figure 6. RPAT characteristics. Representative fields of RPAT pads from CC (**A**), CF (**B**), FC (**C**) and FF (**D**) rats stained with hematoxylin eosin (scale bar: 50 µm; magnification: ×400); Additionally, RPAT mass (**E**) and, adipocyte diameter (**F**) from different groups is displayed. Values are means ± SEM. $n = 10$ CC rats, $n = 6$ CF rats, $n = 6$ FC rats and $n = 6$ FF rats. * $p < 0.05$ *vs.* CC values, [+] $p < 0.05$ *vs.* CF values; [#] $p < 0.05$ *vs.* FF values, based on one-way ANOVA.

4. Discussion

Our results clearly demonstrate a deleterious effect on male offspring's endocrine-metabolic and adiposity functions induced by feeding pregnant rats a FRD. The consequences of this diet intake by the pregnant mother were evident when pups reached 60 days of age. At that time, male offspring showed dyslipidemia, hyperleptinemia, impaired glucose tolerance and adipocyte hypertrophy; several dysfunctions were further aggravated after offspring were re-challenged with FRD for three weeks.

Epidemiological and experimental studies demonstrated a relationship between maternal nutrition and long-term metabolic consequences in the offspring. Under-/malnourishment [31–33] or over-nourishment [34,35] in pregnant mothers induces in their offspring severe endocrine, metabolic and adiposity dysfunctions. In effect, FRD intake during both pre- and early post-natal periods impairs INS and LEP cell signaling, thereby modifying carbohydrate metabolism in the progeny [11,16,19]. Previous studies have shown that mothers consuming a FRD during both gestation and lactation resulted in offspring characterized by dyslipidemia [36] and insulin resistance [37]. Other studies showed that offspring consumption of a rich carbohydrate-milk during lactation increased plasma levels of INS and LEP, and also BW, resulting in pancreatic disorders [12,32,33]. Moreover, FRD-intake by pregnant rats was reported to affect both mother and fetal metabolism by enhancing lipogenesis and hepatic endoplasmic reticulum stress [38]. The deleterious consequences of FRD administration to pregnant mothers have been previously addressed. This diet is able to induce altered glucose tolerance, hyperinsulinemia and reduced placental vascular area, thus leading to high risk for the mother of developing gestational diabetes and preeclampsia [24]; moreover, their fetuses (embryonic day 20) displayed increased BW. Interestingly, these dysfunctions were fully prevented by metformin co-treatment [24], thereby indicating that impaired overall insulin sensitivity in the mother seems to be mainly responsible for these FRD effects.

A relevant observation made throughout the present study is that the detrimental consequences on AT endocrine function seen in F animals (which never consume FRD) are similar to those developed by CF animals. In both situations, a higher basal leptinemia and hypertrophic adipocytes from RPAT were found. However, while FRD administration to the adult offspring is able to enhance adiponectinemia in CF animals, we found that in F animals there was no change in plasma adiponectin concentration. These findings highlight that the AT seems to be the main target for this diet-noxa, and highlight the importance of the perinatal environment for an individual's development.

It is well known that AT endocrine dysfunction associated to obesity is closely related to adipocyte size, rather than to pad mass [39], and hypertrophic adipocytes are characterized by impaired insulin sensitivity [40] and changes in the adipokine secretory pattern, including higher leptin production [39,41]. Therefore, enhanced adipocyte size could well explain the hyperleptinemia found in F animals despite AT mass decrease. Changes in LEP concentration could contribute to impaired peripheral insulin sensitivity [42]. In the present study, the male offspring born to FRD-fed gestating mothers displayed an apparent paradoxical situation; although, they have a lower AT mass it has large adipocytes. These results could indicate a lower number of adipocytes. It has been found that, in both humans and animal models, AT development occurs mainly during late pregnancy and early postnatal life [43–45]. In fact, the ability to generate new adipocytes in adult life is limited; as a consequence, the number of adipocytes remains relatively stable. Therefore, it is possible to speculate that lower adipocyte numbers is a consequence of the alterations in APC determination during the AT development, leading to a decrease in adipocyte generation [43]. Then, considering this unusual situation, we next examined the cellular composition of the RPAT SVF to determine whether cell hypertrophy and low pad mass could be a result of a lower APC number. Interestingly, a low number of APCs, $CD34^+/CD45^-/CD31^-$ [46] was found in F RPAT pads. This diminished APC number could be responsible for an impaired adipogenic potential [45], and therefore leading to the development of hypertrophic adipocytes. To our knowledge, this is the first study that shows changes in APC numbers induced by excessive prenatal fructose intake.

Indeed, malnutrition during perinatal life could trigger changes in DNA methylation and in histone acetylation/methylation, causing transcriptional changes of key factors involved in adipogenesis (C/EBPα, PPARγ) [47,48]. Examples of this emerge from several studies, such as those findings indicating that, during differentiation of 3T3-L1 cells, there is a modification in the DNA methylation degree (*i.e.*, PPAR, C/EBP, LEP, GULT4) [49–52] and in histone methylation/acetylation [53], thus demonstrating the relevance of epigenetic regulation during the adipogenic process. It is reasonable to speculate that, at least partially, AT dysfunction found in offspring born from FRD mothers could be a consequence of epigenetic changes. Further research is needed to better clarify the role of epigenetic modifications in our model. Given the endocrine-metabolic alterations that we found in 60 day-old animals from FRD-fed mothers, we proposed studying the response of these rats to a direct challenge with FRD in adult life. For this purpose, we treated C and F 60 day-old rats with a FRD or a normal diet for three weeks (achieving 81 days of life), which has been widely used as an animal model of the human MS [30,54]. When older (81-day-old) pups were studied, surprisingly, we found a remarkably deteriorated AT function and metabolic state in FC pups. These rats had higher basal plasma levels of TG and GLU than CC rats, despite no changes in insulinemia, whereas offspring's hyperleptinemia and RPAT hypertrophic adipocytes remained. In this regard, it has been previously reported that FRD intake in rats induced severe basal hyperglycemia, with concomitant normoinsulinemia, accompanied by a high risk of cardiovascular events [55]. In our experiments with 81 day-old rats, we noticed that the FRD challenge to control animals (CF), increased circulating levels of TG, LEP and ADIPOQ, as well as RPAT pad mass and adipocyte size, confirming our previous data [30]. Nevertheless, the consequences of direct FRD administration to male offspring born to FRD-fed mothers (FF rats) were even more serious: they showed increased caloric intake, body weight, and plasma levels of GLU, TG and LEP, thus indicating they could be developing diabetes type 2.

Unlike the FC group and similar to findings in the 60-day-old F male offspring, there was no increase in peripheral levels of ADIPOQ. It is well known that ADIPOQ acts as an insulin-sensitizing factor [56]. In fact, ADIPOQ regulates glucose metabolism by improving insulin signaling pathway [57], enhancing liver and muscle glucose uptake, decreasing hepatic glucose output [58,59] and enhancing fatty acid oxidation [60]. Therefore, an increase in ADIPOQ plasma levels observed in 81 day-old control animals challenged with FRD (CF rats in Table 3) might play a protective role in carbohydrate metabolism. These results are in full agreement with those previously reported from our laboratory [30]. The lack of a physiological increase in adiponectin secretion in FF animals is highly indicative of the loss of its protective effect on carbohydrate dys-metabolism, contributing to the worsening of overall metabolic derangements.

5. Conclusions

Overall, the present study shows that maternal consumption of fructose during gestation alters offspring's development causing metabolic and AT dysfunctions. At 60 days of age, rats born to FRD-fed mothers showed impaired insulin sensitivity and profound AT dysfunction, evidenced by hypertrophic adipocytes that secrete *in vitro* larger amounts of LEP, although with decreased AT mass. This paradoxical situation could be the result, at least partially, of the reduced APC number, present in RPAT from F rats. At 81 days old, the results of FC rats corroborate that the impact of FRD on pups worsened the metabolic profile throughout their lifetime, even when they were not directly exposed to this diet. These changes are clearly aggravated when the offspring directly consume FRD during adulthood.

Considering that hypertrophic expansion of AT mass is a key marker for AT dysfunction, we further conclude that high fructose consumption by pregnant mothers primes the first male generation with a high risk of developing MS, obesity and type 2 diabetes. To our knowledge, this study is the first to report changes in adipose precursor cells numbers, induced by *in utero* diet manipulation. However, the impact of high fructose *in utero* on overall developmental programming of individuals requires deeper research.

Acknowledgments: This work was supported by grants from CONICET (PIP 2013-2015-0198), FONCYT (PICT-1415-2012 and PICT-0930-2013), FPREDM (062013) and CICBA. Authors are grateful to Susan H Rogers and Rebecca Doyle for careful manuscript edition/correction. A.A., E.S., G.M. and A.G. are members of the National Research Council of Argentina.

Author Contributions: A.A., E.S., A.G. conceived and designed the experiments; A.A., G.Z., G.M. and A.P. performed the experiments; A.A., E.S. and A.G. analyzed the data and wrote the manuscript.

Conflicts of Interest: The authors declare no conflict of interest.

References

1. World Health Organization. Obesity: Preventing and Managing the Global Epidemic: Report of a WHO Consultation. Available online: http://www.who.int/nutrition/publications/obesity/WHO_TRS_894/en/ (accessed on 14 March 2016).
2. Johnson, R.J.; Segal, M.S.; Sautin, Y.; Nakagawa, T.; Feig, D.I.; Kang, D.-H.; Gersch, M.S.; Benner, S.; Sánchez-Lozada, L.G. Potential role of sugar (fructose) in the epidemic of hypertension, obesity and the metabolic syndrome, diabetes, kidney disease, and cardiovascular disease. *Am. J. Clin. Nutr.* **2007**, *86*, 899–906. [PubMed]
3. Huang, B.-W.; Chiang, M.-T.; Yao, H.-T.; Chiang, W. The effect of high-fat and high-fructose diets on glucose tolerance and plasma lipid and leptin levels in rats. *Diabetes Obes. Metab.* **2004**, *6*, 120–126. [CrossRef] [PubMed]
4. Blakely, S.R.; Hallfrisch, J.; Reiser, S.; Prather, E.S. Long-term effects of moderate fructose feeding on glucose tolerance parameters in rats. *J. Nutr.* **1981**, *111*, 307–314. [PubMed]
5. Nagai, Y.; Nishio, Y.; Nakamura, T.; Maegawa, H.; Kikkawa, R.; Kashiwagi, A. Amelioration of high fructose-induced metabolic derangements by activation of PPARalpha. *Am. J. Physiol. Endocrinol. Metab.* **2002**, *282*, E1180–E1190. [CrossRef] [PubMed]
6. Barker, D.J.P. The origins of the developmental origins theory. *J. Intern. Med.* **2007**, *261*, 412–417. [CrossRef] [PubMed]

7. Armitage, J.A.; Taylor, P.D.; Poston, L. Experimental models of developmental programming: Consequences of exposure to an energy rich diet during development. *J. Physiol.* **2005**, *565*, 3–8. [CrossRef] [PubMed]
8. Bruce, K.D.; Hanson, M.A. The developmental origins, mechanisms, and implications of metabolic syndrome. *J. Nutr.* **2010**, *140*, 648–652. [CrossRef] [PubMed]
9. Stocker, C.J.; Arch, J.R.S.; Cawthorne, M.A. Fetal origins of insulin resistance and obesity. *Proc. Nutr. Soc.* **2007**, *64*, 143–151. [CrossRef]
10. Wells, J.C.K. The thrifty phenotype as an adaptive maternal effect. *Biol. Rev. Camb. Philos. Soc.* **2007**, *82*, 143–172. [CrossRef] [PubMed]
11. Rawana, S.; Clark, K.; Zhong, S.; Buison, A.; Chackunkal, S.; Jen, K.L. Low dose fructose ingestion during gestation and lactation affects carbohydrate metabolism in rat dams and their offspring. *J. Nutr.* **1993**, *123*, 2158–2165. [PubMed]
12. Srinivasan, M.; Dodds, C.; Ghanim, H.; Gao, T.; Ross, P.J.; Browne, R.W.; Dandona, P.; Patel, M.S. Maternal obesity and fetal programming: effects of a high-carbohydrate nutritional modification in the immediate postnatal life of female rats. *Am. J. Physiol. Endocrinol. Metab.* **2008**, *295*, E895–E903. [CrossRef] [PubMed]
13. Alzamendi, A.; Castrogiovanni, D.; Gaillard, R.C.; Spinedi, E.; Giovambattista, A. Increased male offspring's risk of metabolic-neuroendocrine dysfunction and overweight after fructose-rich diet intake by the lactating mother. *Endocrinology* **2010**, *151*, 4214–4223. [CrossRef] [PubMed]
14. Vickers, M.H.; Clayton, Z.E.; Yap, C.; Sloboda, D.M. Maternal fructose intake during pregnancy and lactation alters placental growth and leads to sex-specific changes in fetal and neonatal endocrine function. *Endocrinology* **2011**, *152*, 1378–1387. [CrossRef] [PubMed]
15. Stephan, B.C.M.; Wells, J.C.K.; Brayne, C.; Albanese, E.; Siervo, M. Increased fructose intake as a risk factor for dementia. *J. Gerontol. A. Biol. Sci. Med. Sci.* **2010**, *65*, 809–814. [CrossRef] [PubMed]
16. Fergusson, M.A.; Koski, K.G. Comparison of effects of dietary glucose versus fructose during pregnancy on fetal growth and development in rats. *J. Nutr.* **1990**, *120*, 1312–1319. [PubMed]
17. Mukai, Y.; Kumazawa, M.; Sato, S. Fructose intake during pregnancy up-regulates the expression of maternal and fetal hepatic sterol regulatory element-binding protein-1c in rats. *Endocrine* **2013**, *44*, 79–86. [CrossRef] [PubMed]
18. Zou, M.; Arentson, E.J.; Teegarden, D.; Koser, S.L.; Onyskow, L.; Donkin, S.S. Fructose consumption during pregnancy and lactation induces fatty liver and glucose intolerance in rats. *Nutr. Res.* **2012**, *32*, 588–598. [CrossRef] [PubMed]
19. Jen, K.L.; Rochon, C.; Zhong, S.B.; Whitcomb, L. Fructose and sucrose feeding during pregnancy and lactation in rats changes maternal and pup fuel metabolism. *J. Nutr.* **1991**, *121*, 1999–2005. [PubMed]
20. Chen, C.-Y.O.; Crott, J.; Liu, Z.; Smith, D.E. Fructose and saturated fats predispose hyperinsulinemia in lean male rat offspring. *Eur. J. Nutr.* **2010**, *49*, 337–343. [CrossRef] [PubMed]
21. Rodríguez, L.; Otero, P.; Panadero, M.I.; Rodrigo, S.; Álvarez-Millán, J.J.; Bocos, C. Maternal fructose intake induces insulin resistance and oxidative stress in male, but not female, offspring. *J. Nutr. Metab.* **2015**, *2015*, 158091. [CrossRef] [PubMed]
22. Rodríguez, L.; Panadero, M.I.; Roglans, N.; Otero, P.; Rodrigo, S.; Álvarez-Millán, J.J.; Laguna, J.C.; Bocos, C. Fructose only in pregnancy provokes hyperinsulinemia, hypoadiponectinemia, and impaired insulin signaling in adult male, but not female, progeny. *Eur. J. Nutr.* **2015**, *55*, 665–674. [CrossRef] [PubMed]
23. Lineker, C.; Kerr, P.M.; Nguyen, P.; Bloor, I.; Astbury, S.; Patel, N.; Budge, H.; Hemmings, D.G.; Plane, F.; Symonds, M.E.; *et al.* High fructose consumption in pregnancy alters the perinatal environment without increasing metabolic disease in the offspring. *Reprod. Fertil.Dev.* **2015**. [CrossRef] [PubMed]
24. Alzamendi, A.; Del Zotto, H.; Castrogiovanni, D.; Romero, J.; Giovambattista, A.; Spinedi, E. Oral Metformin Treatment Prevents Enhanced Insulin Demand and Placental Dysfunction in the Pregnant Rat Fed a Fructose-Rich Diet. *ISRN Endocrinol.* **2012**, *2012*, 1–8. [CrossRef] [PubMed]
25. Giovambattista, A.; Piermaría, J.; Suescun, M.O.; Calandra, R.S.; Gaillard, R.C.; Spinedi, E. Direct effect of ghrelin on leptin production by cultured rat white adipocytes. *Obesity* **2006**, *14*, 19–27. [CrossRef] [PubMed]
26. Perello, M.; Castrogiovanni, D.; Giovambattista, A.; Gaillard, R.C.; Spinedi, E. Impairment in insulin sensitivity after early androgenization in the post-pubertal female rat. *Life Sci.* **2007**, *80*, 1792–1798. [CrossRef] [PubMed]

27. Zubiría, M.G.; Fariña, J.P.; Moreno, G.; Gagliardino, J.J.; Spinedi, E.; Giovambattista, A. Excess fructose intake-induced hypertrophic visceral adipose tissue results from unbalanced precursor cell adipogenic signals. *FEBS J.* **2013**, *280*, 5864–5874. [CrossRef] [PubMed]

28. Perelló, M.; Castrogiovanni, D.; Moreno, G.; Gaillard, R.C.; Spinedi, E. Neonatal hypothalamic androgenization in the female rat induces changes in peripheral insulin sensitivity and adiposity function at adulthood. *Neuro Endocrinol. Lett.* **2003**, *24*, 241–248. [PubMed]

29. Giovambattista, A.; Chisari, A.N.; Gaillard, R.C.; Spinedi, E. Food intake-induced leptin secretion modulates hypothalamo-pituitary-adrenal axis response and hypothalamic Ob-Rb expression to insulin administration. *Neuroendocrinology* **2000**, *72*, 341–349. [CrossRef] [PubMed]

30. Alzamendi, A.; Giovambattista, A.; Raschia, A.; Madrid, V.; Gaillard, R.C.; Rebolledo, O.; Gagliardino, J.J.; Spinedi, E. Fructose-rich diet-induced abdominal adipose tissue endocrine dysfunction in normal male rats. *Endocrine* **2009**, *35*, 227–232. [CrossRef] [PubMed]

31. Langley, S.C.; Jackson, A.A. Increased Systolic Blood Pressure in Adult Rats Induced by Fetal Exposure to Maternal Low Protein Diets. *Clin. Sci.* **1994**, *86*, 217–222. [CrossRef] [PubMed]

32. Cambonie, G.; Comte, B.; Yzydorczyk, C.; Ntimbane, T.; Germain, N.; Lê, N.L.O.; Pladys, P.; Gauthier, C.; Lahaie, I.; Abran, D.; *et al.* Antenatal antioxidant prevents adult hypertension, vascular dysfunction, and microvascular rarefaction associated with *in utero* exposure to a low-protein diet. *Am. J. Physiol. Regul. Integr. Comp. Physiol.* **2007**, *292*, R1236–R1245. [CrossRef] [PubMed]

33. Theys, N.; Ahn, M.-T.; Bouckenooghe, T.; Reusens, B.; Remacle, C. Maternal malnutrition programs pancreatic islet mitochondrial dysfunction in the adult offspring. *J. Nutr. Biochem.* **2011**, *22*, 985–994. [CrossRef] [PubMed]

34. Howie, G.J.; Sloboda, D.M.; Kamal, T.; Vickers, M.H. Maternal nutritional history predicts obesity in adult offspring independent of postnatal diet. *J. Physiol.* **2009**, *587*, 905–915. [CrossRef] [PubMed]

35. Ashino, N.G.; Saito, K.N.; Souza, F.D.; Nakutz, F.S.; Roman, E.A.; Velloso, L.A.; Torsoni, A.S.; Torsoni, M.A. Maternal high-fat feeding through pregnancy and lactation predisposes mouse offspring to molecular insulin resistance and fatty liver. *J. Nutr. Biochem.* **2012**, *23*, 341–348. [CrossRef] [PubMed]

36. Ghezzi, A.C.; Cambri, L.T.; Ribeiro, C.; Botezelli, J.D.; Mello, M.A.R. Impact of early fructose intake on metabolic profile and aerobic capacity of rats. *Lipids Health Dis.* **2011**, *10*, 3. [CrossRef] [PubMed]

37. Ching, R.H.H.; Yeung, L.O.Y.; Tse, I.M.Y.; Sit, W.-H.; Li, E.T.S. Supplementation of bitter melon to rats fed a high-fructose diet during gestation and lactation ameliorates fructose-induced dyslipidemia and hepatic oxidative stress in male offspring. *J. Nutr.* **2011**, *141*, 1664–1672. [CrossRef] [PubMed]

38. Clayton, Z.E.; Vickers, M.H.; Bernal, A.; Yap, C.; Sloboda, D.M. Early Life Exposure to Fructose Alters Maternal, Fetal and Neonatal Hepatic Gene Expression and Leads to Sex-Dependent Changes in Lipid Metabolism in Rat Offspring. *PLoS ONE* **2015**, *10*, e0141962. [CrossRef] [PubMed]

39. Skurk, T.; Alberti-Huber, C.; Herder, C.; Hauner, H. Relationship between adipocyte size and adipokine expression and secretion. *J. Clin. Endocrinol. Metab.* **2007**, *92*, 1023–1033. [CrossRef] [PubMed]

40. Franck, N.; Stenkula, K.G.; Ost, A.; Lindström, T.; Strålfors, P.; Nystrom, F.H. Insulin-induced GLUT4 translocation to the plasma membrane is blunted in large compared with small primary fat cells isolated from the same individual. *Diabetologia* **2007**, *50*, 1716–1722. [CrossRef] [PubMed]

41. Wåhlen, K.; Sjölin, E.; Löfgren, P. Role of fat cell size for plasma leptin in a large population based sample. *Exp. Clin. Endocrinol. Diabetes* **2011**, *119*, 291–294. [CrossRef] [PubMed]

42. Walder, K.; Filippis, A.; Clark, S.; Zimmet, P.; Collier, G.R. Leptin inhibits insulin binding in isolated rat adipocytes. *J. Endocrinol.* **1997**, *155*, R5–R7. [CrossRef] [PubMed]

43. Wang, Q.A.; Tao, C.; Gupta, R.K.; Scherer, P.E. Tracking adipogenesis during white adipose tissue development, expansion and regeneration. *Nat. Med.* **2013**, *19*, 1338–1344. [CrossRef] [PubMed]

44. De Oliveira, J.C.; Lisboa, P.C.; de Moura, E.G.; Barella, L.F.; Miranda, R.A.; Malta, A.; Franco, C.C.; Ribeiro, T.A.; Torrezan, R.; Gravena, C.; *et al.* Poor pubertal protein nutrition disturbs glucose-induced insulin secretion process in pancreatic islets and programs rats in adulthood to increase fat accumulation. *J. Endocrinol.* **2013**, *216*, 195–206. [CrossRef] [PubMed]

45. Muhlhausler, B.; Smith, S.R. Early-life origins of metabolic dysfunction: Role of the adipocyte. *Trends Endocrinol. Metab.* **2009**, *20*, 51–57. [CrossRef] [PubMed]

46. Maumus, M.; Sengenès, C.; Decaunes, P.; Zakaroff-Girard, A.; Bourlier, V.; Lafontan, M.; Galitzky, J.; Bouloumié, A. Evidence of in situ proliferation of adult adipose tissue-derived progenitor cells: influence of fat mass microenvironment and growth. *J. Clin. Endocrinol. Metab.* **2008**, *93*, 4098–4106. [CrossRef] [PubMed]

47. Musri, M.M.; Párrizas, M. Epigenetic regulation of adipogenesis. *Curr. Opin. Clin. Nutr. Metab. Care* **2012**, *15*, 342–349. [CrossRef] [PubMed]

48. Masuyama, H.; Hiramatsu, Y. Effects of a high-fat diet exposure *in utero* on the metabolic syndrome-like phenomenon in mouse offspring through epigenetic changes in adipocytokine gene expression. *Endocrinology* **2012**, *153*, 2823–2830. [CrossRef] [PubMed]

49. Lee, J.-E.; Ge, K. Transcriptional and epigenetic regulation of PPARγ expression during adipogenesis. *Cell Biosci.* **2014**, *4*, 29. [CrossRef] [PubMed]

50. Fujiki, K.; Kano, F.; Shiota, K.; Murata, M. Expression of the peroxisome proliferator activated receptor gamma gene is repressed by DNA methylation in visceral adipose tissue of mouse models of diabetes. *BMC Biol.* **2009**, *7*, 38. [CrossRef] [PubMed]

51. Yokomori, N.; Tawata, M.; Onaya, T. DNA demethylation modulates mouse leptin promoter activity during the differentiation of 3T3-L1 cells. *Diabetologia* **2002**, *45*, 140–148. [CrossRef] [PubMed]

52. Yokomori, N.; Tawata, M.; Onaya, T. DNA demethylation during the differentiation of 3T3-L1 cells affects the expression of the mouse GLUT4 gene. *Diabetes* **1999**, *48*, 685–690. [CrossRef] [PubMed]

53. Chatterjee, T.K.; Idelman, G.; Blanco, V.; Blomkalns, A.L.; Piegore, M.G.; Weintraub, D.S.; Kumar, S.; Rajsheker, S.; Manka, D.; Rudich, S.M.; *et al.* Histone deacetylase 9 is a negative regulator of adipogenic differentiation. *J. Biol. Chem.* **2011**, *286*, 27836–27847. [CrossRef] [PubMed]

54. Verma, S.; Bhanot, S.; Yao, L.; McNeill, J.H. Vascular insulin resistance in fructose-hypertensive rats. *Eur. J. Pharmacol.* **1997**, *322*, R1–R2. [CrossRef]

55. Dupas, J.; Goanvec, C.; Feray, A.; Guernec, A.; Alain, C.; Guerrero, F.; Mansourati, J. Progressive Induction of Type 2 Diabetes: Effects of a Reality-Like Fructose Enriched Diet in Young Wistar Rats. *PLoS ONE* **2016**, *11*, e0146821. [CrossRef] [PubMed]

56. Chakraborti, C.K. Role of adiponectin and some other factors linking type 2 diabetes mellitus and obesity. *World J. Diabetes* **2015**, *6*, 1296–1308. [CrossRef] [PubMed]

57. Awazawa, M.; Ueki, K.; Inabe, K.; Yamauchi, T.; Kubota, N.; Kaneko, K.; Kobayashi, M.; Iwane, A.; Sasako, T.; Okazaki, Y.; *et al.* Adiponectin enhances insulin sensitivity by increasing hepatic IRS-2 expression via a macrophage-derived IL-6-dependent pathway. *Cell Metab.* **2011**, *13*, 401–412. [CrossRef] [PubMed]

58. Hajer, G.R.; van Haeften, T.W.; Visseren, F.L.J. Adipose tissue dysfunction in obesity, diabetes, and vascular diseases. *Eur. Heart J.* **2008**, *29*, 2959–2971. [CrossRef] [PubMed]

59. Bastard, J.-P.; Maachi, M.; Lagathu, C.; Kim, M.J.; Caron, M.; Vidal, H.; Capeau, J.; Feve, B. Recent advances in the relationship between obesity, inflammation, and insulin resistance. *Eur. Cytokine Netw.* **2006**, *17*, 4–12. [PubMed]

60. Yoon, M.J.; Lee, G.Y.; Chung, J.-J.; Ahn, Y.H.; Hong, S.H.; Kim, J.B. Adiponectin increases fatty acid oxidation in skeletal muscle cells by sequential activation of AMP-activated protein kinase, p38 mitogen-activated protein kinase, and peroxisome proliferator-activated receptor alpha. *Diabetes* **2006**, *55*, 2562–2570. [CrossRef] [PubMed]

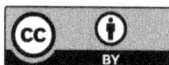

nutrients

MDPI

Article

Long-Term Fructose Intake Increases Adipogenic Potential: Evidence of Direct Effects of Fructose on Adipocyte Precursor Cells

María Guillermina Zubiría [1,2], Ana Alzamendi [1], Griselda Moreno [3], María Amanda Rey [1], Eduardo Spinedi [4] and Andrés Giovambattista [1,2,*]

[1] Neuroendocrinology Laboratory, Multidisciplinary Institute of Cellular Biology
    (IMBICE, CICPBA-CONICET-UNLP), Calles 526 10 y 11, La Plata 1900, Argentina;
    gzubiria@imbice.gov.ar (M.G.Z.); aalzamendi@imbice.gov.ar (A.A.); mamandarey@gmail.com (M.A.R.)
[2] Biology Department, School of Exact Sciences, Universidad Nacional de La Plata, La Plata 1900, Argentina
[3] Institute of Immunological and Physiopathological Research (IIFP, CONICET-UNLP),
    School of Exact Sciences, Universidad Nacional de La Plata, La Plata 1900, Argentina;
    gmoreno@iifp.laplata-conicet.gov.ar
[4] Center of Experimental and Applied Endocrinology (CENEXA, UNLP-CONICET, PAHO/WHO
    Collaborating Center for Diabetes), La Plata Medical School, Universidad Nacional de La Plata,
    La Plata 1900, Argentina; spinedi@cenexa.org
*   Correspondence: agiovamba@imbice.gov.ar; Tel.: +54-221-421-0112

Received: 20 January 2016; Accepted: 22 March 2016; Published: 2 April 2016

Abstract: We have previously addressed that fructose rich diet (FRD) intake for three weeks increases the adipogenic potential of stromal vascular fraction cells from the retroperitoneal adipose tissue (RPAT). We have now evaluated the effect of prolonged FRD intake (eight weeks) on metabolic parameters, number of adipocyte precursor cells (APCs) and *in vitro* adipogenic potential from control (CTR) and FRD adult male rats. Additionally, we have examined the direct fructose effects on the adipogenic capacity of normal APCs. FRD fed rats had increased plasma levels of insulin, triglyceride and leptin, and RPAT mass and adipocyte size. FACS studies showed higher APCs number and adipogenic potential in FRD RPAT pads; data is supported by high mRNA levels of competency markers: PPARγ2 and Zfp423. Complementary *in vitro* experiments indicate that fructose-exposed normal APCs displayed an overall increased adipogenic capacity. We conclude that the RPAT mass expansion observed in eight week-FRD fed rats depends on combined accelerated adipogenesis and adipocyte hypertrophy, partially due to a direct effect of fructose on APCs.

Keywords: retroperitoneal adipose tissue; adipogenesis; SVF cells; precursor cell competency

1. Introduction

In the last few decades, obesity, metabolic syndrome and type 2 diabetes mellitus (DMT2) have become serious problems for health systems, emerging as a worldwide epidemic. These metabolic disorders are multifactorial depending on genetic background as well as environmental and behavioral factors, such as eating habits. The quantity and quality of modern diets, in particular the increase of sugar intake, have been associated with the high incidence of metabolic disorders [1,2]. In fact, high fructose consumption, mainly through sweetened drinks, has been linked to deleterious metabolic consequences, such as insulin resistance, dyslipidemias, increased abdominal adipose tissue (AAT) mass and changes in the pattern of AT adipokine secretion [3,4].

The deleterious metabolic effects of high fructose intake have been related to the activating role in the *de novo* lipogenesis pathway in the liver, and therefore stimulating AT fatty acid uptake. This stimulation of *de novo* lipogenesis is not so markedly increased by other carbohydrates [5], mainly because fructose bypasses the main control point of glycolysis, the phosphofructokinase step, and is converted into trioses [6], precursors of triglyceride synthesis. Although most of the absorbed fructose is extracted and metabolized by the liver [7], a small amount remains in circulation and can be absorbed through its specific cellular transporter GLUT-5 by tissues such as kidney and AT [8,9].

The increase in AAT mass has been considered one of the main disorders associated with fructose overconsumption. AT expansion is the result of two independent processes: hyperplasia and hypertrophy. Dysfunctional AT is correlated with adipocyte size rather than AT mass. In fact, hypertrophic adipocytes are insulin resistant; secrete more leptin and pro-inflammatory cytokines and less adiponectin [10–12]. AT hyperplasia is the consequence of activated adipogenesis; a process involving two stages: the determination of the adipocyte precursor cells (APCs) and terminal cell differentiation, wherein APCs change into adipocytes. The ability of APCs to turn into adipocytes after specific stimulation is known as APCs competency and it is a characteristic of determined cells [13].

As we have previously shown, fructose rich diet (10% w/v, FRD) intake induces several metabolic alterations related to AT mass expansion [14–16]; however the activation or inhibition of adipogenesis in this phenomenon remains unclear. In the 3T3L1 preadipocyte cell line, the addition of fructose to the culture medium stimulates the terminal stage of adipogenesis, a mechanism that is dependent on the specific fructose transporter, GLUT-5 [17,18]. We earlier demonstrated that adult rats fed with FRD for three weeks showed APCs from retroperitoneal AT (RPAT) displaying high levels of competency markers, such as PPARγ2 and Zfp423 [15]. Nevertheless, the *in vivo* impact of FRD intake for a longer period of time and the direct *in vitro* effect of fructose on APCs adipogenic potential and number have not been studied up to now. Our study provides, for the first time, evidence that high fructose intake for eight weeks increases, probably through a direct effect, the number and competency of APCs from RPAT, therefore favoring adipocyte differentiation and contributing to its mass expansion.

2. Material and Methods

2.1. Animals and Treatment

Normal adult male Sprague-Dawley rats (60 days of age) were kept in a temperature-controlled environment (20–22 °C and fixed 12 h light/12 h dark cycle, lights on at 07:00 a.m. and fed *ad libitum* with Purina commercial rat chow. Rats were divided into two groups: one was provided with tap water only (CTR) and, the other, a solution of 10% fructose (w/v, Sigma-Aldrich, St. Louis, MO, USA) in tap water for eight weeks (conventionally called fructose rich diet, FRD). Rats were euthanized under non-fasting conditions (between 08:00 a.m. and 09:00 a.m.) and trunk blood was collected; plasma samples were then frozen (−20 °C) until metabolite measurements were taken. RPAT was aseptically dissected (brown adipose tissue vessels surrounding the kidney were removed and discarded), weighed and kept in sterile Dulbecco's Modified Eagle's Medium-Low Glucose (1 g/L) (DMEM-LG) for further procedures. Animals were euthanized according to protocols for animal use, in agreement with NIH guidelines for the care and use of experimental animals. All experiments were approved by our Institutional Animal Care Committee.

2.2. Peripheral Metabolite Measurements

Plasma levels of leptin (LEP), insulin (INS) and corticosterone (CORT) were determined by specific radioimmunoassays (RIAs) previously developed in our laboratory [19]. Circulating glucose (Glu, Wiener Argentina Lab., Rosario, Argentina) and triacylglycerols (Tg, Wiener, Rosario, Argentina) levels were measured using commercial kits.

2.3. RPAT Stromal Vascular Fraction (SVF) Cell and Adipocyte Isolation

Fresh RPAT pads were dissected, weighed and digested with collagenase as previously reported [20]. Briefly, fat tissue was minced and digested using 1 mg/mL collagenase solution in DMEM (at 37 °C, for 1 h). After centrifugation (1000 rpm, during 15 min), floating mature adipocytes were separated and reserved for later measurement. SVF pellets were filtered (in a 50 μm mesh nylon cloth) and washed with DMEM-LG (×3). SVF cells, containing APCs, were then resuspended in DMEM-LG supplemented with 10% (v/v) fetal bovine serum (FBS), HEPES (20 nM), 100 IU/mL penicillin and 100 μg/mL streptomycin (basal medium).

2.4. Adipocyte Size Analysis

The size of the isolated fat cells was measured as previously described [21], with minor changes. Briefly, a 50–150 μL aliquot from the top layer (floating cells) was added to 450 μL DMEM. 5–10 μL from the cell suspension were placed into a Neubauer chamber and cover-slipped. Five representative pictures from each sample were taken using a Nikon Eclipse 50i microscope equipped with a camera (Nikon Digital Sight D5-U3, Melville, NY, USA). Cell diameter was measured with image analysis software (Image ProPlus6.0, Rockville, MD, USA). Values below 25 μm were discarded as they can be considered lipid droplets. Values were recorded and assigned to groups differing by 10 μm diameter, creating a histogram with 10 μm-bins. Histograms were used to determine whether the distribution of adipocyte diameters was either normal or binomial, and to assess the presence of different sized, adipocyte sub-populations. We measured an average of 500–600 cells per field to calculate average adipocyte size.

2.5. RPAT SVF Cell Culture

RPAT SVF cells from CTR and FRD groups were seeded (2×10^4 cells/cm^2) in 24-well plates (Greiner Bio-One, Kremsmünster, Austria) and cultured in the basal medium at 37 °C in a 5% CO_2-atmosphere [20]. Cells were induced to differentiate and processed for several determinations as described in more detail below (Materials and Methods section: 2.8; 2.9; 2.10; 2.11). Additionally, normal SVF cells from RPAT from control adult male rats were seeded and cultured for 7 days in the basal medium alone (Basal) or supplemented with 1 g/L of fructose (FRU) or 1 g/L glucose (GLU). After this period cells were immediately processed for RNA extraction or FACS analysis, or differentiated to adipocytes for lipid content determination, as described below.

2.6. SVF Cell Composition Analysis by Flow Cytometry (FACS)

Freshly isolated or cultured SVF cells from RPAT pads (at least 2×10^5 cells in 100 μL PBS/0.5% BSA) were incubated with fluorescent antibodies or respective isotype controls for 1 h at 4 °C. After washing steps, flow cytometry was performed using a FACSCalibur flow cytometer (Becton Dickinson Biosciences, San Jose, CA, USA). A combination of cell surface markers were used to identify APCs as: CD34$^+$/CD45$^-$/CD31$^-$ for freshly isolated SVF cells and CD34$^+$/CD31$^-$ for cultured SVF cells [22]. Conjugated monoclonal antibodies used were: anti-rat CD34:PE, anti-rat CD45:FITC, and anti-rat CD31:FITC (1 μg/1×10^6 cells, Santa Cruz Biotechnology Inc., Santa Cruz, CA, USA). Samples were analyzed using CellQuest Pro (Becton-Dickinson, San Jose, CA, USA) and FlowJo softwares (TreeStar, San Carlo, CA, USA).

2.7. Cell Differentiation

Proliferating SVF cells (having reached 70%–80% confluence after 5–6 days of culture) were induced to differentiate by the addition of a differentiation mix containing 5 μg/mL insulin, 0.25 μM DXM, 0.5 mM 3-isobutyl-L-methylxanthine (IBMX) in the basal medium [20]. After 48 h media were removed and replaced with the fresh basal medium containing 5 μg/mL insulin. Cell samples were harvested after 10 days of the induction of differentiation (Dd10) and processed for several determinations, as described below. Medium samples were taken on Dd10 and kept frozen at −20 °C until measurement of leptin concentrations (see below).

2.8. RNA Isolation and Quantitative Real-Time PCR (qRT-PCR)

Total RNA was isolated from cells by the Trizol extraction method (Invitrogen, Life Tech., Carlsbad, CA, USA). Total RNA was reverse-transcribed using random primers (250 ng) and RevertAid Reverse Transcriptase (200 U/µL, Thermo Scientific, Vilnius, Lithuania). Two µL cDNA were amplified with HOT FIRE Pol EvaGreenqPCR Mix Plus (Solis BioDyne, Tartu, Estonia) containing 0.5 µM of each specific primer, using LightCycler Detection System (MJ Mini Opticon, Biorad, CA, USA). PCR efficiency was near 1. Expression levels were analyzed for β-actin (ACTβ, reporter gene), Adiponectin (ADIPOQ), CCAAT/enhancer binding protein alpha (C/EBPα), glucose transporter (GLUT-4), fructose transporter (GLUT-5) glucocorticoid receptor (GR), insulin receptor 1 (IRS-1) and 2 (IRS-2), Leptin (Ob), mineralocorticoid receptor (MR), Peroxisome Proliferator-Activated Receptor gamma 2 (PPAR-γ2), Preadipocyte Factor 1 (Pref-1), wingless-type MMTV integration site family member 10b (WNT-10b) and Zinc finger protein 423 (Zfp423). Designed primers are shown in alphabetical order in Table 1. Relative changes in the expression level of one specific gene (ΔΔCt) were calculated by the ΔCt method.

Table 1. Rat specific primers for qRT-PCR.

	Primers (5′-3′)	GBAN	bp
ACTβ	se, AGCCATGTACGTAGCCATCC as, ACCCTCATAGATGGGCACAG	NM_031144	115
ADIPOQ	se, AATCCTGCCCAGTCATGAAG as, TCTCCAGGAGTGCCATCTCT	NM_144744	159
C/EBPα	se, CTGCGAGCACGAGACGTCTATAG as, TCCCGGGTAGTCAAAGTCACC	NM_012524	159
GLUT-4	se, GCTTCTGTTGCCCTTCTGTC as, TGGACGCTCTCTTTCCAACT	NM_012751.1	166
GLUT-5	se, CTTGCAGAGCAACGATGGAG as, AACTCTGAGGGCGAGTTGAC	NM_031741.1	145
GR	se, TGCCCAGCATGCCGCTATCG as, GGGGTGAGCTGTGGTAATGCTGC	NW_047512	170
IRS-1	se, TGTGCCAAGCAACAAGAAAG as, ACGGTTTCAGAGCAGAGGAA	NM_012969.1	176
IRS-2	se, CTACCCACTGAGCCCAAGAG as, CCAGGGATGAAGCAGGACTA	NM_001168633.1	151
MR	se, TCGCTCCGACCAAGGAGCCA as, TTCGCTGCCAGGCGGTTGAG	NM_013131	193
Ob	se, GAGACCTCCTCCATCTGCTG as, CTCAGCATTCAGGGCTAAGG	NM_013076	192
PPAR-γ2	se, AGGGGCCTGGACCTCTGCTG as, TCCGAAGTTGGTGGGCCAGA	NW_047696	185
Pref-1	se, TGCTCCTGCTGGCTTTCGGC as, CCAGCCAGGCTCACACCTGC	NM_053744	113
Wnt-10b	se, AGGGGCTGCACATCGCCGTTC as, ACTGCGTGCATGACACCAGCAG	NW_047784	175
Zfp423	se, CCGCGATCGGTGAAAGTTG as, CACGGCTGGATTTCCGATCA	NM_053583.2	121

Primers sequences are listed in alphabetical order (se: sense; as: anti-sense; GBAN: GenBank Accession Number; bp: amplicon length in bp).

2.9. Leptin Measurement

Medium leptin concentration was determined by specific RIA [23]. In this assay, the standard curve ranged between 50 and 12,500 pg/mL, coefficients of variation intra- and inter-assay of 4%–7% and 9%–11%, respectively.

2.10. Cellular Lipid Content

On Dd 10, cells were washed with PBS and fixed with 10% formalin (for 10–15 min) in PBS. Then cells were quickly washed with PBS and stained for 1 h with Oil-Red O (ORO) solution (2:3 v/v H_2O:isopropanol, containing 0.5% ORO) [24]. After staining, cells were washed ($\times$3 with PBS) and dye from lipid droplets was extracted by adding isopropanol (10 min). To quantify cell lipid content, sample OD was obtained at 510 nm in a spectrophotometer. Remaining cells were digested with 0.25% Trypsin solution in PBS-EDTA, at 37 °C for 24 h and centrifuged at 8000$\times$ *g* for 15 s. OD of supernatants was read at 260 nm for DNA quantification and cell lipid content (measured by ORO and expressed in OD units) was then expressed by the corresponding cell DNA content.

2.11. Percentages of Cell Differentiation and Maturation

On Dd 10, differentiated cells were fixed with 10% formalin solution for 1 h at room temperature, and then stained using the Papanicolaou technique. The percentage of differentiated cells was calculated by counting the total number of cells and that of cells containing lipid droplets, when visualized in a light microscope (after counting 200–250 total cells per layer, at 40$\times$ magnification). Lipid-containing cells were assigned to one of the 3 graded stages of maturation according to the nucleus position: stage I (central), stage II (between central and peripheral), and stage III (completely peripheral) [25]. Percentages of cells corresponding to each maturation stage were expressed in relation to the total number of differentiated cells. Image analysis was assessed using a light Nikon Microscope and image analysis software (Image ProPlus6.0, Rockville, MD, USA).

2.12. Statistical Analysis

Results are expressed as mean values $\pm$ SEM. Data were analyzed by ANOVA (one-way) followed by Fisher's test. To determine the differential effect of the treatment according to age, ANOVA (two-ways) was performed followed by Bonferroni's test. The non-parametric Mann-Whitney test was used to compare adipocyte size populations between groups. Normal or binomial distribution of adipocyte size data was determined by Kruskall-Wallis test, followed by Mann-Whitney test. *P* values lower than 0.05 were considered statistically significant. All statistical tests were performed using GraphPad Prism 6.0.

3. Results

3.1. Effect of FRD Intake on Metabolic Parameters

FRD rats showed high average of total energy intake from three up to eight weeks of treatment (Figure 1A), although they did not exhibit differences in body weight (Figure 1B). However, FRD intake significantly increased INS, Tg and LEP plasma levels, and also induced a significant increase in RPAT depot (Table 2). When we determined the size distribution of mature adipocytes contained in the RPAT we found two adipocyte populations, one similar to and another larger than CTR adipocyte population (Figure 2). The presence of small adipocytes in FRD rats may suggest that the generation of new adipocytes took place (adipogenesis), whereas large adipocytes could be the result of enlargement of preexisting fat cells, leading to adipocyte hypertrophy.

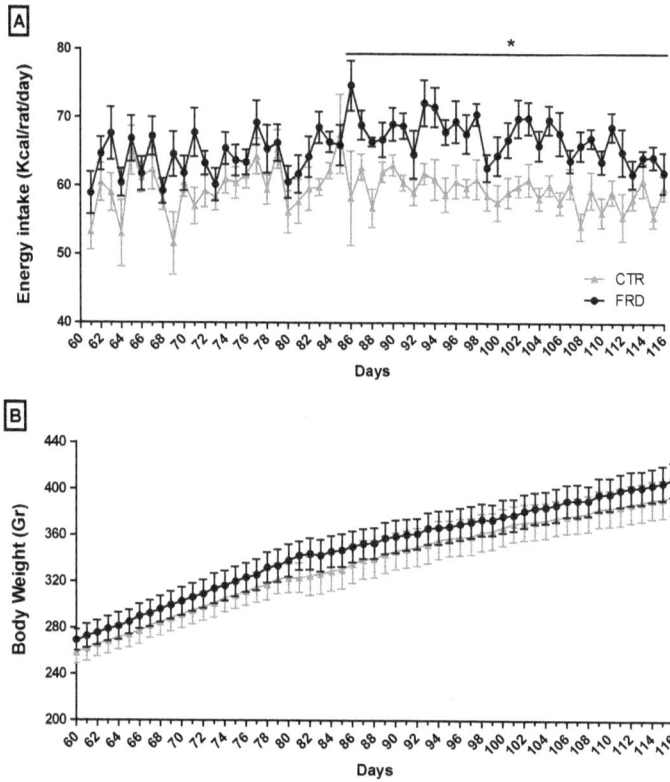

Figure 1. Food-derived energy intake and body weight of CTR and FRD rats. (**A**) Caloric intake and (**B**) body weight of CTR and FRD rats. Values are means $\pm$ SEM (n = 8 rats per group). * $p < 0.05$ *vs.* CTR values on the same day.

Table 2. Metabolic parameters in CTR and FRD rats.

	CTR	FRD
Body Weight (g)	403.87 $\pm$ 10.54	408.69 $\pm$ 10.95
LEP (ng/mL)	5.34 $\pm$ 0.68	9.39 $\pm$ 1.66 *
CORT (nM)	345.21 $\pm$ 32.32	282.67 $\pm$ 23.36
INS (nM)	0.29 $\pm$ 0.04	0.46 $\pm$ 0.03 *
Glu (mM)	6.94 $\pm$ 0.11	7.05 $\pm$ 0.22
Tg (mM)	1.29 $\pm$ 0.09	2.51 $\pm$ 0.16 *
RPAT mass (g)	3.92 $\pm$ 0.29	5.30 $\pm$ 0.51 *
RPAT Adipocyte diameter (µm)	69.24 $\pm$ 0.67	77.36 $\pm$ 0.77 *

Body weight, plasma levels of several metabolites, AT mass and adipocyte size from RPAT in CTR and FRD rats. Values are means $\pm$ SEM (n = 8 rats per group). * $p < 0.05$ *vs.* CTR values.

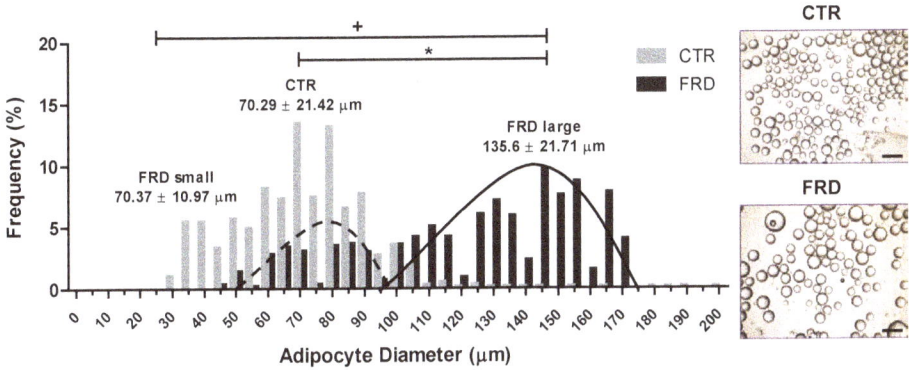

Figure 2. RPAT adipocyte diameter distribution. Dotted and continuous lines represent FRD small and large populations of adipocytes, respectively. Values are means ± SEM (*n* = 3 animals per group). Representative images of CTR and FRD mature adipocytes in cell suspension are shown (right, magnification 10×). Scale bars at 200 μm.

3.2. FRD Modifies APCs Number and Adipogenic Potential

To test the effect of FRD intake on the adipogenic capacity of APCs, we measured the mRNA levels of anti-adipogenic, pro-adipogenic and competency factors expressed by these cells contained in the SVF. Freshly isolated SVF cells from FRD pads expressed significantly ($p < 0.05$ *vs.* CTR cells) higher levels of Zfp423 and PPARγ2 (competency markers), and the pro-adipogenic factor MR (Figure 3A). Conversely, no differences were found in Pref-1 and Wnt-10b mRNA levels (anti-adipogenic factors, Figure 3A).

We also evaluated the expression levels of the specific fructose transporter GLUT-5 in APCs. We found that this gene was expressed in APCs, although no differences were noticed in either group of cells; the same phenomenon occurred when GLUT-4 mRNA expression was quantified. Importantly, the APCs expression levels of GLUT-4 were markedly lower than those of GLUT-5, regardless of the cell-group examined (Figure 3B).

Interestingly, the number of APCs contained in the SVF of RPAT pads, was significantly higher in the FRD rats (Figure 3C). Collectively, these results strongly reveal that high fructose intake affects the adipogenic potential of APCs, changing their ability to respond to the differentiation stimuli and their cell number.

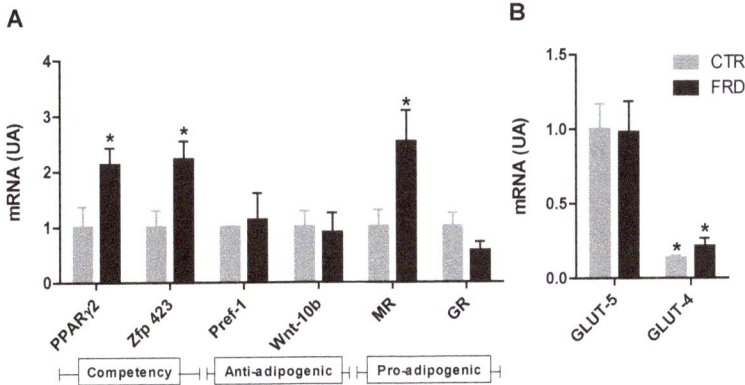

Figure 3. *Cont.*

C

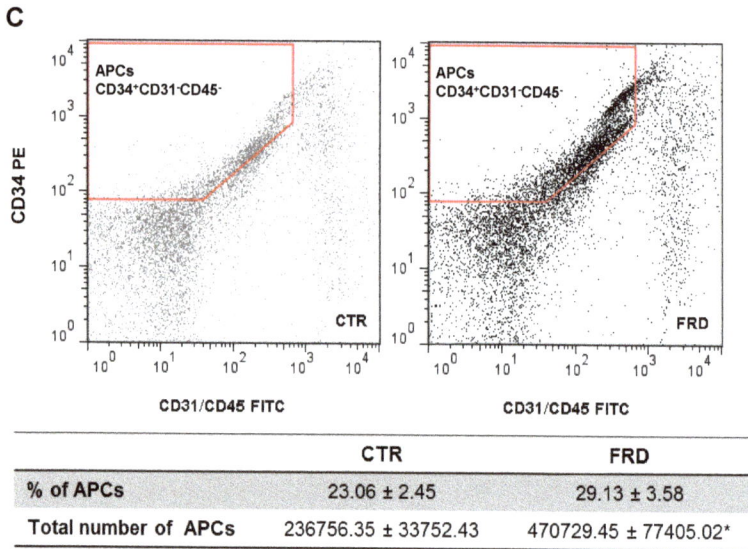

	CTR	FRD
% of APCs	23.06 ± 2.45	29.13 ± 3.58
Total number of APCs	236756.35 ± 33752.43	470729.45 ± 77405.02*

Figure 3. Effect of FRD intake on the APCs adipogenic potential and number. (**A**) Gene expression levels of cell competency (PPAR-γ2 and Zfp423), anti-adipogenic (Pref-1 and Wnt-10b) and pro-adipogenic (GR and MR) markers. * $p < 0.05$ *vs.* CTR values; (**B**) Gene expression levels of the specific fructose (GLUT-5) and glucose (GLUT-4) transporters in SVF cells in RPAT from CTR and FRD rats. Relative values to GLUT-5 expression in CTR cells. (AU: arbitrary units). Values are means ± SEM ($n = 4$ different experiments). * $p < 0.05$ *vs.* GLUT-5 values from each group; (**C**) APCs number in SVF in RPAT from CTR and FRD rats. APCs were identified by FACS analysis using CD34$^+$CD45$^-$CD31$^-$ profile (indicated in red borders). Fluorescence profiles obtained for IgG isotype controls are shown in Figure S1 (Supplementary materials) FITC: fluorescein isothiocyanate; PE: phycoerythrin. Values are means ± SEM ($n = 3/4$ different experiments).

3.3. In vitro Adipocyte Differentiation

We measured two classical differentiation parameters, such as leptin release and intracellular lipid content in order to determine whether the impact of FRD on APCs adipogenic potential affected, in turn, terminal adipocyte differentiation. We found that while intracellular lipid content increased on Dd 10 (Figure 4A) in FRD cells, leptin release was not modified (Figure 4B). Additionally, the mRNA levels of fully differentiated adipocyte markers indicate that the expression levels of C/EBPα, IRS-1, IRS-2, and Ob genes were higher in FRD than in CTR cells (Figure 4C).

Finally, we evaluated the percentage of differentiated cells and maturation degrees to determine the extent of adipogenesis. Interestingly, we noticed a higher percentage of differentiated adipocytes in RPAT from FRD, whereas the maturation degree in both groups remained the same (Figure 4E,F). These results strongly support that higher APCs competency and number, described above, caused the differentiation increase recorded in FRD adipocytes.

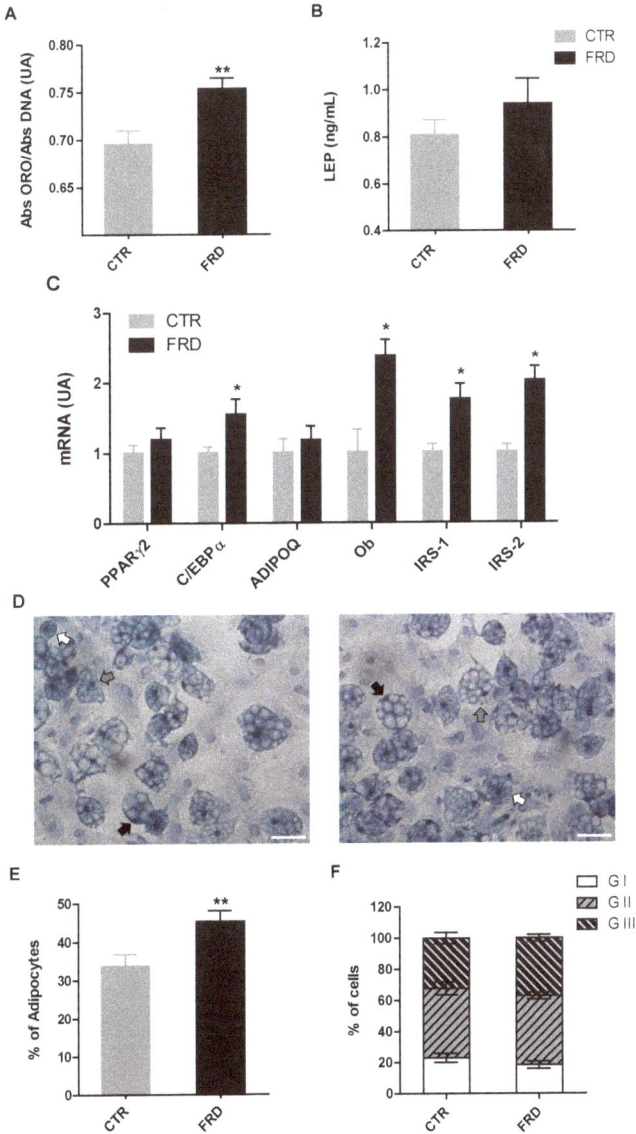

Figure 4. Parameters of terminal adipocyte differentiation. (**A**) Quantification of intracellular lipid accumulation and (**B**) leptin cell secretion ($n = 5$ different experiments with 12 wells per experiment); (**C**) Gene expression of fully-differentiated adipocyte markers (PPAR-γ2, C/EBPα, Adipoq and Ob, IRS-1 and IRS-2) on Dd 10 in cells isolated from CTR and FRD RPAT pads ($n = 5/6$ different experiments; AU: arbitrary units); (**D**) Representative fields containing *in vitro* differentiated CTR and FRD adipocytes (stained on Dd 10, magnification 40×), displaying different degrees of maturation depending on the nucleus position: GI, central (white arrows); GII, displaced from the center (gray arrows); and GIII: fully peripheral (black arrows). Scale bars at 50 μm; (**E**) Percentage of differentiated cells according to the presence of lipid droplets; (**F**) Percentages of cells according to the maturation stage. ($n = 4/5$ different experiments; data from 200/250 cells were recorded 1 in each experiment). Values are means ± SEM. * $p < 0.05$ *vs.* CTR values.

3.4. Direct Effect of Fructose Exposure on the Adipogenic Potential of Normal APCs

To examine whether the effect of FRD on normal RPAT APCs was caused, at least in part, by a direct cell exposure to fructose, cells were cultured with FRU and then the APCs adipogenic potential was determined. Our results indicate that normal cells exposed to either FRU or GLU expressed higher levels (*vs.* basal levels) of PPARγ2, without any change in those of Zfp423 (Figure 5A). We also evaluated the mRNA expression level of GLUT-5, which was similarly expressed regardless of the culture conditions, *i.e.*, basal, FRU or GLU (Figure 5B). Similarly to that found in SVF cells (see above), the mRNA expression of GLUT-4 was markedly lower than that of GLUT-5, regardless of FRU or GLU condition. Again, APCs GLUT-4 mRNA levels were similar in all incubation conditions studied (Figure 5B). Interestingly, MR expression level was higher only in FRU-exposed cells, whereas GR expression levels were lower in both FRU- and GLU-exposed cells (Figure 5B).

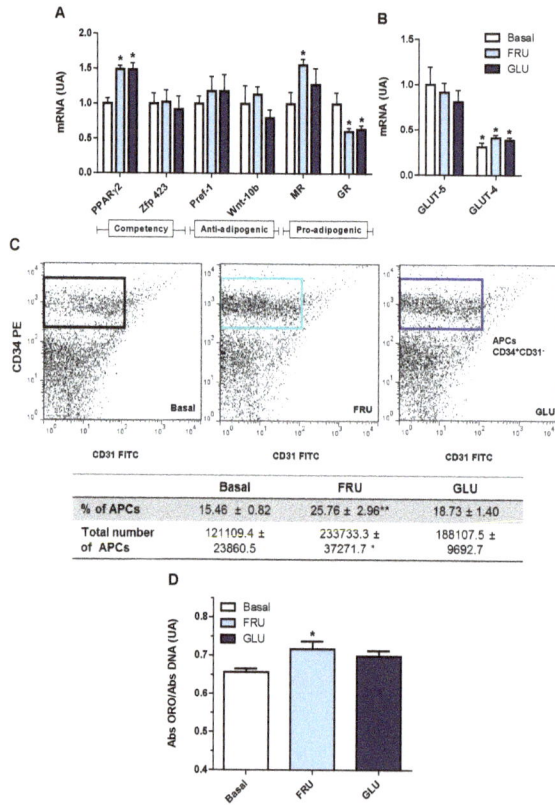

Figure 5. Direct effects of fructose on cultured APCs. (**A**) APCs gene expression of competency (PPAR-γ2 and Zfp423), anti-adipogenic (Pref-1 and Wnt-10b) and pro-adipogenic (GR and MR) markers. * $p < 0.05$ *vs.* CTR values; (**B**) APCs gene expression of specific fructose (GLUT-5) and glucose (GLUT-4) transporters, in Basal and FRU or GLU conditions, in cells from normal rats (AU: arbitrary units). Values are means ± SEM ($n = 4$ different experiments). * $p < 0.05$ *vs.* GLUT-5 values in each group; (**C**) Number of APCs in FRU- and GLU-exposed cells. APCs were identified by FACS analysis using the CD34+CD31− profile (boxes). Fluorescence profiles obtained for IgG isotype controls are shown in Figure S2 (Supplementary materials). FITC: fluorescein isothiocyanate; PE: phycoerythrin; (**D**) Intracellular lipid accumulation on Dd10 ($n = 5$ different experiments with 12 wells per experiment). Values are means ± SEM ($n = 4$ different experiments). * $p < 0.05$ *vs.* Basal values.

Additionally we quantified the number of APCs after either FRU or GLU condition. Interestingly, we found that APCs number increased in FRU- but not in GLU-exposed cells (Figure 5C), similarly to what we observed in APCs from FRD-fed rats. It is important to highlight that after seven days of culture, the presence of immune cells was undetectable (Figure S2, Supplementary Materials), and for that reason CD45 was not used in the FACS analysis. Finally, in order to assess whether these APCs changes might increase adipocyte differentiation, we analyzed the *in vitro* intracellular lipid accumulation on Dd 10. We found that FRU-exposed, but not GLU-exposed, cells showed a significantly higher lipid accumulation than that found in cells cultured in basal condition (Figure 5D). Taken together, these results strongly suggest that a direct effect of fructose on the adipogenic potential of APCs might be responsible, at least in part, for the subsequent increase in adipocyte differentiation.

4. Discussion

High-fructose feeding has been widely used in animal models to induce similar dysfunctions to those seen in human obesity and metabolic syndrome phenotypes. We previously used FRD intake in rats (10% p/v fructose in drinking water for three weeks) and found numerous metabolic disorders, including peripheral insulin resistance, AAT adipocyte hypertrophy and high oxidative stress, and others [14,15,26]. In the present study the rats were fed a FRD for eight weeks, which was only hyper-caloric during the last five weeks of the experiment. The switch from iso- to hyper-caloric intake could be the result of modifications in the peripheral hormone levels (e.g., ghrelin, leptin and peptide YY (PYY)) and hypothalamic factors (e.g., neuropeptide Y (NPY), pro-opiomelanocortin (POMC)) involved in appetite control, leading to an increase in the caloric intake. It has been suggested that the time required for the establishment of these changes in appetite regulation depends on the amount of fructose ingested [27,28]. Similarly to our previous studies [14,15,26], eight-week FRD intake induced several alterations, including increased plasma levels of INS, LEP and Tg.

The impact of FRD on the development of abdominal obesity has been studied in rodents and humans [15,29]. We have now observed that eight-week FRD intake contributes to abdominal obesity by increasing the RPAT, one of the most representatives AT depots in the rat abdominal cavity. AT depot remodeling after fructose feeding has been reported in a previous study describing larger abdominal adipocytes in contrast to smaller subcutaneous ones [30]. Our results agree with those findings; indeed, adipocyte size analyses from RPAT showed that FRD adipocytes were hypertrophic compared to CTR adipocytes. Besides, adipocyte size distribution showed two adipocyte populations in RPAT from FRD rats: one similar and other larger than CTR adipocyte population, respectively, thus suggesting that RPAT mass expansion in FRD rats may occur from both the combination of newly generated adipocytes through adipogenesis and the hypertrophy of existing adipocytes, respectively.

It is accepted that adipogenesis involves two sequential steps: commitment of mesenchymal stem cells (MSCs) into APCs, acquiring the adipogenic potential and restricting them to the adipocyte linage, followed by terminal adipocyte differentiation [13]. In the first step APCs begin to express CD34, a cell surface antigen that distinguishes between adipogenic and non-adipogenic cell subpopulations [31]. This CD34$^+$ cell subpopulation expresses almost exclusively the transcriptional factor Zfp423 [32], which in turn activates the basal expression of PPAR-γ2, a key pro-adipogenic signal that assures APCs conversion into adipocytes [33]. The differential expression of both transcriptional factors determines the competency of APCs, in other words, a cell's ability to differentiate into adipocytes upon the action of adipogenic stimulus [13]. Finally, in response to the adipogenic stimulus, APCs differentiate into mature adipocytes, cells mainly characterized by intracellular lipid storage and insulin responsiveness.

We were able to assess how the eight-week FRD intake affects competency of APCs from RPAT pads. For this purpose we evaluated the mRNA expression levels of PPARγ2 and Zfp423 in freshly isolated SVF cells. We found that APCs from FRD rats showed an increase in both competency markers, which have also been found after shorter periods of high fructose intake [15], indicating that high APCs competency is maintained between three and eight weeks of FRD intake. This phenomenon might be responsible for the small new adipocyte population observed in FRD rats, as discussed above. FRD intake also induced an increase in APCs MR gene expression without any change in that of GR, both receptors being natural mediators of the pro-adipogenic effects of glucocorticoids [34,35]. However, FRD intake did not modify APCs expression of two anti-adipogenic factors Pref-1 and Wnt10b, thus suggesting that the main FRD effect could be due to the change in APCs competency.

The cell expression pattern of both competency and pro-adipogenic factors in FRD-fed rats reveals an increased APC ability to differentiate into mature adipocytes. Indeed, FRD differentiated adipocytes also showed higher lipid intracellular content, differentiation percentage and expression levels of C/EBPα, Ob and IRS-1/-2 than CTR adipocytes. Collectively, these results indicate that APCs from FRD rats have a greater ability to become mature adipocytes. It is reasonable to speculate that some of the alterations observed in FRD APCs could be due to, in some degree , a direct fructose effect on these cells; in fact, after intestinal absorption a percentage of fructose enters into the systemic circulation and is metabolized by extrahepatic tissues, such as the AT [36]. Both 3T3-L1 preadipocytes and adipocytes express the specific fructose transporter GLUT-5 [17,37]. It has been described that GLUT-5 gene expression is higher in undifferentiated than differentiated 3T3-L1 cells [17], in which it is practically undetectable [17,38], thus indicating that adipocyte precursors are a better target for fructose action than mature adipocytes. Our results showed that cell GLUT-5 expression was not modified by either FRD intake (*in vivo* experiments) or direct fructose treatment (*in vitro* experiments). These results correspond with other reports describing that GLUT-5 is not modulated by an increase in substrate supply [39,40]. However, other authors have shown the opposite [18]. On the other hand, as previously reported [17], we found that GLUT-5 gene expression in both fresh SVF cells and cultured APCs, was greater than that of GLUT-4. Further studies are needed to evaluate any effect on other glucose transporters, such as GLUT-10 and GLUT-12, which are also expressed in adipocytes and SVF cells [41]. There are few available reports regarding direct fructose effects on adipogenesis that have only focused on the terminal differentiation stage of 3T3-L1 preadipocytes [17]. The presence of fructose (55–5500 μM) during adipocyte differentiation induced an increase in PPARγ2, C/EBPα among other pro-adipogenic factors, and either GLUT-5 knockdown or overexpression reduced or increased this effect, respectively [17]. GLUT-5−/− mice have diminished EAT mass compared with wild-type mice, and mouse embryonic fibroblasts derived from GLUT-5−/− mice exhibited impaired adipocyte differentiation [17]. Also, fructose in the culture medium increased lipolysis and the activity of 11-β hydroxysteroid dehydrogenase-1 in differentiated 3T3-L1 cells [18]. To our knowledge, the present work is the first that evaluates direct fructose effects on the early stages of adipogenesis; *i.e.*, before inducing cell differentiation. To this purpose, APCs were grown in presence of FRU for seven days. In this condition APCs expressed higher mRNA levels of PPARγ2 without any change in Zfp423, indicating a greater APCs competency. A similar result was found when cells were cultured with a comparable concentration of GLU. As found in the APCs from FRD rats, FRU did not modify the gene expression of Pref-1 and WNT10b. It has been proposed that the balance between MR/GR plays a key role in the pro-adipogenic effects of glucocorticoids. We found that the APCs grown in the presence of FRU had higher MR and lower GR mRNA levels. Interestingly, no GLU effect on cell MR expression was found. In agreement with this data, it has been described that fructose decreases GR gene expression in adipocytes [42]. Interestingly, when the FRU-exposed APCs were differentiated they accumulated high lipid content. Taken together, these *in vitro* results are quite similar to those we observed in freshly isolated SVF cells from FRD rats.

Another factor that can influence the adipogenic potential in each AT depot is its APCs number. It is generally accepted that subcutaneous AT contains more APCs than AAT [43]. High fat diet intake increases the number of APCs in different AT depots [43,44]. Interestingly, we have previously reported that three-week FRD intake does not induce any change in the number of APCs in RPAT [15]. However, in the present study we evaluated whether a longer period of FRD intake (eight weeks) might alter RPAT APCs number, quantified by using the CD34+CD31−CD45− FACS pattern [15]. Our results showed an increase in the number of APCs present in RPAT SVF cells from FRD rats. This fact, together with their higher APC competency, clearly indicates a greater differentiation capacity of the RPAT from

FRD rats. Additionally, we evaluated the direct effect of fructose on APCs number. Our results showed that FRU directly induced an increase in both CD34$^+$CD31$^-$ cell number and percentage. However, these results were not observed by using GLU, thus indicating a fructose-specific effect.

5. Conclusions

The present study demonstrates that long-term FRD intake altered the RPAT APCs by enhancing their adipogenic potential. Indeed, eight weeks of FRD intake were able to modulate APCs competency and number. Although we previously reported that three weeks of FRD intake modified APCs competency [15], the effect of FRD on APCs number is a novel observation. Moreover and importantly, it has now been assessed that FRU directly modulates the adipogenic competency and number of APCs. In addition, it is important to highlight that the fructose-induced changes in the number/competency of the APCs were not observed with glucose, which agree with the highest GLUT-5 compared with GLUT-4 expression levels in the APCs. It is more than likely that, after both direct and indirect fructose effects, APCs are more capable of generating new adipocytes, which subsequently and as a result of the positive energy balance, will become hypertrophic and contribute to an unhealthy AT mass expansion.

In conclusion, although we demonstrated that fructose intake can activate the adipogenic process in the RPAT, overall the activation of the hyperplasia would not be enough to counteract the hypertrophy. Therefore, predominant hypertrophic RPAT expansion could lead to the development of adiposity dysfunctions, and consequently to the endocrine-metabolic alterations also seen in the human metabolic syndrome/obese phenotype.

Acknowledgments: This work was supported by grants from CONICET (PIP-2013-2015-0198), FONCYT (PICT-2012-1415 and PICT-2013-0930) and FPREDM (062013). Authors are grateful to Rebecca Doyle for careful manuscript edition/correction. A.A., G.M., E.S. and A.G. are researchers from the National Research Council of Argentina (CONICET).

Author Contributions: A.G., M.G.Z. and E.S. conceived and designed the experiments. M.G.Z. performed research. A.A. and M.A.R. participated in cell culture and qPCR assays and analyses. G.M. participated in FACS experiments and analyses. A.G. and M.G.Z. analyzed all data and wrote the manuscript. E.S. participated in the critical revision and correction of the final manuscript. All authors read and approved the final manuscript.

Conflicts of Interest: The authors declare no conflicts of interest.

References

1. Malik, V.S.; Popkin, B.M.; Bray, G.A.; Després, J.-P.; Willett, W.C.; Hu, F.B. Sugar-sweetened beverages and risk of metabolic syndrome and type 2 diabetes: A meta-analysis. *Diabetes Care* **2010**, *33*, 2477–2483. [CrossRef] [PubMed]

2. Høstmark, A.T. The Oslo health study: Soft drink intake is associated with the metabolic syndrome. *Appl. Physiol. Nutr. Metab.* **2010**, *35*, 635–642. [CrossRef] [PubMed]

3. Johnson, R.J.; Segal, M.S.; Sautin, Y.; Nakagawa, T.; Feig, D.I.; Kang, D.-H.; Gersch, M.S.; Benner, S.; Sánchez-Lozada, L.G. Potential role of sugar (fructose) in the epidemic of hypertension, obesity and the metabolic syndrome, diabetes, kidney disease, and cardiovascular disease. *Am. J. Clin. Nutr.* **2007**, *86*, 899–906. [PubMed]

4. Tappy, L.; Lê, K.A.; Tran, C.; Paquot, N. Fructose and metabolic diseases: New findings, new questions. *Nutrition* **2010**, *26*, 1044–1049. [CrossRef] [PubMed]

5. Parks, E.J.; Skokan, L.E.; Timlin, M.T.; Dingfelder, C.S. Dietary sugars stimulate fatty acid synthesis in adults. *J. Nutr.* **2008**, *138*, 1039–1046. [PubMed]

6. Samuel, V.T. Fructose induced lipogenesis: From sugar to fat to insulin resistance. *Trends Endocrinol. Metab.* **2011**, *22*, 60–65. [CrossRef] [PubMed]

7. Douard, V.; Ferraris, R.P. Regulation of the fructose transporter GLUT5 in health and disease. *Am. J. Physiol. Endocrinol. Metab.* **2008**, *295*, E227–E237. [CrossRef] [PubMed]

8. Litherland, G.J.; Hajduch, E.; Gould, G.W.; Hundal, H.S. Fructose transport and metabolism in adipose tissue of Zucker rats: Diminished GLUT5 activity during obesity and insulin resistance. *Mol. Cell. Biochem.* **2004**, *261*, 23–33. [CrossRef] [PubMed]

9. Björkman, O.; Felig, P. Role of the kidney in the metabolism of fructose in 60-hour fasted humans. *Diabetes* **1982**, *31*, 516–520. [CrossRef] [PubMed]
10. Skurk, T.; Alberti-Huber, C.; Herder, C.; Hauner, H. Relationship between adipocyte size and adipokine expression and secretion. *J. Clin. Endocrinol. Metab.* **2007**, *92*, 1023–1033. [CrossRef] [PubMed]
11. Franck, N.; Stenkula, K.G.; Ost, A.; Lindström, T.; Strålfors, P.; Nystrom, F.H. Insulin-induced GLUT4 translocation to the plasma membrane is blunted in large compared with small primary fat cells isolated from the same individual. *Diabetologia* **2007**, *50*, 1716–1722. [CrossRef] [PubMed]
12. Wåhlen, K.; Sjölin, E.; Löfgren, P. Role of fat cell size for plasma leptin in a large population based sample. *Exp. Clin. Endocrinol. Diabetes* **2011**, *119*, 291–294. [CrossRef] [PubMed]
13. Cristancho, A.G.; Lazar, M.A. Forming functional fat: A growing understanding of adipocyte differentiation. *Nat. Rev. Mol. Cell Biol.* **2011**, *12*, 722–734. [CrossRef] [PubMed]
14. Alzamendi, A.; Giovambattista, A.; Raschia, A.; Madrid, V.; Gaillard, R.C.; Rebolledo, O.; Gagliardino, J.J.; Spinedi, E. Fructose-rich diet-induced abdominal adipose tissue endocrine dysfunction in normal male rats. *Endocrine* **2009**, *35*, 227–232. [CrossRef] [PubMed]
15. Zubiría, M.G.; Fariña, J.P.; Moreno, G.; Gagliardino, J.J.; Spinedi, E.; Giovambattista, A. Excess fructose intake-induced hypertrophic visceral adipose tissue results from unbalanced precursor cell adipogenic signals. *FEBS J.* **2013**, *280*, 5864–5874. [CrossRef] [PubMed]
16. Fariña, J.P.; García, M.E.; Alzamendi, A.; Giovambattista, A.; Marra, C.A.; Spinedi, E.; Gagliardino, J.J. Antioxidant treatment prevents the development of fructose-induced abdominal adipose tissue dysfunction. *Clin. Sci.* **2013**, *125*, 87–97. [CrossRef] [PubMed]
17. Du, L.; Heaney, A.P. Regulation of adipose differentiation by fructose and GluT5. *Mol. Endocrinol.* **2012**, *26*, 1773–1782. [CrossRef] [PubMed]
18. Legeza, B.; Balázs, Z.; Odermatt, A. Fructose promotes the differentiation of 3T3-L1 adipocytes and accelerates lipid metabolism. *FEBS Lett.* **2014**, *588*, 490–496. [CrossRef] [PubMed]
19. Perelló, M.; Gaillard, R.C.; Chisari, A.; Spinedi, E. Adrenal enucleation in MSG-damaged hyperleptinemic male rats transiently restores adrenal sensitivity to leptin. *Neuroendocrinology* **2003**, *78*, 176–184. [PubMed]
20. Giovambattista, A.; Gaillard, R.C.; Spinedi, E. Ghrelin gene-related peptides modulate rat white adiposity. *Vitam. Horm.* **2008**, *77*, 171–205. [PubMed]
21. Tchoukalova, Y.D.; Harteneck, D.A.; Karwoski, R.A.; Tarara, J.; Jensen, M.D. A quick, reliable, and automated method for fat cell sizing. *J. Lipid Res.* **2003**, *44*, 1795–1801. [CrossRef] [PubMed]
22. Maumus, M.; Sengenès, C.; Decaunes, P.; Zakaroff-Girard, A.; Bourlier, V.; Lafontan, M.; Galitzky, J.; Bouloumié, A. Evidence of in situ proliferation of adult adipose tissue-derived progenitor cells: Influence of fat mass microenvironment and growth. *J. Clin. Endocrinol. Metab.* **2008**, *93*, 4098–4106. [CrossRef] [PubMed]
23. Giovambattista, A.; Piermaría, J.; Suescun, M.O.; Calandra, R.S.; Gaillard, R.C.; Spinedi, E. Direct effect of ghrelin on leptin production by cultured rat white adipocytes. *Obesity* **2006**, *14*, 19–27. [CrossRef] [PubMed]
24. Chen, J.; Dodson, M.V.; Jiang, Z. Cellular and molecular comparison of redifferentiation of intramuscular- and visceral-adipocyte derived progeny cells. *Int. J. Biol. Sci.* **2010**, *6*, 80–88. [CrossRef] [PubMed]
25. Grégoire, F.; Todoroff, G.; Hauser, N.; Remacle, C. The stroma-vascular fraction of rat inguinal and epididymal adipose tissue and the adipoconversion of fat cell precursors in primary culture. *Biol. Cell Auspices Eur. Cell Biol. Organ.* **1990**, *69*, 215–222.
26. Alzamendi, A.; Giovambattista, A.; García, M.E.; Rebolledo, O.R.; Gagliardino, J.J.; Spinedi, E. Effect of pioglitazone on the fructose-induced abdominal adipose tissue dysfunction. *PPAR Res.* **2012**, *2012*, 259093. [CrossRef] [PubMed]
27. Lowette, K.; Roosen, L.; Tack, J.; Vanden Berghe, P. Effects of high-fructose diets on central appetite signaling and cognitive function. *Front. Nutr.* **2015**, *2*, 5. [CrossRef] [PubMed]
28. Lindqvist, A.; Baelemans, A.; Erlanson-Albertsson, C. Effects of sucrose, glucose and fructose on peripheral and central appetite signals. *Regul. Pept.* **2008**, *150*, 26–32. [CrossRef] [PubMed]
29. Stanhope, K.L.; Schwarz, J.M.; Keim, N.L.; Griffen, S.C.; Bremer, A.A.; Graham, J.L.; Hatcher, B.; Cox, C.L.; Dyachenko, A.; Zhang, W.; et al. Consuming fructose-sweetened, not glucose-sweetened, beverages increases visceral adiposity and lipids and decreases insulin sensitivity in overweight/obese humans. *J. Clin. Investig.* **2009**, *119*, 1322–1334. [CrossRef] [PubMed]
30. Crescenzo, R.; Bianco, F.; Coppola, P.; Mazzoli, A.; Valiante, S.; Liverini, G.; Iossa, S. Adipose tissue remodeling in rats exhibiting fructose-induced obesity. *Eur. J. Nutr.* **2014**, *53*, 413–419. [CrossRef] [PubMed]

31. Sengenès, C.; Lolmède, K.; Zakaroff-Girard, A.; Busse, R.; Bouloumié, A. Preadipocytes in the human subcutaneous adipose tissue display distinct features from the adult mesenchymal and hematopoietic stem cells. *J. Cell. Physiol.* **2005**, *205*, 114–122. [CrossRef] [PubMed]

32. Gupta, R.K.; Arany, Z.; Seale, P.; Mepani, R.J.; Ye, L.; Conroe, H.M.; Roby, Y.A.; Kulaga, H.; Reed, R.R.; Spiegelman, B.M. Transcriptional control of preadipocyte determination by Zfp423. *Nature* **2010**, *464*, 619–623. [CrossRef] [PubMed]

33. Tontonoz, P.; Spiegelman, B.M. Fat and beyond: the diverse biology of PPARgamma. *Annu. Rev. Biochem.* **2008**, *77*, 289–312. [CrossRef] [PubMed]

34. Caprio, M.; Fève, B.; Claës, A.; Viengchareun, S.; Lombès, M.; Zennaro, M.-C. Pivotal role of the mineralocorticoid receptor in corticosteroid-induced adipogenesis. *FASEB J.* **2007**, *21*, 2185–2194. [CrossRef] [PubMed]

35. Lee, M.-J.; Fried, S.K. The glucocorticoid receptor, not the mineralocorticoid receptor, plays the dominant role in adipogenesis and adipokine production in human adipocytes. *Int. J. Obes.* **2014**, *38*, 1228–1233. [CrossRef] [PubMed]

36. Bray, G.A. How bad is fructose? *Am. J. Clin. Nutr.* **2007**, *86*, 895–896. [PubMed]

37. Hajduch, E.; Darakhshan, F.; Hundal, H.S. Fructose uptake in rat adipocytes: GLUT5 expression and the effects of streptozotocin-induced diabetes. *Diabetologia* **1998**, *41*, 821–828. [CrossRef] [PubMed]

38. Romero, M.; del, M.; Sabater, D.; Fernández-López, J.A.; Remesar, X.; Alemany, M. Glycerol Production from Glucose and Fructose by 3T3-L1 Cells: A Mechanism of Adipocyte Defense from Excess Substrate. *PLoS ONE* **2015**, *10*, e0139502. [CrossRef] [PubMed]

39. Darakhshan, F.; Hajduch, E.; Kristiansen, S.; Richter, E.A.; Hundal, H.S. Biochemical and functional characterization of the GLUT5 fructose transporter in rat skeletal muscle. *Biochem. J.* **1998**, *336*, 361–366. [CrossRef] [PubMed]

40. Robubi, A.; Huber, K.R.; Krugluger, W. Extra fructose in the growth medium fuels lipogenesis of adipocytes. *J. Obes.* **2014**, *2014*, 647034. [CrossRef] [PubMed]

41. Wood, I.S.; Hunter, L.; Trayhurn, P. Expression of Class III facilitative glucose transporter genes (GLUT-10 and GLUT-12) in mouse and human adipose tissues. *Biochem. Biophys. Res. Commun.* **2003**, *308*, 43–49. [CrossRef]

42. Kovačević, S.; Nestorov, J.; Matić, G.; Elaković, I. Dietary fructose-related adiposity and glucocorticoid receptor function in visceral adipose tissue of female rats. *Eur. J. Nutr.* **2014**, *53*, 1409–1420. [CrossRef] [PubMed]

43. Joe, A.W.B.; Yi, L.; Even, Y.; Vogl, A.W.; Rossi, F.M. V Depot-specific differences in adipogenic progenitor abundance and proliferative response to high-fat diet. *Stem Cells* **2009**, *27*, 2563–2570. [CrossRef] [PubMed]

44. Macotela, Y.; Emanuelli, B.; Mori, M.A.; Gesta, S.; Schulz, T.J.; Tseng, Y.-H.; Kahn, C.R. Intrinsic Differences in Adipocyte Precursor Cells From Different White Fat Depots. *Diabetes* **2012**, *61*, 1691–1699. [CrossRef] [PubMed]

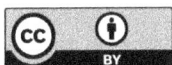

Section 4:
Diet and Obesity

nutrients

MDPI

Article

Apple-Derived Pectin Modulates Gut Microbiota, Improves Gut Barrier Function, and Attenuates Metabolic Endotoxemia in Rats with Diet-Induced Obesity

Tingting Jiang [1,†], Xuejin Gao [1,†], Chao Wu [1], Feng Tian [1], Qiucheng Lei [1,2], Jingcheng Bi [1], Bingxian Xie [3], Hong Yu Wang [3], Shuai Chen [3,*] and Xinying Wang [1,*]

[1]   Department of General Surgery, Jinling Hospital, Medical School of Nanjing University, Nanjing 210002, China; jiangtingting08med@163.com (T.J.); xuejingao870214@163.com (X.G.); wuchao0008@163.com (C.W.); tianfeng_nju@163.com (F.T.); lqiuchenggd@163.com (Q.L.); ahbijingcheng@163.com (J.B.)
[2]   Department of General Surgery, South Medical University, Guangzhou 510515, China
[3]   State Key Laboratory of Pharmaceutical Biotechnology and MOE Key Laboratory of Model Animal for Disease Study, Model Animal Research Center, Nanjing University, Pukou District, Nanjing 210061, China; xiebx@nicemice.cn (B.X.); wanghy@nicemice.cn (H.Y.W.)
*   Correspondence: schen6@163.com (S.C.); wxinying@263.net (X.W.); Tel.: +86-25-5864-1552 (S.C.); +86-139-1302-8866 (X.W.)
†   These authors contributed equally to this work.

Received: 18 December 2015; Accepted: 22 February 2016; Published: 29 February 2016

Abstract: This study was aimed at determining potential effects of apple-derived pectin on weight gain, gut microbiota, gut barrier and metabolic endotoxemia in rat models of diet-induced obesity. The rats received a standard diet (control; Chow group; n = 8) or a high-fat diet (HFD; n = 32) for eight weeks to induce obesity. The top 50th percentile of weight-gainers were selected as diet induced obese rats. Thereafter, the Chow group continued on chow, and the diet induced obese rats were randomly divided into two groups and received HFD (HF group; n = 8) or pectin-supplemented HFD (HF-P group; n = 8) for six weeks. Compared to the HF group, the HF-P group showed attenuated weight gain (207.38 ± 7.96 g *vs.* 283.63 ± 10.17 g, $p < 0.01$) and serum total cholesterol level (1.46 ± 0.13 mmol/L *vs.* 2.06 ± 0.26 mmol/L, $p < 0.01$). Compared to the Chow group, the HF group showed a decrease in Bacteroidetes phylum and an increase in Firmicutes phylum, as well as subordinate categories ($p < 0.01$). These changes were restored to the normal levels in the HF-P group. Furthermore, compared to the HF group, the HF-P group displayed improved intestinal alkaline phosphatase (0.57 ± 0.20 *vs.* 0.30 ± 0.19, $p < 0.05$) and claudin 1 (0.76 ± 0.14 *vs.* 0.55 ± 0.18, $p < 0.05$) expression, and decreased Toll-like receptor 4 expression in ileal tissue (0.76 ± 0.58 *vs.* 2.04 ± 0.89, $p < 0.01$). The HF-P group also showed decreased inflammation (TNFα: 316.13 ± 7.62 EU/mL *vs.* 355.59 ± 8.10 EU/mL, $p < 0.01$; IL-6: 51.78 ± 2.35 EU/mL *vs.* 58.98 ± 2.59 EU/mL, $p < 0.01$) and metabolic endotoxemia (2.83 ± 0.42 EU/mL *vs.* 0.68 ± 0.14 EU/mL, $p < 0.01$). These results suggest that apple-derived pectin could modulate gut microbiota, attenuate metabolic endotoxemia and inflammation, and consequently suppress weight gain and fat accumulation in diet induced obese rats.

Keywords: obesity; apple-derived pectin; gut microbiota; gut barrier function; metabolic endotoxemia

1. Introduction

In recent years, obesity and related metabolic disorders have emerged as major health concerns [1,2]. Obesity is associated with increased risks for developing type 2 diabetes mellitus (T2DM), hyperlipidemia, hypertension, coronary heart disease (CHD), stroke, and cancer. Development of these diseases can also lead to psychological and psychiatric illnesses, adding to the societal burden associated with these diseases [3–5].

Obesity and related metabolic disorders are attributable to a combination of genetics, unhealthy diet and lifestyle. Recent studies have demonstrated that disturbance of gut microbiota, especially the ratio of Bacteriodetes to Firmicutes phylum, is closely related to obesity and metabolic disorders [6–11]. In addition, obese subjects exhibit systemic chronic inflammation and a high level of serum endotoxins (lipopolysaccharides (LPS), a key component of the cell wall of gram-negative bacteria), termed "metabolic endotoxemia", which associates with gut barrier dysfunction [12–16].

Gut microbiota in the lumen is normally isolated by the intestinal epithelium from lamina propria and deeper layers [17,18], and LPS derived from gut microbiota is confined to the gut lumen and does not penetrate healthy intestinal epithelium [19]. However, a damaged intestinal epithelium or other gut barrier dysfunction can lead to disturbance of gut microbiota [16], allow for LPS permeation and cause metabolic endotoxemia [20–22]. Recognition of LPS by Toll-like receptor 4 (TLR4) of host cells triggers downstream inflammatory events [23,24] that contributes to the development of obesity and metabolic disorders such as insulin resistance [10,25].

Tight junctions are key components for maintaining gut barrier integrity [17,26]. Another important protein for gut barrier function is intestinal alkaline phosphatase (IAP) that is a type of glycoprotein anchored in the apical membrane of enterocytes. IAP has multiple roles in maintenance of gut barrier, including detoxification of LPS via its dephosphorylation, remission of systemic inflammation, protection of gut barrier function and modulation of gut microbiota [27,28].

Although various approaches are recommended for obesity management [29], such as dieting, behavior therapy, exercise, pharmacotherapy, and bariatric surgery, they are often defective [29,30]. Here, we consider that modification of gut microbiota, protection of gut barrier, remission of metabolic endotoxemia, and relief of systemic inflammation may provide a novel strategy for the treatment of obesity and related metabolic disorders.

Dietary fiber consists of non-digestible carbohydrates that derived from plants. Recent animal experiments and clinical trials have shown that dietary fiber, such as whole-grain cereal, grape skin extract, yellow pea fiber and wheat-derived arabinoxylan oligosaccharides, has hypolipidemic and hypoglycemic effects and may contribute to weight loss [31–35]. Apple-derived pectin is the main soluble fiber in apples and can be fermented by gut microbiota in the colon to produce metabolites with local intestinal and systemic effects. Apple-derived pectin may also help to maintain the balance of gut microbiota [36].

The aim of the present study was to assess potential effects of apple-derived pectin on diet-induced obesity in rats. We found that apple-derived pectin could modulate gut microbiota, preserve gut barrier function, and alleviate metabolic endotoxemia and inflammation in diet-induced obese rats. Our findings suggest that apple-derived pectin may be useful for the clinical management of obesity.

2. Materials and Methods

2.1. Animals

Male Sprague-Dawley rats were obtained from the Medical Experiment Animal Center of the Jinling Hospital, Nanjing, China, at 4 weeks of age with an initial weight of 90 ± 10 g. Rats were housed in individual cages in an optimum environment at 23 ± 2 °C and a relative air humidity of 55% ± 10% with a 12 h light/dark cycle. Animals had free access to a standard chow diet (10% kcal% fat; D12450J, Research Diets, New Brunswick, NJ, USA) or a high fat diet (60% kcal% fat; D12492, Research Diets) and water throughout the experiment. This study was approved by the Animal Care and Use Committee of Nanjing University and Jinling Hospital and complied with the principles of laboratory animal care (NIH publication No. 86–23, revised 1985).

2.2. Diet and Study Design

Rats were randomized into two groups and received either a standard chow diet (Chow group, $n = 8$) as a control or a HFD ($n = 32$) to induce obesity for 8 weeks. Body weight and food intake were recorded every week.

After high fat feeding, diet induced obese rats were selected as previously described [37], wherein the top 50th percentile of weight gainers were randomized for the following interventions. Sixteen were randomized to receive either a HFD (HF group, $n = 8$) or a HFD supplemented with pectin (5% wt/wt) (HF-P group, $n = 8$) for 6 weeks. The Chow group continued a standard chow diet for 6 weeks. Body weight and food intake were recorded every week.

2.3. Sample Collection

All animals were anesthetized by intraperitoneal administration of ketamine (0.3 mL/100 g body weight). Blood (about 3 mL) was immediately collected in a dry tube without heat source. Blood samples were allowed to clot for 2 h at room temperature and were then centrifuged for 15 min at 3000 rpm at 4 °C. Serum was removed, and the samples were stored at −80 °C until further analysis.

After blood collection, a part of the liver, distal ileum, mesentery adipose, and the whole part of epididymal fat pad were collected, weighed, wrapped, and immediately put into liquid nitrogen. This process took no longer than 3 min after sacrifice of the animal. All samples were stored frozen at −80 °C until further analysis.

2.4. Body Weight and Adipose Tissue Wet Weight

Body weight and adipose tissue wet weight were measured using an electronic scale. Body weight was measured once a week and adipose tissue wet weight was measured after the rats were sacrificed.

2.5. Blood Parameters

Serum glucose, triglycerides, and total cholesterol concentrations were measured by enzyme linked immunosorbent assay (ELISA) kits in accordance with the manufacturer's instructions (Labassay™ Wako kit, Wako Pure Chemical Industries, Ltd., Osaka, Japan). Serum insulin concentrations were measured using an ELISA kit (Millipore Corp., Billerica, MA, USA).

2.6. Measurement of Serum LPS

Serum LPS concentration was determined by Chromogenic End-point Tachypleus Amebocyte Lysate (CE TAL) assay (Chinese Horseshoe Crab Reagent Manufactory, Co., Ltd., Xiamen, China). In this assay, color intensity is directly proportional to endotoxin levels. Serum was diluted 1/10 with pyrogen-free pipes to avoid interference in the reaction. Endotoxin in the serum activates a cascade of enzymes in the assay, and the activated enzyme splits the synthetic substrate, producing a yellow product with maximum absorbance at 405 nm. The yellow product can further react with diazo reagents to form a purple product with maximum absorbance at 545 nm. Every sample was treated in duplicate for determination. The limit of detection ranged from 0.1 to 1.0 EU/mL. An internal control for LPS recovery was included in the calculation. Every reaction in the kit was done in duplicate.

2.7. Western Blot

Proteins of ileum or liver samples were separated by sodium dodecyl sulfate (SDS)-polyacrylamide gel electrophoresis and transferred to polyvinylidene fluoride (PVDF) membranes. After blocking with skim milk (BioRad, Hercules, CA, USA), membranes were incubated at 4 °C overnight using the antibodies indicated. Band density was detected by horseradish-peroxidase conjugated secondary antibodies (Promega, Madison, WI, USA) and ECL (enhanced chemiluminescence reagent; GE Healthcare, Chalfont St. Giles, UK). Bands located in a predicted molecular weight were used to verify targeted proteins. β-actin or glyceraldehyde-3-phosphate dehydrogenase (GAPDH) was used as an internal control to adjust the density of bands on multiple membranes. For quantification of signals, the images were quantified by an Image J software (Wayne Rasband, National Institutes of Health, Bethesda, MD, USA).

2.8. Quantitative RT-PCR Analysis

mRNA levels of TNF α, IL-6, IL-10, and TLR4 were measured by quantitative real-time polymerase chain reaction (qPCR). The primers are listed in Table 1.

Table 1. Primer for quantitative real-time polymerase chain reaction.

Primer	Sequence
TNFa Forward	AAATGGGCTCCCTCTCATCAGTTC
TNFa Reverse	TCTGCTTGGTGGTTTGCTACGAC
IL6 Forward	AGCCAGAGTCATTCAGAGCA
IL6 Reverse	AGAGCATTGGAAGTTGGGGT
IL10 Forward	GTTGCCAAGCCTTGTCAGAA
IL10 Reverse	GGGAGAAATCGATGACAGCG
TLR4 Forward	TTCCTTTCCTGCCTGAGACC
TLR4 Reverse	CATGCCATGCCTTGTCTTCA
βactin Forward	GAGAGGGAAATCGTGCGTGACA
βactin Reverse	GTTTCATGGATGCCACAGGAT
36B4 Forward	TAAAGACTGGAGACAAGGTG
36B4 Reverse	GTGTACTCAGTCTCCACAGA

mRNA extraction and RT-PCR were performed according to the manufacturer's instructions as described in the PrimeScript RT reagent Kit (TaKaRa Bio, Tokyo, Japan). Q RT-PCR was performed by SYBR Select Master Mix System (Applied Biosystems, Foster City, CA, USA). The levels of mRNA expression were measured by StepOne Realtime PCR system with a ΔCt relative quantification model. The mRNA expression of βactin and 36B4, two reference genes, were calculated and used for normalization. In our study, mRNA expression of the tested genes displayed similar results with either reference gene, thus we used βactin as the reference gene for normalization in this manuscript.

2.9. Hematoxylin and Eosin (H & E) Staining

The ileal tissues were processed (Tissue-Tek VIP; Sakura Finetek, Tokyo, Japan), embedded in paraffin wax, and cut into 5-μm thick slices. Paraffin embedding, slicing, and H & E staining were performed according to the standard procedure.

2.10. Immunohistochemistry (IHC) Staining

IHC staining was used to detect the location of IAP. After antigen retrieval with buffered citrate and blocking with 5% bovine serum albumin (BSA), ileum tissues were incubated with primary antibodies against IAP (Abcam, Cambridge, UK, 1:200) overnight at 4 °C. The sections were then processed using the DAB Kit (ZSGB-Bio, Beijing, China) according to the manufacturer's instructions. Hematoxylin staining was performed at the end to counterstain nuclei. The cover slips were fixed with 50% glycerin.

2.11. 16S rRNA Pyrosequencing

2.11.1. Collection and Transportation of Samples

Cecum content was collected from every rat, stored in liquid nitrogen, transported to BGI laboratory (Shenzhen, China), packed with dry ice, and then immediately stored in a −80 °C refrigerator before extraction of total DNA.

2.11.2. Detection of Samples

Detection of samples included concentration and sample integrity. Concentration was detected by a fluorometer or microplate Reader, while sample integrity was detected by agarose gel electrophoresis (concentration of agarose gel: 1%; voltage: 150 V; electrophoresis Time: 40 min).

2.11.3. Library Construction

Total DNA was normalized to 30 ng per reaction, and then V4 Dual-index Fusion PCR Primer Cocktail and PCR Master Mix were added to run PCR (melting temperature: 56 °C, PCR cycle: 30). Subsequently, AmpureXP beads (AGENCOURT) were added to the PCR products to remove unspecific products.

2.11.4. Library Validation

The final library was quantitated by real-time quantitative PCR (EvaGreen™, Hayward, CA, USA).

2.11.5. Library Sequencing

Library sequencing was conducted by pair end on MiSeq System, with sequencing strategy PE250 (PE251 + 8 + 8 + 251) (MiSeq Reagent Kit, Illumina Hong Kong Limited, Hong Kong, China). Mothur pipeline and QIIME pipeline were used to analyze the data.

2.12. Statistical Analysis

Data are presented as the mean ± standard deviation (SD), and significant difference among groups was analyzed by one-way analysis of variance (ANOVA) followed by Dunnett's *post hoc* test (SPSS 21.0, IBM, New York, NY, USA). Significant difference of the body weight among groups was analyzed by repeated measures analysis of variance (SPSS 21.0). Statistical significance was set at $p < 0.05$.

3. Results

3.1. Apple-Derived Pectin Protected Rats from High Fat Diet Induced Obesity

In the intervention stage, rats in the high fat diet (HF) group gained more body weight than rats in the Chow group (283.63 ± 10.17 g *vs.* 161.00 ± 2.88 g, $p < 0.01$). Importantly, rats in the HF supplemented with pectin (HF-P) group gained significantly less weight than rats in the HF group (207.38 ± 7.96 g *vs.* 283.63 ± 10.17 g, $p < 0.01$) (Figure 1). Rats in the HF group developed adipose tissue more rapidly than the Chow group (epididymal, 23.44 ± 2.36 g *vs.* 14.86 ± 2.04 g, $p < 0.01$; subcutaneous, 18.44 ± 2.36 g *vs.* 11.99 ± 1.21 g, $p < 0.01$) (Figure 1). Pectin supplementation significantly suppressed the development of adipose tissue in the HF-P group as compared with the HF group (epididymal, 17.90 ± 1.55 g *vs.* 23.44 ± 2.36 g, $p < 0.01$; subcutaneous, 15.02 ± 1.44 g *vs.* 18.44 ± 2.36 g, $p < 0.01$) (Figure 1).

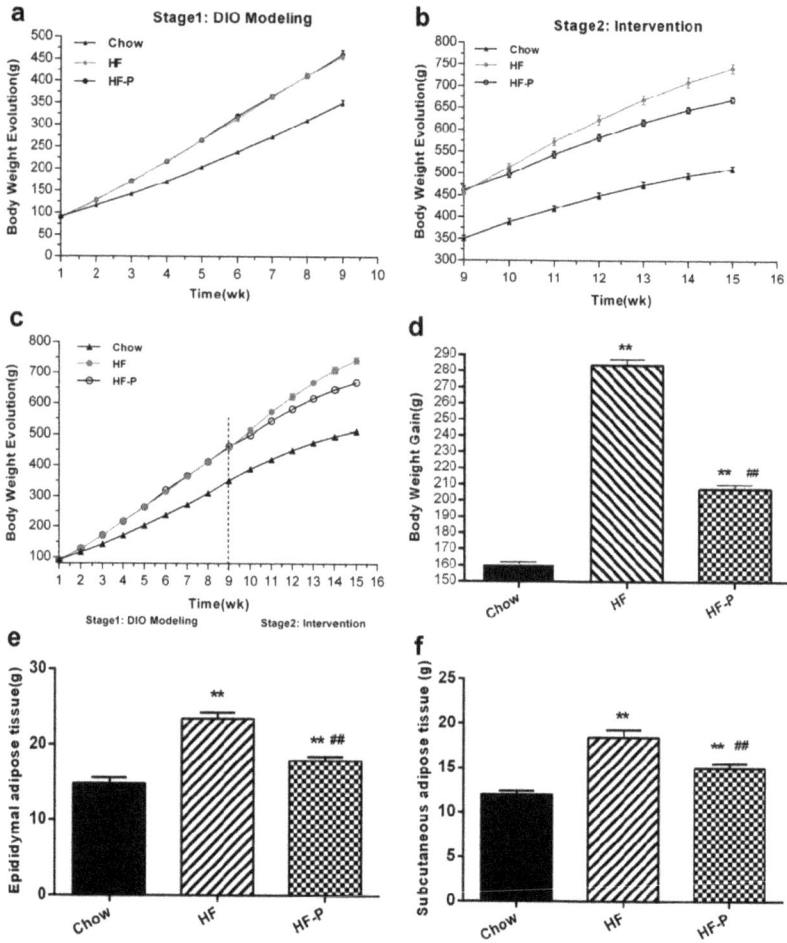

Figure 1. Apple-derived pectin suppresses body weight gain and development of adipose tissue in rats fed a high fat diet. (**a–c**) Growth curves; (**d**) body weight gain; (**e**) weight of epididymal adipose tissue; and (**f**) weight of subcutaneous adipose tissue of rats in Chow, high fat diet (HF), and high fat diet supplemented with pectin (HF-P) groups (** $p < 0.01$ *vs.* Chow, ## $p < 0.01$ *vs.* HF, one way analysis of variance (ANOVA)).

3.2. Apple-Derived Pectin Alleviated High Fat Diet Induced Hypercholesterolemia

Rats in the HF group exhibited higher levels of serum total cholesterol, triglycerides, glucose, and insulin than those in the Chow group (total cholesterol, 2.06 ± 0.26 mmol/L *vs.* 1.43 ± 0.16 mmol/L, $p < 0.01$; triglycerides, 1.31 ± 0.41 mmol/L *vs.* 0.57 ± 0.294 mmol/L, $p < 0.01$; glucose, 15.14 ± 3.85 mmol/L *vs.* 10.18 ± 0.35 mmol/L, $p < 0.01$; insulin, 6.49 ± 1.82 mmol/L *vs.* 3.07 ± 1.14 mmol/L, $p < 0.01$). Total cholesterol levels were significantly decreased in rats of the HF-P group as compared with those in the HF group (1.46 ± 0.13 mmol/L, $p < 0.01$), while serum triglycerides, fasting serum glucose, and insulin levels showed only a trend of decrease within the duration of the study (triglycerides, 1.02 ± 0.65 mmol/L *vs.* 1.31 ± 0.41 mmol/L, $p = 0.669$; glucose, 13.37 ± 1.32 mmol/L *vs.* 15.14 ± 3.85 mmol/L, $p = 0.607$; insulin, 3.75± 3.00 mmol/L *vs.* 6.49 ± 1.82 mmol/L, $p = 0.167$) (Figure 2).

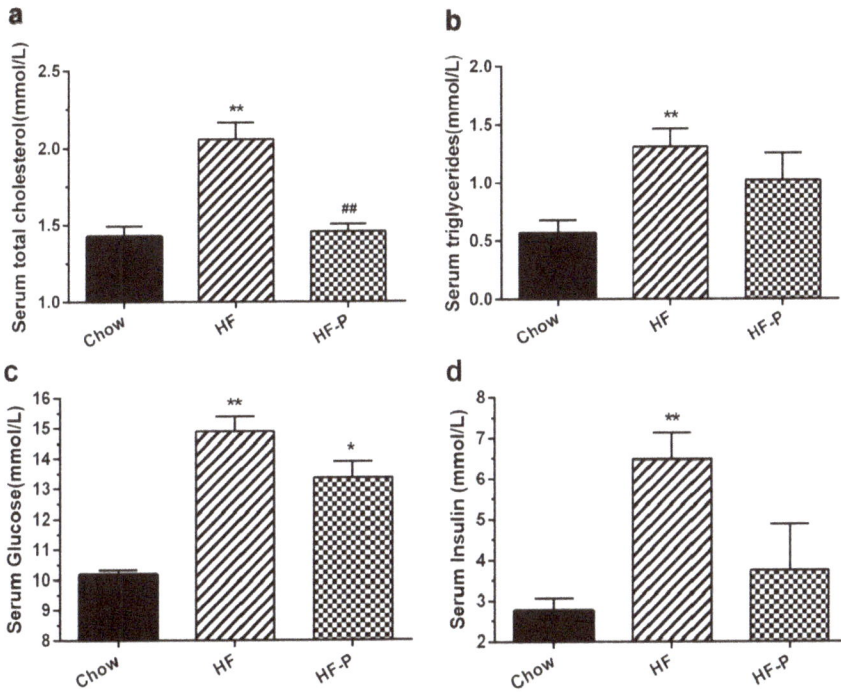

Figure 2. Effects of apple-derived pectin on HFD-induced changes in blood chemistry: (**a**) serum total cholesterol; (**b**) triglycerides; (**c**) glucose; and (**d**) insulin in Chow, HF, and HF-P groups. (** $p < 0.01$ *vs.* Chow, * $p < 0.05$ *vs.* Chow, ## $p < 0.01$ *vs.* HF, one way ANOVA).

3.3. Apple-Derived Pectin Prevented HFD-Induced Alterations of Gut Microbiota

Gut microbiota was analyzed by 16S rDNA pyrosequencing at the levels of phylum, class, order, family, genus and species (Figure 3). The number of reads per sample and raw data can be found in Supplementary Materials (Table S1).

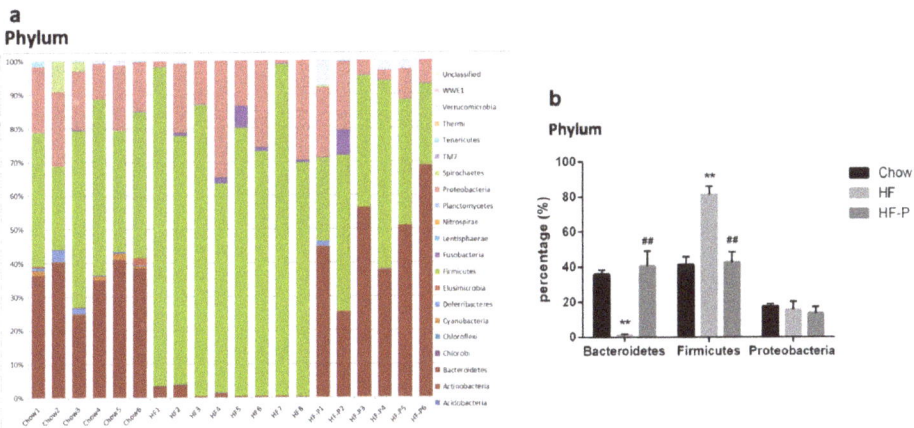

Figure 3. *Cont.*

c
Class

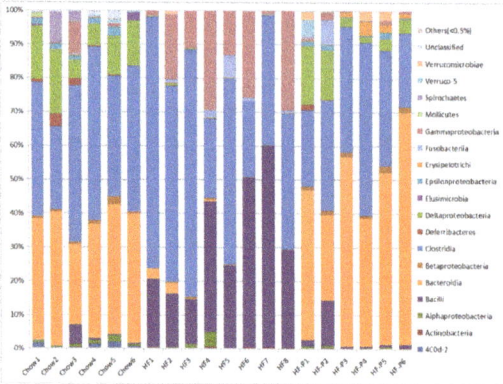

d
Class

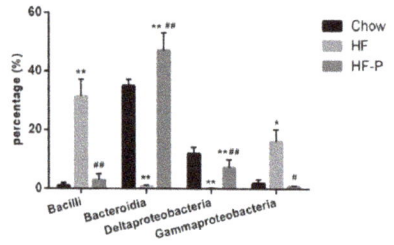

e
Order

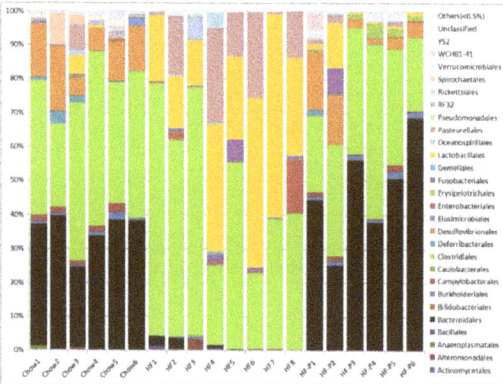

f
Order

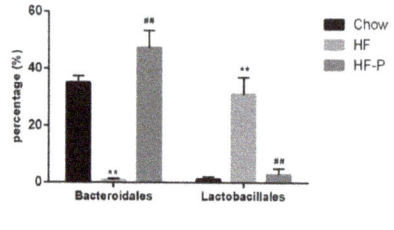

g
Family

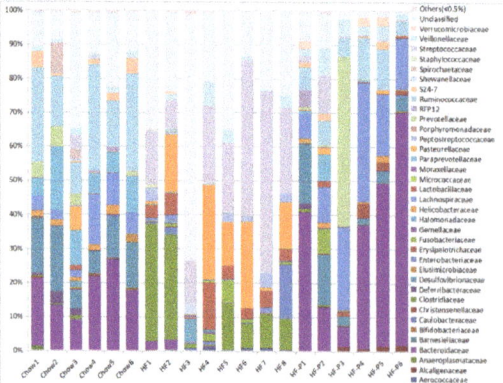

h
Family

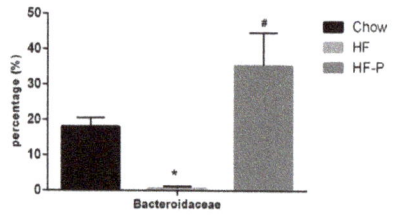

Figure 3. *Cont.*

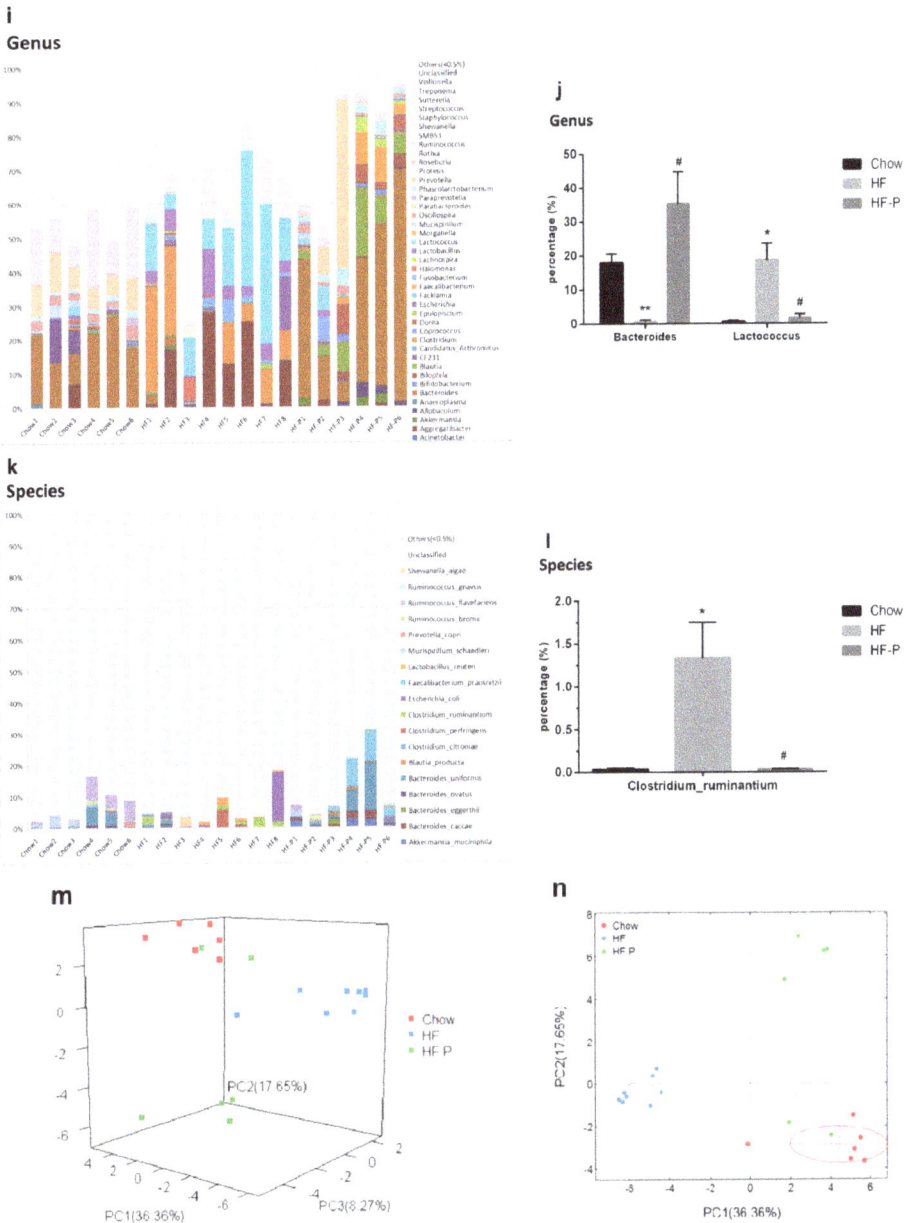

Figure 3. Composition analysis of gut microbiota at the: (**a**,**b**) phylum; (**c**,**d**) class; (**e**,**f**) order; (**g**,**h**) family; (**i**,**j**) genus; and (**k**,**l**) species level in Chow, HF, and HF-P groups; (**m**) Principal component analysis (PCA) and (**n**) clustering analysis of gut microbiota in Chow, HF, and HF-P groups (** $p < 0.01$ *vs.* Chow, * $p < 0.05$ *vs.* Chow, ## $p < 0.01$ *vs.* HF, # $p < 0.05$ *vs.* HF, one way ANOVA).

At the phylum level, rats in the HF group had a significantly lower level of Bacteroidetes and a higher level of Firmicutes than the Chow group. However, in the HF-P groups, these changes were restored to similar levels as the Chow group. There was no significant difference in the level of Proteobacteria among the three groups.

At the class level, rats in the HF group presented a significantly higher level of Bacilli (a class of Firmicutes phylum) and Gammaproteobacteria (a class of Proteobacteria phylum) as well as a significantly lower level of Bacteroidia (a class of Bacteroidetes phylum) and Deltaproteobacteria (a class of Proteobacteria phylum). The percentage levels of the above four classes of bacteria were reverted to normal in the HF-P group (Chow group as reference).

At the order level, we observed a significantly lower level of Bacteroidales (an order of Bacteroidia class, Bacteroidetes phylum) and a higher level of Lactobacillales (an order of Bacilli class, Firmicutes phylum) in the HF group than in the Chow group. After pectin supplementation for six weeks, the levels of the above two orders of bacteria in the HF-P group were similar to those in the Chow group.

At the family level, we observed a significantly lower level of Bacteroidaceae (a family of Bacteroidales order, Bacteroidia class, Bacteroidetes phylum) in the HF group than in the Chow group, and these decreases were restored to normal levels in the HF-P group.

At the genus level, we observed a dramatically lower level of *Bacteroides* (a genus of Bacteroidaceae family, Bacteroidales order, Bacteroidia class, Bacteroidetes phylum) and a higher level of *Lactococcus* (a genus of Streptococcaceae Family, Lactobacillales Order, Bacilli Class, Firmicutes Phylum) in the HF group than in the Chow group. Again, pectin supplementation prevented these changes induced by high fat diet.

At the species level, *Clostridium ruminantium* (a species of *Clostridium* Genus, Clostridiaceae Family, Clostridiales Order, Clostridia Class, Firmicutes Phylum) was the only species that displayed a significant increase upon high fat diet and became normal with pectin supplementation.

Accordingly, principal component analysis (PCA, Figure 3m) and clustering analysis (Figure 3n) illustrated both similarity and variance among the Chow, HF, and HF-P groups, where the first three components explained 62.28% of the total variance (36.36%, 17.65%, and 8.27% for PC1, PC2, and PC3, respectively). The score plot showed that diversity of gut microbiota was similar between the Chow and HF-P groups but different from the HF group.

Taken together, these data indicated that rats in the HF group exhibited a lower level of Bacteroidetes phylum and a higher level of Firmicutes phylum than those in the Chow group. Importantly, both of these changes were restored to normal levels in the HF-P group. At the downstream level, we found some changes consistent with the phylum level, such as higher levels in the HF group of the Bacilli class, Lactobacillales order, *Lactococcus* genus, *Clostridium ruminantium* species (belonging to the Firmicutes phylum), and a significantly lower level of Bacteroidia class, Bacteroidales order, Bacteroidaceae family, and *Bacteroides* genus (belonging to Bacteroidetes phylum). Supplementation of apple-derived pectin brought these changes back to normal levels (Chow group as reference).

3.4. Apple-Derived Pectin Restored the Expression of Intestinal Alkaline Phosphatase (IAP) in the Ileal Tissueof Rats on High Fat Diet

We measured the protein levels of IAP via immunoblotting and found that the expression of IAP in the ileal tissue of rats in the HF group was significantly lower than that in the Chow group (0.30 ± 0.19 *vs.* 1.00 ± 0.25, $p < 0.01$). Supplementation of pectin significantly increased the level of IAP in the ileal tissue of rats as compared with high fat diet alone (0.57 ± 0.20 *vs.* 0.30 ± 0.19, $p < 0.05$) (Figure 4).

Consist with the immunoblotting analysis of IAP, IHC analysis of IAP in the ileum also revealed that high fat diet reduced the expression of IAP in comparison with chow diet while supplementation of pectin could attenuate this reduction.

a

b

c

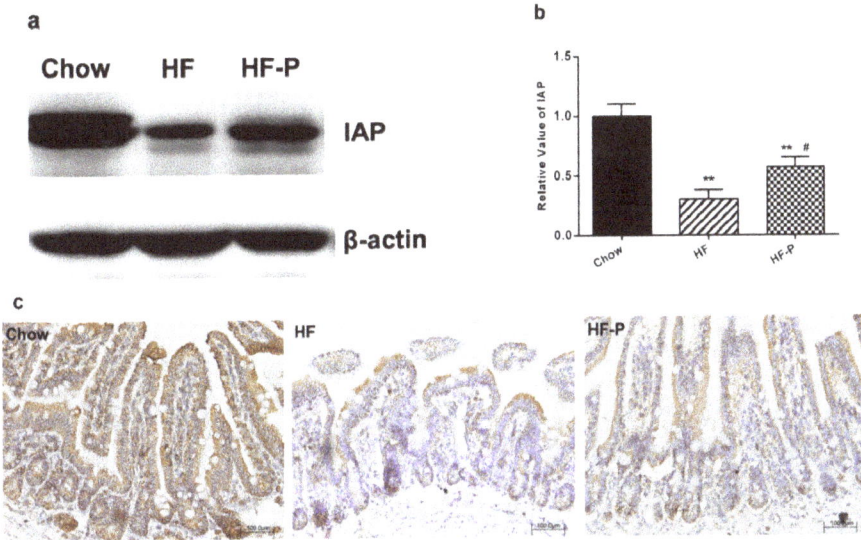

Figure 4. Expression of intestinal alkaline phosphatase (IAP) in the ileum of rats: (**a**) representative immunoblots for IAP and β-actin; (**b**) quantitation of IAP in the Chow, HF, and HF-P groups (** $p < 0.01$ vs. Chow, # $p < 0.05$ vs. HF, one way ANOVA); and (**c**) immunological histological chemistry analysis of IAP in Chow, HF, and HF-P groups. Original magnification: 20×.

3.5. Apple-Derived Pectin Prevented the High Fat Diet Induced mRNA Expression of TLR4 in the Ileal Issue

TLR4 mRNA levels in the ileal tissue of rats in the HF group were higher than those in the Chow group (2.04 ± 0.89 vs. 1.00 ± 0.49, $p < 0.05$). Pectin supplementation blunted this high fat diet induced increase of TLR4 mRNA in the HF-P group (0.76 ± 0.58 vs. 2.04 ± 0.89, $p < 0.01$) (Figure 5).

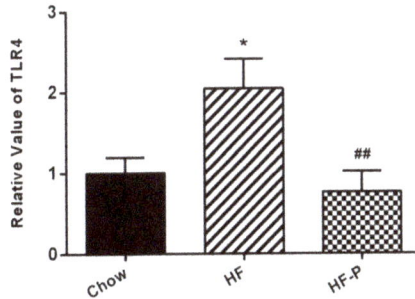

Figure 5. TLR4 mRNA expression in the ileal tissue of rats in the Chow, HF, and HF-P groups (* $p < 0.05$ vs. Chow, ## $p < 0.01$ vs. HF, one way ANOVA).

3.6. Apple-Derived Pectin Alleviated High Fat Diet Induced Ileal Inflammation in Rats

The levels of pro-inflammation markers were significantly higher in the ileal issue of the HF group than in the Chow group (tumor necrosis factor alpha (TNFα), 3.48 ± 0.71 vs. 1.00 ± 0.27, $p < 0.01$; interleukin (IL)-6, 2.59 ± 0.45 vs. 1.00 ± 0.25, $p < 0.01$). The level of anti-inflammation cytokine IL-10 in the ileal issue was significantly lower in the HF group than that in the Chow group (IL-10, 0.25 ± 0.04 vs. 1.00 ± 0.20, $p < 0.01$) (Figure 6). The levels of TNFα and IL-6 were significantly decreased in the HF-P group as compared with the HF group (TNFα, 1.55 ± 0.37 *vs.* 3.48 ± 0.71, *p* < 0.01; IL-6, 1.02 ± 0.17 *vs.* 2.59 ± 0.45, *p* < 0.01), and the level of IL-10 in the ileal tissue was significantly increased in the HF-P group as compared with the HF group (0.60 ± 0.054 *vs.* 0.25 ± 0.04, *p* < 0.01) (Figure 6).

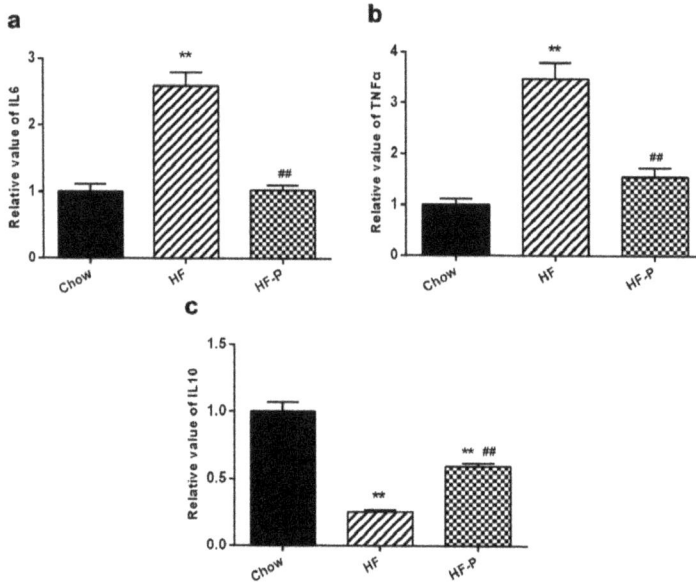

Figure 6. The mRNA levels of (**a**) tumor necrosis factor alpha (TNFα); (**b**) interleukin (IL)-6 and (**c**) IL-10 in the ileal tissue in Chow, HF, and HF-P groups (** *p* < 0.01 *vs.* Chow, ## *p* < 0.01 *vs.* HF, one way ANOVA).

3.7. Apple-Derived Pectin Preserved Gut Barrier (Tight Junction) Function in Rats

The expression levels of claudin1, occludin and zonula occludens-1 (ZO-1) proteins in rats of the HF group were significantly lower than those in the Chow group (claudin1, 0.55 ± 0.18 *vs.* 1.00 ± 0.22, *p* < 0.01; occludin, 0.36 ± 0.11 *vs.* 1.00 ± 0.23, *p* < 0.01; ZO-1, 0.24 ± 0.15 *vs.* 1.00 ± 0.40, *p* < 0.05). Supplementation of pectin significantly improved the level of claudin1 but only caused a tendency of increase in the levels of occludin and ZO-1 as compared with the high fat diet alone (claudin1, 0.76 ± 0.14 *vs.* 0.55 ± 0.18, *p* < 0.05; occludin, 0.57 ± 0.21 *vs.* 0.36 ± 0.11, *p* = 0.060; ZO-1, 0.52 ± 0.25 *vs.* 0.24 ± 0.15, *p* = 0.172) (Figure 7).

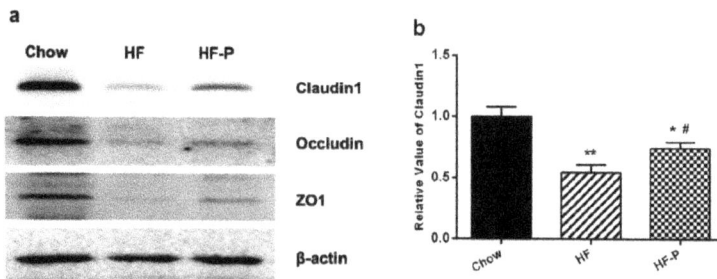

Figure 7. *Cont.*

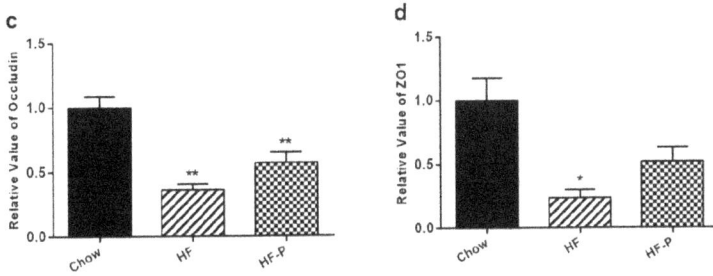

Figure 7. Expression levels of the tight junction proteins claudin1, occludin, and ZO-1. (a) Representative Western blots of claudin 1, occludin, and ZO1 with β-actin as a loading control; Quantitation of: (b) claudin 1; (c) occludin; and (d) ZO1 (** $p < 0.01$ *vs.* Chow, * $p < 0.05$ *vs.* Chow, # $p < 0.05$ *vs.* HF, one way ANOVA).

3.8. Apple-Derived Pectin Decreased High Fat Diet Induced Metabolic Endotoxemia

High fat diet caused a significant increase in the serum level of LPS as compared with chow diet (HF 2.83 ± 0.42 EU/mL *vs.* Chow 0.68 ± 0.14 EU/mL, $p < 0.01$) while supplementation of apple-derived pectin significantly decreased high fat diet induced LPS appearance in the serum (HF-P 2.09 ± 0.24 EU/mL *vs.* HF 2.83 ± 0.42 EU/mL, $p < 0.01$) (Figure 8).

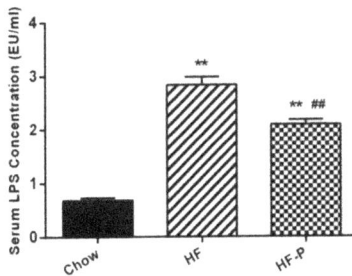

Figure 8. Serum LPS concentration (EU/mL) in Chow, HF, and HF-P groups. (** $p < 0.01$ *vs.* Chow, ## $p < 0.01$ *vs.* HF, one way ANOVA).

3.9. Apple-Derived Pectin Alleviated High Fat Diet Induced Systemic Inflammation in Rats

The levels of pro-inflammation cytokines (TNFα and IL-6) in the portal serum of rats in the HF group were higher than those in the Chow group (TNFα: 355.59 ± 8.10 EU/mL *vs.* 283.16 ± 7.28 EU/mL, $p < 0.01$; IL-6: 58.98 ± 2.59 EU/mL *vs.* 44.56 ± 3.67 EU/mL, $p < 0.01$). Serum TNFα and IL-6 in the HF-P group were decreased compared with those in the HF group (TNFα: 316.13 ± 7.62 EU/mL *vs.* 355.59 ± 8.10 EU/mL, $p < 0.01$; IL-6: 51.78 ± 2.35 EU/mL *vs.* 58.98 ± 2.59 EU/mL, $p < 0.01$) (Figure 9).

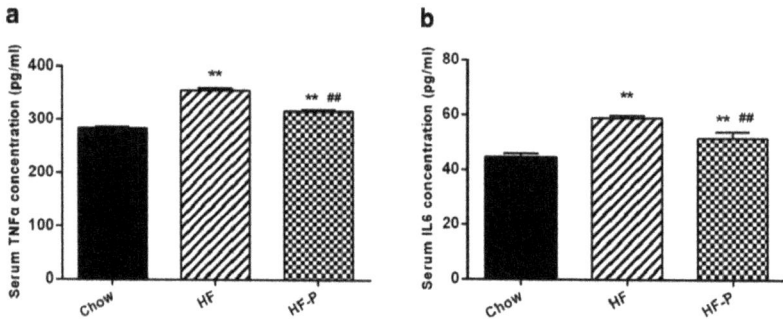

Figure 9. Portal serum levels of (**a**) TNFα and (**b**) IL-6 in Chow, HF, and HF-P groups (** $p < 0.01$ *vs.* Chow, ## $p < 0.01$ *vs.* HF, one way ANOVA).

4. Discussion

In this study, we found that rats fed with a high fat diet exhibited obvious increases of body weight and adipose tissue, disturbance of gut microbiota, gut barrier dysfunction, systemic chronic inflammation, and metabolic endotoxemia. However, these changes could be restored to normal levels by dietary supplementation with pectin. To the best of our knowledge, no previous study has investigated the potential effects of apple-derived pectin on obesity and how apple-derived pectin could modulate gut microbiota, gut barrier function, metabolic endotoxemia, and systemic inflammation in diet-induced obese rats.

Many studies have demonstrated that various types of dietary fiber play roles in anti-obesity and have hypoglycemic and hypolipidemic effects [31–35]. Similarly, we found in this study that supplementation with apple-derived pectin could significantly suppress weight gain and fat deposition in HFD fed rats. In addition, dyslipidemia, hyperglycemia, and hyperinsulinism caused by HFD were also alleviated with pectin supplementation to different extents.

In 2004, Gordon *et al.* first reported that gut microbiota modulated lipid metabolism, suppressed activity of genes involved in fat consumption, and improved the activity of genes involved in fat synthesis, which led to excessive fat synthesis and fat accumulation in mice. They also found that the presence of gut microbiota was necessary for obesity occurrence, as germ free animals did not get obese even when fed a HFD [37]. Since then, additional studies have demonstrated that gut microbiota is an important factor when assessing risk factors associated with obesity and related disorders, such as dyslipidemia, hyperglycemia, inflammation and diabetes. Thus, modulation of gut microbiota might be a novel approach to manage body weight and metabolic disorders [35,38–44].

Here, we found that Bacteroidetes phylum, a principal component of gut microbiota, as well as subordinate Bacteroidia class, Bacteroidales order, Bacteroidaceae family, and *Bacteroides* genus, decreased sharply in rats fed with a high fat diet as compared to rats fed a normal diet. However, Firmicutes phylum, another principal component of gut microbiota, as well as subordinate Bacilli class, Lactobacillales order, *Lactococcus* genus and *Clostridium ruminantium* species, increased significantly in the HF group. Supplementation with apple-derived pectin in HFD fed rats restored bacteria levels to normal ranges (Chow group as reference).

Interestingly, Gammaproteobacteria and Deltaproteobacteria, two classes from the Proteobacteria phylum, presented different alteration trends, where the former increased and the latter decreased in the HF group as compared to the Chow group. As a result, the total level of Proteobacteria at the phylum level was similar among the three groups. Nevertheless, both Gammaproteobacteria and Deltaproteobacteria were restored to normal levels after supplementation with pectin.

Although not unanimously recognized, obesity is generally characterized by an increased ratio of Firmicutes to Bacteroidetes [45,46]. Similarly, we found here an increased level of Firmicutes and a lower level of Bacteroidetes. A previous study showed that some Lactobacillus species were associated with normal weight *(Bifidobacterium animalis* (B. animalis)) while others *(Lactobacillus reuteri* (L. reuteri)) were associated with obesity [47]. In this study, we observed changes in the level of *L. reuteri* in Bacilli class, Lactobacillales order and *Lactococcus* genus, which were restored with pectin supplementation. In addition, we report here for the first time changes in *Clostridium ruminantium* species in rats fed with HFD and attenuation with pectin supplementation. This finding needs to be investigated further for verification.

In previous studies, the expression of IAP and the activation of TLR4 were increased in the ileal tissue of obese rats, showing that activation of TLR4 could alter tight junctions and increase intestinal permeability [48]. IAP is a type of glycoprotein anchored in the apical membrane of intestine by a glycosyl-phosphatidyl-inositol linkage, which plays an important role in gut barrier function, including detoxification of bacterial LPS and free nucleotides [49,50], remission of intestinal inflammation [27,51], and modulation of gut microbiota [52–55]. Intercellular tight junctions play an important role in the permeability properties of the gut barrier [17,26]. Tight junctions consist of transmembrane proteins (occludin, claudins, and junctional adhesion molecule (JAM)), junctional complex proteins (such as ZO-1, zonula occludens-2 (ZO-2), Symplekin, and cingulin), and actin cytoskeleton [56]. Transmembrane proteins act as a mediator in adhesion, gut barrier formation, selective paracellular diffusion, interaction with junctional complex proteins, and actin cytoskeleton, which is significant for the regulation of the permeability of gut barrier [26].

In this study, we observed that increased expression of TLR4 mRNA in the ileum tissue of HFD fed rats was blunted upon pectin supplementation (Figure 5). We also observed that expression of IAP as well as the tight junction proteins claudin 1, occludin, and ZO-1 were significantly reduced in comparison with the chow group (Figure 4). Notably, supplementation with pectin restored claudin 1 and IAP to normal levels, and caused a tendency of increase in the levels of occludin and ZO-1. One possible explanation for this ineffectiveness of pectin to restore occludin and ZO-1 is that the duration of HFD was too long so that the damage was irreversible. Taken together, our data suggest that apple-derived pectin improves gut barrier function and maintains the integrity of intestine.

In previous studies, inulin-type fructan and wheat-derived arabinoxylan oligosaccharides were shown to modulate gut microbiota in cecal content and increase integrated gut barrier function, leading to improvements in metabolic endotoxemia and inflammation [9,35,57]. In the present study, we observed that the level of endotoxin in the portal serum was significantly reduced with pectin supplementation (Figure 3). In addition, we observed that two pro-inflammatory factors, namely TNFα and IL-6, were downregulated in the portal serum upon pectin supplementation. The HFD-induced increase in TNFα and IL-6 mRNA in the ileal tissue was also blunted with pectin. Meanwhile, pectin upregulated the mRNA expression of the anti-inflammatory factor IL-10 in the ileal tissue of obese rats, increasing the anti-inflammatory effect. In accordance with a decrease in metabolic endotoxemia, we propose that the lower inflammatory tone observed upon pectin supplementation was due to modulation of inflammatory factors.

It is well known that inflammatory cytokines TNFα and IL-6 could cause insulin resistance [58–60]. Consist with the effects on TNFα and IL-6, pectin supplementation could mildly alleviate insulin resistance in HFD fed rats as evidenced by changes in serum total cholesterol, triglycerides, glucose and insulin ($p < 0.01$ for total cholesterol, however, only a trend for triglycerides, glucose, and insulin). These findings are consistent with other studies that showed consumption of different kinds of dietary fiber, such as fractionated yellow pea fiber, oligofructose, and grape skin extract could lower blood glucose levels in human subjects and rodents [33,34,61–63].

It is known that insulin functions to promote fat synthesis, transfer glucose into cells, and promote glycogen synthesis. In a state of hyperinsulinism and glycemia, more fat deposition occurs, leading to obesity. In accordance with our hypothesis, the increases in body weight and fat pad weight in the HF group were blunted with pectin supplementation.

This study demonstrated a complex link between obesity and gut microbiota, gut barrier, inflammation, and metabolic endotoxemia. The sequence of events could possibly occur as follows: modulation of gut microbiota, expression of IAP and TLR4, intestinal inflammation, altered gut barrier function (especially tight junction), change in serum LPS concentration, and, finally, increases in weight gain and development of adipose tissue (see Figure 10).

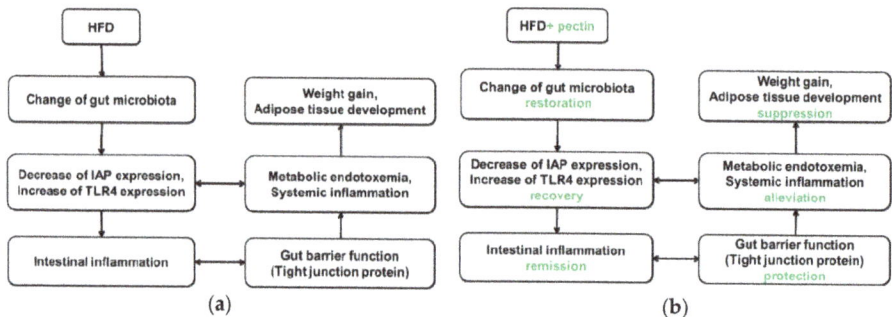

(a)   (b)

Figure 10. (a) Proposed model by which HFD leads to weight gain and adipose development. HFD leads to disturbance of gut microbiota, possibly by decreasing IAP expression and increasing TLR4 expression, which may result in metabolic endotoxemia and intestinal and systemic inflammation. Intestinal inflammation results in altered gut barrier function and promotes penetration of LPS from the lumen to the lamina propria. The precise mechanism by which metabolic endotoxemia leads to weight gain and adipose tissue development is not clear; (b) Proposed model by which supplementation of apple-derived pectin suppresses weight gain and adipose development. Pectin supplementation maintains gut microbiota, promoting recovery of IAP and TLR4 levels, which may alleviate metabolic endotoxemia and intestinal and systemic inflammation. Thus, gut barrier function is protected and penetration of LPS from the lumen to the lamina propria is suppressed. These events lead to suppression of weight gain and adipose development.

However, there are some limitations associated with our study, which warrants precautions in interpretation of the data. For instance, gut microbiota are different in human and rats, and our conclusion in rats may not be readily translatable into human. Given our positive results in rats, it is worthwhile to carry out clinical trials to properly address whether apple-derived pectin also has such beneficial effects in human. Moreover, since we did not transplant the possible "obesity-causing" microbiota to sterile rats for further verification, we could not establish causality between gut microbiota and obesity development. We also realize the potential limitation of our method for measurement of serum LPS. This method determines the bio-reactivity of LPS rather than its absolute quantity. Although the bio-reactivity of LPS in different groups of rats correlated with the changes in gut barrier function, we cannot rule out the possibility that changes in gut microbiota might directly cause the differences in the bio-reactivity of LPS in serum. Nevertheless, apple-derived pectin could alleviate HFD-induced metabolic endotoxemia.

5. Conclusions

In conclusion, this study demonstrated that apple-derived pectin could modulate gut microbiota, as previously shown for inulin-type fructan and wheat-derived arabinoxylan oligosaccharides [35,64]. Concomitantly, pectin supplementation alleviated HFD-induced body weight gain, fat mass development, dyslipidemia, hyperglycemia, hyperinsulinism, metabolic endotoxemia, and systemic inflammation in obese rats. In addition, expression of IAP and gut barrier function (tight junctions) were improved with pectin supplementation. These results indicate that apple-derived pectin might play a protective role with prebiotic properties in the prevention of obesity and associated metabolic and inflammatory disorders. Prospectively, it might become a useful tool for clinical management of patients with metabolic disorders.

Supplementary Materials: The following are available online at http://www.mdpi.com/2072-6643/8/3/126/s1, Table S1: Total pairs read number and raw data per sample.

Acknowledgments: We thank BGI laboratory for expert guidance in 16S rRNA Pyrosequencing and data analysis. We thank Jingcheng Bi, Qiaoli Chen, Liang Chen, Min Li, Chao Quan and Yang Sheng for their expert help with animal and biology experimentations. Thanks to the National Natural Science Foundation in China (81470797) and the Ministry of Science and Technology of China (Grant No. 2014BAI02B01 (the National Key Scientific Research Program of China)) for financial support.

Author Contributions: Tingting Jiang, Xuejin Gao, Chao Wu, Feng Tian, Qiucheng Lei and Xinying Wang conceived and designed the experiments. Tingting Jiang, Xuejin Gao, Chao Wu, Qiucheng Lei, Jingcheng Bi, and Bingxian Xie performed the experiment. Tingting Jiang and Feng Tian analyzed the data. Tingting Jiang and Xuejin Gao drafted the manuscript. Hong Yu Wang, Xinying Wang and Shuai Chen reviewed the manuscript. All authors read and approved the manuscript.

Conflicts of Interest: The authors declare no conflict of interest.

Abbreviations

The following abbreviations are used in this manuscript:

ANOVA	Analysis of variance
CHD	Coronary heart disease
HFD	High-fat diet
HF-P	High-fat diet supplemented with pectin
IAP	Intestinal alkaline phosphatase
IL	Interleukin
LPS	Lipopolysaccharide
T2DM	Type 2 diabetes mellitus
TLR4	Toll-like receptor 4
TNF	Tumor necrosis factor alpha

References

1. Hoyt, C.L.; Burnette, J.L.; Auster-Gussman, L. "Obesity is a disease": Examining the self-regulatory impact of this public-health message. *Psychol. Sci.* **2014**, *25*, 997–1002. [CrossRef]
2. Sassi, F.; Devaux, M.; Cecchini, M.; Rusticelli, E. *The Obesity Epidemic: Analysis of Past and Projected Future Trends in Selected OECD Countries*; Oecd Health Working Papers; Organisation for Economic Cooperation and Development (OECD): Paris, France, 2009.
3. Jensen, M.D.; Ryan, D.H.; Donato, K.A.; Apovian, C.M.; Ard, J.D.; Comuzzie, A.G.; Hu, F.B.; van Hubbard, S.; Jakicic, J.M.; Kushner, R.F.; *et al.* Executive summary: Guidelines (2013) for the management of overweight and obesity in adults. *Obesity* **2014**, *22*, S5–S39.
4. Yoshimoto, S.; Loo, T.M.; Atarashi, K.; Kanda, H.; Sato, S.; Oyadomari, S.; Iwakura, Y.; Oshima, K.; Morita, H.; Hattori, M.; *et al.* Obesity-induced gut microbial metabolite promotes liver cancer through senescence secretome. *Nature* **2013**, *499*, 97–101. [CrossRef] [PubMed]
5. Osborn, O.; Olefsky, J.M. The cellular and signaling networks linking the immune system and metabolism in disease. *Nat. Med.* **2012**, *18*, 363–374. [CrossRef] [PubMed]
6. Miele, L.; Valenza, V.; la Torre, G.; Montalto, M.; Cammarota, G.; Ricci, R.; Mascianà, R.; Forgione, A.; Gabrieli, M.L.; Perotti, G.; *et al.* Increased intestinal permeability and tight junction alterations in nonalcoholic fatty liver disease. *Hepatology* **2009**, *49*, 1877–1887. [CrossRef] [PubMed]
7. Backhed, F.; Manchester, J.K.; Semenkovich, C.F.; Gordon, J.I. Mechanisms underlying the resistance to diet-induced obesity in germ-free mice. *Proc. Natl. Acad. Sci. USA* **2007**, *104*, 979–984. [CrossRef] [PubMed]

8. Dumas, M.E.; Barton, R.H.; Toye, A.; Cloarec, O.; Blancher, C.; Rothwell, A.; Fearnside, J.; Tatoud, R.; Blanc, V.; Lindon, J.C.; *et al.* Metabolic profiling reveals a contribution of gut microbiota to fatty liver phenotype in insulin-resistant mice. *Proc. Natl. Acad. Sci. USA* **2006**, *103*, 12511–12516. [CrossRef] [PubMed]

9. Cani, P.D.; Neyrinck, A.M.; Fava, F.; Knauf, C.; Burcelin, R.G.; Tuohy, K.M.; Gibson, G.R.; Delzenne, N.M. Selective increases of bifidobacteria in gut microflora improve high-fat-diet-induced diabetes in mice through a mechanism associated with endotoxaemia. *Diabetologia* **2007**, *50*, 2374–2383. [CrossRef] [PubMed]

10. Cani, P.D.; Amar, J.; Iglesias, M.A.; Poggi, M.; Knauf, C.; Bastelica, D.; Neyrinck, A.M.; Fava, F.; Tuohy, K.M.; Chabo, C.; *et al.* Metabolic endotoxemia initiates obesity and insulin resistance. *Diabetes* **2007**, *56*, 1761–1772. [CrossRef] [PubMed]

11. Vijay-Kumar, M.; Aitken, J.D.; Carvalho, F.A.; Cullender, T.C.; Mwangi, S.; Srinivasan, S.; Sitaraman, S.V.; Knight, R.; Ley, R.E.; Gewirtz, A.T. Metabolic syndrome and altered gut microbiota in mice lacking Toll-like receptor 5. *Science* **2010**, *328*, 228–231. [CrossRef] [PubMed]

12. Frazier, T.H.; DiBaise, J.K.; McClain, C.J. Gut microbiota, intestinal permeability, obesity-induced inflammation, and liver injury. *JPEN J. Parenter. Enter. Nutr.* **2011**, *35* (Suppl. 5), 14S–20S. [CrossRef]

13. Teixeira, T.F.S.; Collado, M.C.; Ferreira, C.L.L.F.; Bressan, J.; Peluzio, M.D.C.G. Potential mechanisms for the emerging link between obesity and increased intestinal permeability. *Nutr. Res.* **2012**, *32*, 637–647. [CrossRef] [PubMed]

14. Jayashree, B.; Bibin, Y.S.; Prabhu, D.; Shanthirani, C.S.; Gokulakrishnan, K.; Lakshmi, B.S.; Mohan, V.; Balasubramanyam, M. Increased circulatory levels of lipopolysaccharide (LPS) and zonulin signify novel biomarkers of proinflammation in patients with type 2 diabetes. *Mol. Cell. Biochem.* **2014**, *388*, 203–210. [CrossRef] [PubMed]

15. Horton, F.; Wright, J.; Smith, L.; Hinton, P.J.; Robertson, M.D. Increased intestinal permeability to oral chromium (51 Cr)-EDTA in human Type 2 diabetes. *Diabet. Med.* **2014**, *31*, 559–563. [CrossRef] [PubMed]

16. Yang, P.J.; Yang, W.S.; Nien, H.C.; Chen, C.N.; Lee, P.H.; Yu, L.C.; Lin, M.T. Duodenojejunal bypass leads to altered gut microbiota and strengthened epithelial barriers in rats. *Obes. Surg.* **2015**. [CrossRef] [PubMed]

17. Turner, J.R. Intestinal mucosal barrier function in health and disease. *Nat. Rev. Immunol.* **2009**, *9*, 799–809. [CrossRef] [PubMed]

18. Ma, T.Y.; Anderson, J.M. Tight junctions and the intestinal barrier—Physiology of the gastrointestinal tract (fourth edition)—Chapter 61. *Physiol. Gastrointest. Tract.* **2006**, 1559–1594.

19. Ge, Y.; Ezzell, R.M.; Warren, H.S. Localization of endotoxin in the rat intestinal epithelium. *J. Infect. Dis.* **2000**, *182*, 873–881. [CrossRef] [PubMed]

20. Andreasen, A.S.; Krabbe, K.S.; Krogh-Madsen, R.; Taudorf, S.; Pedersen, B.K.; MøLler, K. Human endotoxemia as a model of systemic inflammation. *Curr. Med. Chem.* **2008**, *15*, 1697–1705. [CrossRef] [PubMed]

21. Marshall, J.C.; Walker, P.M.; Foster, D.M.; Harris, D.; Ribeiro, M.; Paice, J.; Romaschin, A.D.; Derzko, A.N. Measurement of endotoxin activity in critically ill patients using whole blood neutrophil dependent chemiluminescence. *Crit. Care* **2002**, *6*, 342–348. [CrossRef] [PubMed]

22. Hurley, J.C. Endotoxemia: Methods of detection and clinical correlates. *Clin. Microbiol. Rev.* **1995**, *8*, 268–292. [PubMed]

23. Manuel, F.R.J.; Montserrat, B.; Cristóbal, R.; Joan, V.; Abel, L.B.; Wifredo, R. CD14 monocyte receptor, involved in the inflammatory cascade, and insulin sensitivity. *J. Clin. Endocrinol. Metab.* **2003**, *88*, 1780–1784.

24. Sweet, M.J.; Hume, D.A. Endotoxin signal transduction in macrophages. *J. Leukoc. Biol.* **1996**, *60*, 8–26. [PubMed]

25. Cani, P.D.; Rodrigo, B.; Claude, K.; Aurélie, W.; Neyrinck, A.M.; Delzenne, N.M.; Burcelin, R. Changes in gut microbiota control metabolic endotoxemia-induced inflammation in high-fat diet-induced obesity and diabetes in mice. *Diabetes* **2008**, *57*, 1470–1481. [CrossRef] [PubMed]

26. Matter, K.; Aijaz, S.; Tsapara, A.; Balda, M.S. Mammalian tight junctions in the regulation of epithelial differentiation and proliferation. *Curr. Opin. Cell Biol.* **2005**, *17*, 453–458. [CrossRef] [PubMed]

27. Lalles, J.P. Intestinal alkaline phosphatase: Multiple biological roles in maintenance of intestinal homeostasis and modulation by diet. *Nutr. Rev.* **2010**, *68*, 323–332. [PubMed]

28. Hamarneh, S.R.; Mohamed, M.M.R.; Economopoulos, K.P.; Morrison, S.A.; Tanit, P.; Tantillo, T.J.; Gul, S.S.; Gharedaghi, M.H.; Tao, Q.; Kaliannan, K.; *et al.* A novel approach to maintain gut mucosal integrity using an oral enzyme supplement. *Ann. Surg.* **2014**, *260*, 706–715. [CrossRef] [PubMed]

29. Apovian, C.M.; Aronne, L.J.; Bessesen, D.H.; Nnell, M.E.; Hassan, M.M.; Uberto, P.; Ryan, D.H.; Still, C.D. Pharmacological management of obesity: An endocrine society clinical practice guideline. *J. Clin. Endocrinol. Metab.* **2015**, *100*, 342–362. [CrossRef] [PubMed]

30. National Institute for Health and Care Excellence. *Obesity Identification, Assessment and Management of Overweight and Obesity in Children, Young People and Adults*; National Institute for Health and Care Excellence (UK): London, UK, 2014.

31. Melanson, K.J.; Angelopoulos, T.J.; Nguyen, V.T.; Martini, M.; Zukley, L.; Lowndes, J.; Dube, T.J.; Fiutem, J.J.; Yount, B.W.; Rippe, J.M. Consumption of whole-grain cereals during weight loss: Effects on dietary quality, dietary fiber, magnesium, vitamin B-6, and obesity. *J. Am. Diet. Assoc.* **2006**, *106*, 1380–1388. [CrossRef] [PubMed]

32. Woo, M.N.; Bok, S.H.; Lee, M.K.; Kim, H.J.; Jeon, S.M.; Do, G.M.; Shin, S.K.; Ha, T.Y.; Choi, M.S. Anti-obesity and hypolipidemic effects of a proprietary herb and fiber combination (S & S PWH) in rats fed high-fat diets. *J. Med. Food.* **2008**, *11*, 169–178. [PubMed]

33. Shelly, H.; Corene, C.; Shi, S.; Xiuxiu, S.; Hoda, K.; Kequan, Z. Dietary supplementation of grape skin extract improves glycemia and inflammation in diet-induced obese mice fed a Western high fat diet. *J. Agric. Food Chem.* **2011**, *59*, 3035–3041.

34. Eslinger, A.J.; Eller, L.K.; Ra, R. Yellow pea fiber improves glycemia and reduces *Clostridium leptum* in diet-induced obese rats. *Nutr. Res.* **2014**, *34*, 714–722. [CrossRef] [PubMed]

35. Neyrinck, A.M.; van Hee, V.F.; Piront, N.; de Backer, F.; Toussaint, O.; Cani, P.D.; Delzenne, N.M. Wheat-derived arabinoxylan oligosaccharides with prebiotic effect increase satietogenic gut peptides and reduce metabolic endotoxemia in diet-induced obese mice. *Nutr. Diabetes* **2012**, *2*. [CrossRef] [PubMed]

36. Licht, T.R.; Hansen, M.; Bergstrom, A.; Poulsen, M.; Krath, B.N.; Markowski, J.; Dragsted, L.O.; Wilcks, A. Effects of apples and specific apple components on the cecal environment of conventional rats: Role of apple pectin. *BMC Microbiol.* **2010**, *10*, 13. [CrossRef] [PubMed]

37. Bäckhed, F.; Ding, H.; Wang, T.; Hooper, L.V.; Koh, G.Y.; Nagy, A.; Semenkovich, C.F.; Gordon, J.I. The gut microbiota as an environmental factor that regulates fat storage. *Proc. Natl. Acad. Sci. USA* **2004**, *101*, 15718–15723. [CrossRef] [PubMed]

38. Ley, R.E. Obesity and the human microbiome. *Curr. Opin. Gastroenterol.* **2010**, *26*, 5–11. [PubMed]

39. Delzenne, N.M.; Neyrinck, A.M.; Backhed, F.; Cani, P.D. Targeting gut microbiota in obesity: Effects of prebiotics and probiotics. *Nat. Rev. Endocrinol.* **2011**, *7*, 639–646. [CrossRef] [PubMed]

40. Delzenne, N.M.; Neyrinck, A.M.; Cani, P.D. Modulation of the gut microbiota by nutrients with prebiotic properties: Consequences for host health in the context of obesity and metabolic syndrome. *Microb. Cell Fact.* **2011**, *10* (Suppl. 1), S10.

41. Bäckhed, F.; Crawford, P.A. Coordinated regulation of the metabolome and lipidome at the host-microbial interface. *BBA Mol. Cell Biol. Lipids* **2010**, *1801*, 240–245.

42. Caesar, R.; Fak, F.; Backhed, F. Effects of gut microbiota on obesity and atherosclerosis via modulation of inflammation and lipid metabolism. *J. Intern. Med.* **2010**, *268*, 320–328. [CrossRef] [PubMed]

43. Diamant, M.; Blaak, E.E.; de Vos, W.M. Do nutrient-gut-microbiota interactions play a role in human obesity, insulin resistance and type 2 diabetes? *Obes. Rev.* **2011**, *12*, 272–281. [PubMed]

44. Geurts, L.; Lazarevic, V.; Derrien, M.; Everard, A.; van, R.M.; Knauf, C.; Valet, P.; Girard, M.; Muccioli, G.G.; François, P.; et al. Altered gut microbiota and endocannabinoid system tone in obese and diabetic leptin-resistant mice: Impact on apelin regulation in adipose tissue. *Front. Microbiol.* **2011**, *2*, 149. [PubMed]

45. Ley, R.E.; Backhed, F.; Turnbaugh, P.; Lozupone, C.A.; Knight, R.D.; Gordon, J.I. Obesity alters gut microbial ecology. *Proc. Natl. Acad. Sci. USA* **2005**, *102*, 11070–11075. [CrossRef] [PubMed]

46. Ley, R.E.; Turnbaugh, P.J.; Klein, S.; Gordon, J.I. Microbial ecology: Human gut microbes associated with obesity. *Nature* **2006**, *444*, 1022–1023. [CrossRef] [PubMed]

47. Million, M.; Maraninchi, M.; Henry, M.; Armougom, F.; Richet, H.; Carrieri, P.; Valero, R.; Raccah, D.; Vialettes, B.; Raoult, D. Obesity-associated gut microbiota is enriched in *Lactobacillus reuteri* and depleted in Bifidobacterium animalis and Methanobrevibacter smithii. *Int. J. Obes.* **2012**, *36*, 817–825. [CrossRef] [PubMed]

48. Kohler, H.; McCormick, B.A.; Walker, W.A. Bacterial-enterocyte crosstalk: Cellular mechanisms in health and disease. *J. Pediatr. Gastroenterol. Nutr.* **2003**, *36*, 175–185. [CrossRef] [PubMed]

49. Bentala, H.; Verweij, W.R.; der Vlag, A.H.-V.; van Loenen-Weemaes, A.M.; Meijer, D.K.; Poelstra, K. Removal of phosphate from lipid A as a strategy to detoxify lipopolysaccharide. *Shock* **2002**, *18*, 561–566. [CrossRef] [PubMed]

50. Rietschel, E.T.; Seydel, U.; Zähringer, U.; Schade, U.F.; Brade, L.; Loppnow, H.; Feist, W.; Wang, M.H.; Ulmer, A.J.; Flad, H.D.; *et al.* Bacterial endotoxin: Molecular relationships between structure and activity. *Infect. Dis. Clin. N. Am.* **1992**, *5*, 753–579.

51. Chen, K.T.; Malo, M.S.; Beasley-Topliffe, L.K.; Poelstra, K.; Millan, J.L.; Mostafa, G.; Alam, S.N.; Ramasamy, S.; Warren, H.S.; Hohmann, E.L.; *et al.* A role for intestinal alkaline phosphatase in the maintenance of local gut immunity. *Digestive Dis. Sci.* **2011**, *56*, 1020–1027. [CrossRef] [PubMed]

52. Bates, J.M.; Akerlund, J.; Mittge, E.; Guillemin, K. Intestinal alkaline phosphatase detoxifies lipopolysaccharide and prevents inflammation in zebrafish in response to the gut microbiota. *Cell Host Microbe* **2007**, *2*, 371–382. [CrossRef] [PubMed]

53. Lalles, J.P. Intestinal alkaline phosphatase: Novel functions and protective effects. *Nutr. Rev.* **2014**, *72*, 82–94. [CrossRef] [PubMed]

54. Bates, J.M.; Mittge, E.J.; Baden, K.N.; Cheesman, S.E.; Guillemin, K. Distinct signals from the microbiota promote different aspects of zebrafish gut differentiation. *Dev. Biol.* **2006**, *297*, 374–386. [CrossRef] [PubMed]

55. Goldberg, R.F.; Austen, W.G.; Xiaobo, Z.; Gitonga, M.; Golam, M.; Shaluk, B.; McCormack, M.; Eberlin, K.R.; Nguyen, J.T.; Tatlidede, H.S.; *et al.* Intestinal alkaline phosphatase is a gut mucosal defense factor maintained by enteral nutrition. *Proc. Natl. Acad. Sci. USA* **2008**, *105*, 3551–3556. [CrossRef] [PubMed]

56. Visser, J.; Rozing, J.; Sapone, A.; Lammers, K.; Fasano, A. Tight junctions, intestinal permeability, and autoimmunity: Celiac disease and type 1 diabetes paradigms. *Ann. N. Y. Acad. Sci.* **2009**, *1165*, 195–205. [CrossRef] [PubMed]

57. Cani, P.D.; Possemiers, S.; van de Wiele, T.; Guiot, Y.; Everard, A.; Rottier, O.; Geurts, L.; Naslain, D.; Neyrinck, A.; Lambert, D.M.; *et al.* Changes in gut microbiota control inflammation in obese mice through a mechanism involving GLP-2-driven improvement of gut permeability. *Gut* **2009**, *58*, 1091–1103. [CrossRef] [PubMed]

58. Ouchi, N. Adipokines in inflammation and metabolic disease. *Nat. Rev. Immunol.* **2011**, *11*, 85–97. [CrossRef] [PubMed]

59. Cai, D.; Yuan, M.; Frantz, D.F.; Melendez, P.A.; Hansen, L.; Lee, J.; Shoelson, S.E. Local and systemic insulin resistance due to hepatic activation of IKK- and NF-kB. *Nat. Med.* **2005**, *11*, 183–190. [PubMed]

60. Dandona, P.; Aljada, A.; Bandyopadhyay, A. Inflammation: the link between insulin resistance, obesity and diabetes. *Trends Immunol.* **2004**, *25*, 4–7. [PubMed]

61. Marinangeli, C.P.; Jones, P.J. Whole and fractionated yellow pea flours reduce fasting insulin and insulin resistance in hypercholesterolaemic and overweight human subjects. *Br. J. Nutr.* **2011**, *105*, 110–117. [CrossRef] [PubMed]

62. Galvao Candido, F.; Silva Ton, W.T.; Alfenas, R.C.G. Addition of dietary fiber sources to shakes reduces postprandial glycemia and alters food intake. *Nutr. Hosp.* **2014**, *31*, 299–306. [PubMed]

63. Bomhof, M.R.; Saha, D.C.; Reid, D.T.; Paul, H.A.; Reimer, R.A. Combined effects of oligofructose and Bifidobacterium animalis on gut microbiota and glycemia in obese rats. *Obesity* **2014**, *22*, 763–771. [PubMed]

64. Roberfroid, M.; Gibson, G.R.; Hoyles, L.; McCartney, A.L.; Rastall, R.; Rowland, I.; Wolvers, D.; Watzl, B.; Szajewska, H.; Stahl, B.; *et al.* Prebiotic effects: metabolic and health benefits. *Br. J. Nutr.* **2010**, *104* (Suppl. 2), S1–S63. [CrossRef] [PubMed]

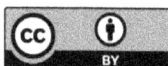

nutrients

MDPI

Article

Allomyrina Dichotoma Larvae Regulate Food Intake and Body Weight in High Fat Diet-Induced Obese Mice Through mTOR and Mapk Signaling Pathways

Jongwan Kim [1], Eun-Young Yun [2], Seong-Won Park [3], Tae-Won Goo [4,*] and Minchul Seo [2,*]

[1] Department of Anatomy, Graduate School of Dongguk University College of Medicine, Gyeongju 38066, Korea; kimjw3189@naver.com
[2] Department of Agricultural Biology, National Academy of Agricultural Science, RDA, Wanju-gun 55365, Korea; yuney@korea.kr
[3] Department of Biotechnology, Catholic University of Daegu, Daegu 38430, Korea; microsw@cu.ac.kr
[4] Department of Biochemistry, Dongguk University College of Medicine, Gyeongju 38066, Korea
* Correspondence: gootw@dongguk.ac.kr (T.-W.G.); nansmc@hanmail.net (M.S.); Tel.: +82-54-703-7801 (T.-W.G.); +82-63-238-2980 (M.S.)

Received: 22 December 2015; Accepted: 4 February 2016; Published: 18 February 2016

Abstract: Recent evidence has suggested that *the Korean horn beetle (Allomyrina dichotoma)* has anti-hepatofibrotic, anti-neoplastic, and antibiotic effects and *is* recognized as a traditional medicine. In our previous works, *Allomyrina dichotoma* larvae (ADL) inhibited differentiation of adipocytes both *in vitro* and *in vivo*. However, the anorexigenic and endoplasmic reticulum(ER) stress-reducing effects of ADL in obesity has not been examined. In this study, we investigated the anorexigenic and ER stress-reducing effects of ADL in the hypothalamus of diet-induced obese (DIO) mice. Intracerebroventricular (ICV) administration of ethanol extract of ADL (ADE) suggested that an antagonizing effect on ghrelin-induced feeding behavior through the mTOR and MAPK signaling pathways. Especially, ADE resulted in strong reduction of ER stress both *in vitro* and *in vivo*. These findings strongly suggest that ADE and its constituent bioactive compounds are available and valuable to use for treatment of various diseases driven by prolonged ER stress.

Keywords: *Allomyrina dichotoma* larvae; diet-induced obesity; ER stress; hypothalamus; appetite

1. Introduction

Obesity is widely recognized as the largest and fastest growing public health problem in the world. Obesity is caused by an imbalance between energy intake and expenditure and results in major comorbidities, including metabolic syndrome, hypertension, type 2 diabetes, stroke, cancer, and dyslipidemia [1–3]. Although anti-obesity drugs were heralded as an answer to the obesity problem in the past, they have demonstrated inconsistency and side effects. Therefore, new treatments for obesity that are both better tolerated and more efficacious are urgently needed. For decades, bioactive products have been identified and isolated from a variety of sources such as living organisms and are widely used in traditional medicine and the food industry [4,5]. Among them, insects have gained attention as a source of effective bioactive products [6]. Although there is a lack of scientific evidence regarding the safety and beneficial effects of insects, numerous insect species are used as a traditional food or medicine in many countries.

Allomyrinal dichotoma (A. dichotoma) is a species of rhinoceros beetle and widely used in traditional medicine for its anti-diabetic, anti-hepatofibrotic, anti-neoplastic, and anti-obesity effects [4,5,7,8]. The Food and Agriculture Organization of the United Nations (FAO) reported the possibility of using edible insects in human dietary supplements in the future. Despite growing interest in insect-based bioactive products, the biological activities of insect-based products have rarely been studied. In previous studies, we reported that *A. dichotoma* larvae (ADL) inhibit *in vitro* and *in vivo* differentiation of adipocytes via downregulation of transcription factors, peroxisome proliferator-activated receptor-γ (PPARγ), and CCAAT/enhancer binding protein-α (C/EBPα) [7,9].

The hypothalamus plays a central role in the regulation of feeding behavior and energy balance by controlling appetite regulatory neuropeptides and specific neuronal excitations [10,11]. However, disruption of these physiological functions of the hypothalamus has been implicated in various diseases, such as diabetes mellitus, neurodegenerative disease, ischemia, prion disease, and cystic fibrosis [12,13]. In particular, hypothalamic ER stress has been suggested to cause feeding behavior disorder and glucose dysregulation for promotion of obesity and diabetes [14–16]. Therefore, sustaining the functional roles of hypothalamic neurons may be beneficial for hypothalamic regulation of energy balance.

In the present study, we investigated the appetite regulatory effect of natural products extracted from *A. dichotoma* larvae (ADE) on the hypothalamus, a section of the brain responsible for homeostasis, of high-fat-induced obese mice since there has been no study elucidating the direct effect of ADE on appetite control in the hypothalamus. We determined food intake, body weight, appetite regulatory neuropeptides, and ER stress in mice fed high-fat diets with or without ADE. Our results demonstrate the potential of ADE as a novel treatment option for anorexigenic function in high-fat-induced obese mice via reduction of ER stress.

2. Materials and Methods

2.1. Reagents and Cells

DMSO was purchased from Sigma-Aldrich (Sigma-Aldrich, St Louis, MO, USA). QGreenTM 2X SybrGreen qPCR Master Mix was purchased from CellSafe (CellSafe, Suwon, Korea). Mouse hypothalamic GT1-7 cells were maintained in Dulbecco's modified Eagle's media (Gibco, Rockville, MD, USA) supplemented with 10% heat-inactivated fetal bovine serum (FBS) (Gibco, Grand Island, NY, USA), 100 U/mL of penicillin, and 100 μg/mL of streptomycin (Gibco, Grand Island, NY, USA).

2.2. Preparation of Allomyrina Dichotoma Larvae Extract (ADE)

Freeze-dried ADL (fdADL), ground to a powder and sterilized, was provided by World Way Co. (Yeongi, Korea). fdADL was mixed with ethanol (1 g of fdADL/mL of ethanol) and incubated at RT for 30 min after ultrasonication (250 J, 10 s, two times). After incubation, the supernatant was filtered and completely dried using a rotary evaporator. Dried ethanol extract of ADL was dissolved in 20% DMSO.

2.3. MTT Assay

Cell viability was determined by 3-(4,5-dimet hylthiazol-2-yl)-2,5-diphenyltetrazolium bromide (MTT) assay. Hypothalamic neuronal GT1-7 cells were seeded in triplicate at a density of 1×10^4 cells per well on a 96-well plate. After treatment, culture media were removed and MTT (0.5 mg/mL) added, followed by incubation at 37 °C for 2 h in a CO_2 incubator. After dissolving the insoluble crystals that formed in DMSO, absorbance was measured at 570 nm using a microplate reader (Anthos Labtec Instruments, Wals, Austria).

2.4. Mice

Male C57BL/6J mice (7 weeks of age) were obtained from Japan SLC (Hamamatsu, Japan). Mice were allowed free access to standard chow diet and water for 1 week. To generate diet-induced obesity (DIO), 8-week-old mice were fed a high-fat diet (HFD, 60% fat, D12492; Research Diets, New Brunswick, NJ, USA) for 8 weeks. Lean control mice were fed a low-fat diet (LFD, 10% fat, D12450B; Research Diets) for the same period. The mice were placed in a controlled temperature room (23 °C) with a 12-h light/12-h dark cycle with free access to food and water. All procedures followed the Principles of Laboratory Animal Care (NIH, Washington, DC, USA) and were approved by the Institution Animal Care and Use Committee of College of Medicine, Dongguk University.

2.5. Intracerebro-Ventricular Cannulation and ADE Administration

Mice were implanted with a 26-gauge stainless guide cannular (5 mm bellow pedestal; C315G, Plastics one, Roanoke, VA, USA) into the third ventricle under stereotaxic control using a stereotaxic apparatus (coordinates from Bregma: anteroventral, -1.8 mm; lateral, 0.0 mm; dorsoventral, 5.0 mm) through a hole created in the skull with a micro driller. The cannula was secured to the skull with dental cement and capped with a dummy cannular (C315DC, Plastic one) that extended 0.5 mm below the guide cannular. Animals were weighed daily, and any animal showing signs of illness or weight loss was removed from the study and euthanized. At 7 days after ICV cannulation, HFD ($n = 20$) and LFD ($n = 20$) mice were divided into two groups. The first group of HFD ($n = 10$) and LFD mice ($n = 10$) was infused with 1 μL of 20% DMSO as a vehicle, whereas the second group of HFD ($n = 10$) and LFD ($n = 10$) mice was infused with 1 μL of ADE (10 mg/mL). All ICV injections were made using a 33-gauge internal cannular (C315I, Plastic one) that extended 0.5 mm below the guide cannular, connected by a cannular connector to a 5 μL Hamilton syringe and infused over 5 min. At 12 h after ADE infusion, hypothalamus were dissected and flash frozen in liquid nitrogen and kept in $-80\ ^\circ$C until further processing.

2.6. Western Blot Analysis

Tissue or cells were lysed in RIPA lysis buffer (50 mM Tris-HCl, pH 8.0, 150 mM NaCl, 0.02% sodium azide, 0.1% SDS, 1% NP-40, 0.5% sodium deoxycholate, and 1 mM phenylmethylsulfonyl fluoride). Protein concentrations of cell lysates were measured using a Bio-Rad protein assay kit (Bio-Rad, Hercules, CA, USA). Equal amounts of protein were separated by 8% or 12% SDS-PAGE and transferred to PVDF membranes (Bio-rad, Hercules, CA, USA). Membranes were blocked with 5% skim milk and sequentially incubated with primary antibodies (mouse monoclonal anti-CHOP antibody (1:1000; Cell Signaling Technology, Danvers, MA, USA); rabbit polyclonal anti-phospho-eIF2α antibody (1:1000; Cell Signaling Technology, Danvers, MA, USA); rabbit polyclonal anti-eIF2α antibody (1:1000; Cell Signaling Technology, Danvers, MA, USA); mouse monoclonal anti-Ero1L antibody (1:1000; Abnova, Taipei, Taiwan); mouse monoclonal anti-PDI antibody (1:1000; Enzo Life Sciences, Inc., Plymouth Meeting, PA, USA); rabbit monoclonal anti-phospho-Stat3 (Tyr705) (1:1000; Cell Signaling Technology, Danvers, MA, USA); mouse monoclonal anti-Stat3 (1:1000; Cell Signaling Technology, Danvers, MA, USA); rabbit polyclonal anti-SOCS3 antibody (1:1000; Cell Signaling Technology, Danvers, MA, USA); α-tubulin antibody (1:2000; Sigma-Aldrich, St Louis, MO, USA), and HRP-conjugated secondary antibody (1:10,000; anti-mouse and rabbit-IgG antibody; Amersham Biosceinces, Piscataway, NJ, USA)), followed by detection using an ECL detection kit (Invitrogen, Waltham, MA, USA).

2.7. Reverse Transcription-PCR

Total RNA was extracted from tissue or cells with an RNeasy Mini Kit (Qiagen, Hilden, Germany), according to the manufacturer's instructions. An aliquot of RNA was subjected to 1% agarose gel electrophoresis to confirm integrity. cDNA was synthetized with M-MLV Reverse Transcriptase (Promega, Madison, WI, USA) and oligo(dT) primers after DNase I treatment (Invitrogen, Life Technologies). Real-time PCR was performed using the specific primer set in Table 1. Traditional PCR amplification was carried out at an annealing temperature of 60 $^\circ$C for 27 cycles using the specific primer set in Table 1. For analysis of PCR products, 10 μL of each PCR product was electrophoresed on a 1%–2.5% agarose gel and detected under UV light. Gapdh was used as an internal control.

Table 1. DNA primers for PCR.

Mouse cDNAs	Primer Sequences	GenBank Accession No.
	For Real-time PCR	
Xbp-1s	Forward, 5′-AGGCTTGGTGTATACATGG-3′ Reverse, 5′-GGTCTGCTGAGTCCGCAGCAGG-3′	NM_013842
Atf4	Forward, 5′-GCAAGGAGGATGCCTTTTC-3′ Reverse, 5′-GTTTCCAGGTCATCCATTCG-3′	NM_009716
Chop	Forward, 5′-CCACCACACCTGAAAGCAGAA-3′ Reverse, 5′-AGGTGAAAGGCAGGGACTCA-3′	NM_007837
Grp78	Forward, 5′-GGCCTGCTCCGAGTCTGCTTC-3′ Reverse, 5′-CCGTGCCCACATCCTCCTTCT-3′	NM_022310
Erdj4	Forward, 5′-CCCCAGTGTCAAACTGTACCAG-3′ Reverse, 5′-AGCGTTTCCAATTTTCCATAAATT-3′	NM_013760
Agrp	Forward, 5′-TAGATCCACAGAACCGCGAGT-3′ Reverse, 5′-GAAGCGGCAGTAGCACGTA-3′	NM_007427
Npy	Forward, 5′-CTCCGCTCTGCGACACTAC-3′ Reverse, 5′-AGGGTCTTCAAGCCTTGTTCT-3′	NM_023456
Pomc	Forward, 5′-CTGGAGACGCCCGTGTTTC-3′ Reverse, 5′-TGGACTCGGCTCTGGACTG-3′	NM_001278584
Socs3	Forward, 5′-GAGTACCCCCAAGAGAGCTTACTA-3′ Reverse, 5′-CTCCTTAAAGTGGAGCATCATACTG-3′	NM_007707
Gapdh	Forward, 5′-CTTCAACAGCAACTCCCACTCTTCC-3′ Reverse, 5′-TGGGTGGTCCAGGGTTTCTTACTCCTT-3′	NM_001289726
	For Traditional PCR	
Xbp-1	Forward, 5′-CAACCAGGAGTTAAGAACACG-3′ Reverse, 5′-AGGCAACAGTGTCAGAGTCC-3′	NM_013842
Atf4	Forward, 5′-GACCTGGAAACCATGCCAGA-3′ Reverse, 5′-TGGCTGCTGTCTTGTTTTGC-3′	NM_009716
Chop	Forward, 5′-TCCCCAGGAAACGAAGAGGA-3′ Reverse, 5′-TTGAGCCGCTCGTTCTCTTC-3′	NM_007837
Gapdh	Forward, 5′-GACCACAGTCCATGCCATCA-3′ Reverse, 5′-CATTGAGAGCAATGCCAGCC-3′	NM_001289726

2.8. Data Analysis

All data are presented as the means ± SDs. Comparisons between two groups were performed using the Student's *t*-test. Comparisons between three or more groups were analyzed using one-way ANOVA with Dunnett experiments. SPSS version 18.0 K (SPSS Inc., Chicago, IL, USA) was used for the analysis, and *p* value differences of < 0.05 were considered statistically significant.

3. Results

3.1. High Fat Diet-Induced Obesity Induces Hypothalamic Endoplasmic Reticulum Stress

To examine whether obesity induces ER stress in hypothalamus, we fed male C57BL/6J mice a high-fat diet (HFD; 60% kcal from fat) and low-fat diet (LFD; 10% kcal from fat) for 8 weeks (Figure 1A). Body weight significantly increased in high-fat-diet-induced mice during the study period compared with low-fat-diet-induced mice (Figure 1B). We then performed quantitative PCR analysis of ER stress responsive markers, such as spliced X-box binding protein 1 (*Xbp-1s*), activating transcription factor 4 (*Atf4*), c/EBP-homologous protein (*Chop*), 78 kDa glucose-regulated protein (*Grp78*), and ER *DnaJ* homolog 4 (*Erdj4*), after mRNA isolation from the hypothalamus of mice fed a high-fat diet or low-fat diet for 8 weeks. The expression levels of ER stress responsive markers were dramatically upregulated in high-fat-diet-induced mice (Figure 1C). Taken together, these results indicate that the persistence of obesity gradually induces ER stress, followed by activation of the UPR signaling pathway in the hypothalamus.

3.2. Central Administration of ADE Reduces Food Intake and Body Weight through Regulation of Appetite-Related Neuropeptides in High Fat Diet-Induced Mice

To examine the possibility that ADE as a natural food supplement can regulate appetite, we tested cytotoxicity of ADE before central administration using hypothalamic neuronal GT1-7 cells. The cytotoxicity of ADE was determined by 3-(4,5-dimethylthiazol-2-yl)-2,5-diphenyltetrazolium bromide (MTT) assay after treatment with various concentrations of ADE (0.01–5 mg/mL). As a result, up to 5 mg/mL of ADE showed no cytotoxic effect on hypothalamic neuronal GT1-7 cells [17]. To determine whether or not central administration of ADE regulates food intake and body weight in high-fat-diet-induced mice, we administrated a single dose of ADE (1 μL of 10 mg/mL ADE) into the third ventricle. Administration of ADE significantly reduced food intake and body weight during 24 h compared to the vehicle control, which was evident 2 h after infusion and was consistent after 24 h (Figure 2A,B, Supplementary Figure S1A,B). Next, we evaluated whether or not the anorexigenic action of ADE is associated with changes in ARC-derived neuropeptides. As shown in Figure 2C, central administration of ADE decreased the mRNA expression levels of *Agrp* and *Npy*, whereas *Pomc* expression increased in high-fat-diet-induced mice. However, low-fat-diet-induced mice showed no changes (Supplementary Figure S1C).

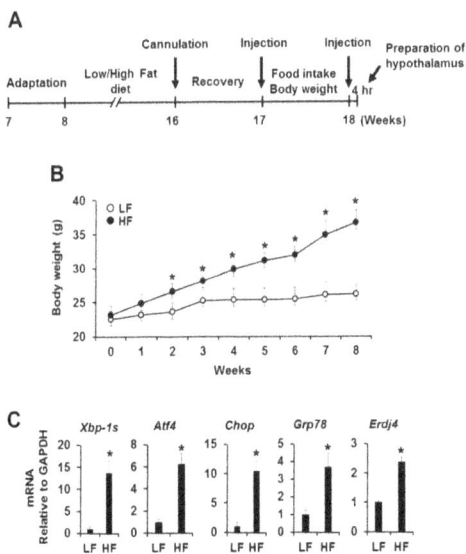

Figure 1. Increased hypothalamic ER stress in mice fed a high-fat diet. (**A**) Experimental timeline of the experimental procedure; (**B**) Time dependence of body weight in low fat and high-fat-diet-induced mice. At 8 weeks of age, mice fed a high-fat diet showed a 43% increase in body weight compared with those fed a low-fat diet. The results are means ± SDs (*n* = 10); * *p* values of < 0.05 indicate significant difference from low-fat diet-induced mice; (**C**) mRNA expression levels of ER stress responsive markers in low fat and high-fat-diet-induced mice. mRNA expression levels of ER stress responsive markers were dramatically upregulated in high-fat-diet-induced obese mice. The results are means ± SDs (*n* = 10); * *p* values of < 0.05 indicate significant difference from low-fat-diet-induced mice. LF, low-fat diet. HF, high-fat diet.

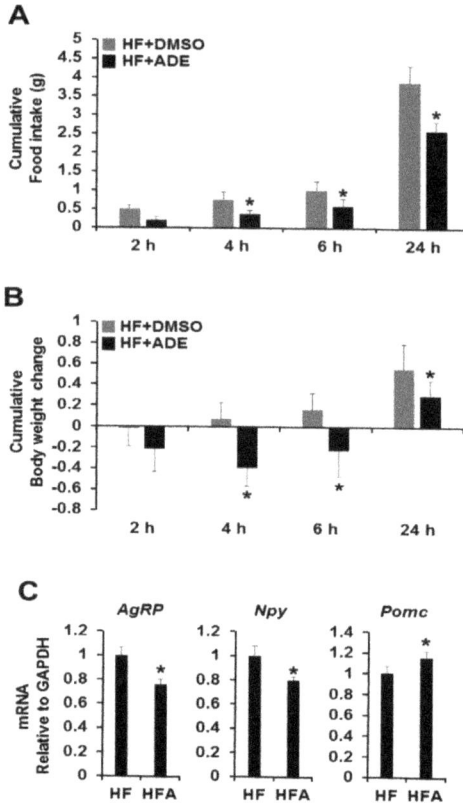

Figure 2. Effects of central administration of ADE on food intake and body weight. The average cumulative food intake (**A**) and body weight (**B**) were measured in high-fat-diet-induced mice ICV administration with ADE (1 µL of 10 mg/mL) or DMSO (1 µL of 20% DMSO) during the experimental period. The results are means ± SDs (*n* = 10 per group); * *p* values of < 0.05 indicate significant difference from administration with DMSO (1 µL of 20% DMSO). (**C**) Effects of ICV administration of ADE (1 µL of 10 mg/mL) on hypothalamic mRNA expression levels of neuropeptides. The results are means ± SDs (*n* = 10 per group); * *p* values of < 0.05 indicate significant difference from administration with DMSO (1 µL of 20% DMSO). ADE, ethanol extract of *Allomyrina dichotoma* larvae. HF, high-fat diet with DMSO. HFA, high-fat diet with ADE.

3.3. Central Administration of ADE Reduces Hypothalamic Endoplasmic Reticulum Stress

In previous works, under diet-induced obesity (DIO) conditions, orexigenic neuropeptides (AgRP and NPY) were induced while anorexigenic neuropeptides (α-MSH) were reduced by hypothalamic ER stress [18–20]. To examine whether or not ADE can regulate hypothalamic ER stress in high-fat-diet-induced mice, we administrated ADE and vehicle control into the third ventricle of high fat or low-fat-diet-induced obese mice. Expression levels of ER stress responsive markers (phosphor-eIF2a and CHOP) and ER chaperone/foldases (Bip, Ero1L, and PDI) were dramatically reduced in the hypothalamus in high fat diet-induced obese mice (Figure 3A). Furthermore, mRNA expression levels of ER stress responsive genes (*Xbp-1s*, *Atf4*, *Chop*, *Grp78*, and *Erdj4*) were significantly reduced in ADE-administrated high fat diet-induced obese mice compared with vehicle control (Figure 3B). However, low-fat-diet-induced mice showed no changes due to lack of ER stress

(Supplementary Figures S2A,B and S3). These results indicate that ADE can forcefully reduce ER stress induced by a high-fat diet in the hypothalamus.

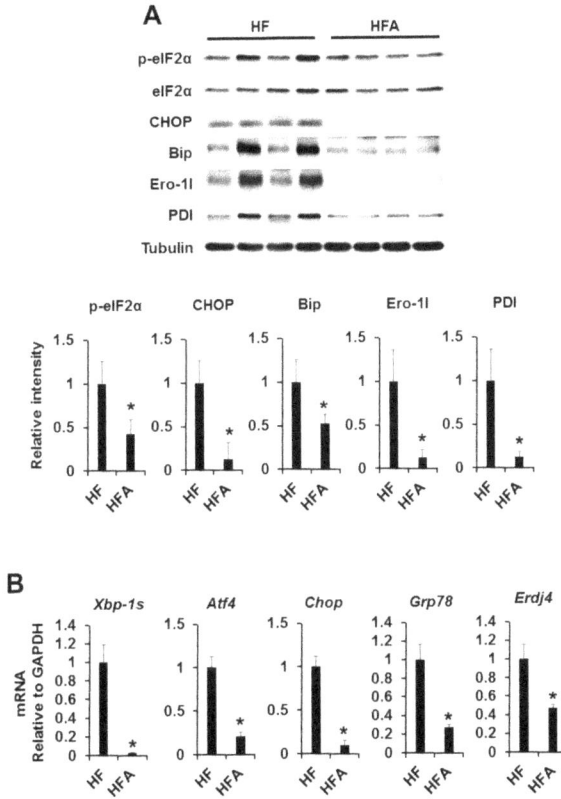

Figure 3. Effects of central administration of ADE on ER stress responsive markers and ER chaperone/foldases expression. (**A**) Effects of ICV administration of ADE (1 μL of 10 mg/mL) on hypothalamic ER stress responsive markers and ER chaperone/foldases. The results of densitometric analysis (*lower*) are means ± SDs (*n* = 10); * *p* values of < 0.05 indicate significant difference from administration with DMSO (1 μL of 20% DMSO); (**B**) Effects of ICV administration of ADE (1 μL of 10 mg/mL) on hypothalamic mRNA expression levels of hypothalamic ER stress responsive markers. The results are means ± SDs (*n* = 10 per group); * *p* values of < 0.05 indicate significant difference from administration with DMSO (1 μL of 20% DMSO). HF, high-fat diet with DMSO. HFA, high-fat diet with ADE.

3.4. Central Administration of ADE Regulates Appetite through MAPK and mTOR Signaling

Recent evidence has demonstrated that hypothalamic mammalian target of rapamycin (mTOR), a highly conserved serine-threonine kinase, signaling plays a role in modulation of feeding behavior by acting as a cellular sensor of changes in energy balance, nutrients, and growth factors [21,22]. Leptin and ghrelin seem to be powerful factors in the regulation of food intake and body weight. In the hypothalamus, activation of leptin or ghrelin receptor initiates different signaling cascades regulating food intake [23–26]. mTOR and MAPKs (ERK and p38) signaling has been previously associated with ghrelin [27–31]. For example, central administration of ghrelin has been reported to activate mTOR and ERK signaling to induce food intake. Therefore, we determined which signaling cascades are linked to appetite control after central administration of ADE. Firstly, we investigated leptin signaling with phospho-Stat3, -JAK2, and SOCS3 antibody. However, phosphorylation or expression of these proteins was unchanged. Secondly, we determined ghrelin signaling downstream of mTOR (phospho-S6K1 and -S6) and MAPKs (phospho-ERK and -p38) (Figure 4 and Supplementary Figure S4). As shown in Figure 4, S6K1, S6, and ERK phosphorylation levels were significantly reduced after administration of ADE compared with vehicle control. However, phosphorylation of p38MAPK was elevated after ADE administration in mice fed a high-fat diet. These results assume that ADE reduces appetite by antagonizing ghrelin signaling cascades rather than leptin signaling, and mTOR and MAPK signaling pathways were necessary for appetite regulation of ADE in the hypothalamus.

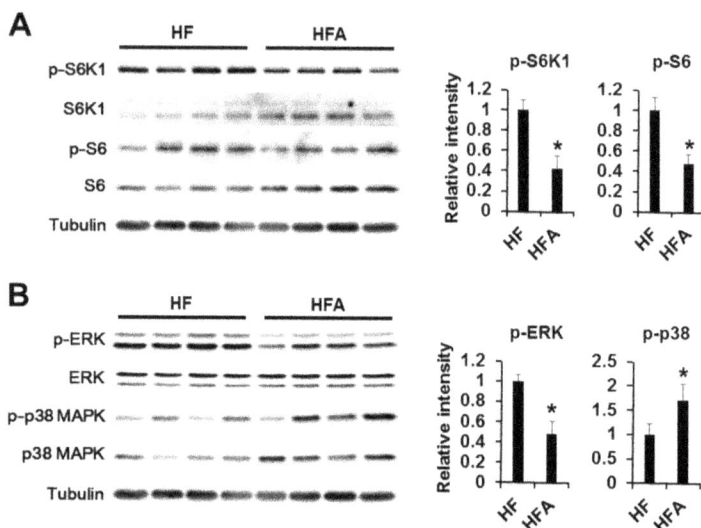

Figure 4. Central administration of ADE reduces ghrelin signaling through mTOR and ERK signaling pathways in mice fed a high-fat diet. (**A**) Effects of ICV administration of ADE (1 μL of 10 mg/mL) on mTOR signaling pathways. The results of densitometric analysis (right) are means ± SDs ($n = 10$ per group); * p values of < 0.05 indicate significant difference from administration with DMSO (1 μL of 20% DMSO); (**B**) Effects of ICV administration of ADE (1 μL of 10 mg/mL) on MAPK signaling pathways. The results of densitometric analysis (right) are means ± SDs ($n = 10$); * p values of < 0.05 indicate significant difference from administration with DMSO (1 μL of 20% DMSO). HF, high-fat diet with DMSO. HFA, high-fat diet with ADE.

4. Discussion

The hypothalamus is considered a key player in the regulation of food intake and body weight, although hypothalamic dysfunction may occur in a chronic energy excess state [20,32]. Under obese conditions induced by pharmacologic or genetic causes, endoplasmic reticulum (ER) stress in the hypothalamus causes central leptin and insulin resistance, resulting in increased food intake, hypertension, and glucose intolerance, whereas reduction of ER stress significantly attenuates these metabolic derangements [33,34]. Beetle species, a very well-known insect, is widely used in Oriental medicine to treat various diseases such as diabetes and hepatofibrosis in Asian countries [8,35]. Insects can be used as a health food supplement or functional food, as they are rich in protein, vitamins, minerals, fiber, and unsaturated fatty acids [36–38]. Previous works reported that several kinds of insect extracts could be used as anti-obesity and liver disease treatment agents [7,9,39].

In this study, we demonstrated the functional effects of ADE on ER stress and appetite regulatory neuropeptide processing in obesity. In diet-induced obesity (DIO), the appetite regulatory α-melanocyte-stimulating hormone (α-MSH) is downregulated, whereas appetite-inducing neuropeptide Y (NPY) and aqouti-related protein (AgRP) are induced [18–20]. To study the effects of ADE on appetite control, ADE was injected with ICV, and food intake and body weight changes were measured (Figure 2A,B). As a result, food intake and body weight were markedly reduced after ADE administration compared with vehicle control, which was evident 2 h after infusion and was consistent after 24 h. Furthermore, we quantified the mRNA expression levels of *Npy*, *Agrp*, and *Pomc* by quantitative PCR. As shown in Figure 2C, *Npy* and *Agrp* mRNA expression levels were reduced, whereas *Pomc* mRNA level increased after ADE administration. From these results, we assume that the appetite reducing effect of ADE is mediated by restoration of DIO-induced leptin resistance accompanied by reduction of ER stress on the hypothalamus. Thus, we investigated expression levels of ER stress markers and chaperones using Western blot analysis or quantitative PCR. As shown in Figure 3, ER stress markers and chaperones were dramatically downregulated upon ADE infusion, whereas leptin resistance was not restored.

Ghrelin expression was elevated upon fasting and reduced upon feeding in normal and genetically obese rodents [40–42]. Based on these findings, we speculate that reduction of food intake and body weight by ADE may be due to antagonization of ghrelin function. In previous works, ICV injection of ghrelin induced orexigenic action by increasing mTOR and ERK signaling pathways [27,28,43,44]. Additionally, ghrelin was shown to inhibit p38 MAPK activation in oligodendrocytes and other types of cells [30,31]. Therefore, we determined levels of S6K1 and S6 phosphorylation, downstream signaling cascades of mTOR, and phosphorylation of MAPKs (ERK and p38) (Figure 4). Central administration of ADE significantly downregulated phosphorylation of S6K1, S6, and ERK as well as upregulation of p38 MAPK in mice fed a high-fat diet. However, low-fat-diet-induced mice showed no changes (Supplementary Figure S4). These result indicate that ADE reduces appetite by antagonizing ghrelin signaling cascades rather than leptin signaling, and mTOR and ERK signaling are necessary for appetite regulation of ADE in the hypothalamus in mice fed a high-fat diet.

In summary, our most significant finding is that ethanol extract of *Allomyrina dichotoma* larvae (ADE) has an anorexigenic effect through regulation of mTOR and MAPK pathways, resulting in reduced food intake and body weight changes accompanied by reduced ER stress. We speculate that the anorexigenic effect of ADE is due to antagonization of ghrelin-induced feeding behavior. Furthermore, ADE showed the strongest reducing effect on ER stress both *in vitro* and *in vivo* (Figure 3 and Supplementary Figure S2). Accumulating evidence suggests that chronic activation of ER stress contributes to the pathogenesis of many diseases, including neurodegenerative diseases, bipolar disorder, diabetes mellitus, atherosclerosis, inflammation, ischemia, heart diseases, liver and kidney disease, and cancer [45,46]. As research on ER stress-related diseases has recently increased, these results strongly suggest that ADE is available and valuable to use for treatment of various diseases driven by prolonged ER stress. This study demonstrates the anorexigenic and ER stress-reducing effects of ADE in the central nervous system and provides a strong possibility for the implications of insect-derived multiple compounds for the therapeutic purposes in patients. However, this study was limited to the administration of ADE, an anti-obesity drug, via the third ventricle, which grants further investigation to validate the effects via other routes of administration including oral. Furthermore, fractionation of ADE is also warranted to examine the proper components of the ADE responsible for these effects, as well as to provide strong evidence of the anorexigenic and ER stress-reducing effects of ADE on hypothalamic ER stress-driven metabolic disorders.

5. Conclusions

Intracerebroventricular (ICV) administration of the ADE had an antagonizing effect on ghrelin-induced feeding behavior through mTOR and MAPK signaling pathways. These findings strongly suggest that ADE and its constituent bioactive compounds are available and valuable to use for treatment of various diseases driven by prolonged ER stress

Supplementary Materials: The following are available online at http://www.mdpi.com/2072-6643/8/2/100/s1: Figure S1: Effects of central administration of ADE on food intake and body, Figure S2: Effects of ADE on ER stress responsive marker expression, Figure S3: Effects of central administration of ADE on ER stress responsive markers and ER chaperone/foldases expression in mice fed a low-fat diet, Figure S4: Central administration of ADE reduces ghrelin signaling through mTOR and ERK signaling pathways in mice fed a low-fat diet.

Acknowledgments: This study was supported by the Bio-industry Technology Development Program (315030-3), Ministry for Food, Agriculture, Forestry and Fisheries, Republic of Korea.

Author Contributions: J.K. and M.S. performed the experiments, analyzed the data, and prepared the manuscript. E.Y.Y., T.W.G., and S.W.P. provided reagents and analyzed the data. M.S. and T.W.G directed the study and were involved in all aspects of the experimental design, data analysis and manuscript preparation. All authors critically reviewed the text and figures.

Conflicts of Interest: The authors declare no conflict of interest.

References

1. Guzman, A.K.; Ding, M.; Xie, Y.; Martin, K.A. Pharmacogenetics of obesity drug therapy. *Curr. Mol. Med.* **2014**, *14*, 891–908. [CrossRef] [PubMed]

2. Rodgers, R.J.; Tschop, M.H.; Wilding, J.P. Anti-obesity drugs: Past, present and future. *Dis. Models Mech.* **2012**, *5*, 621–626. [CrossRef] [PubMed]

3. Flegal, K.M.; Graubard, B.I.; Williamson, D.F.; Gail, M.H. Cause-specific excess deaths associated with underweight, overweight, and obesity. *Jama* **2007**, *298*, 2028–2037. [CrossRef] [PubMed]

4. Sagisaka, A.; Miyanoshita, A.; Ishibashi, J.; Yamakawa, M. Purification, characterization and gene expression of a glycine and proline-rich antibacterial protein family from larvae of a beetle, *Allomyrina dichotoma*. *Insect Mol. Biol.* **2001**, *10*, 293–302. [CrossRef] [PubMed]

5. Miyanoshita, A.; Hara, S.; Sugiyama, M.; Asaoka, A.; Taniai, K.; Yukuhiro, F.; Yamakawa, M. Isolation and characterization of a new member of the insect defensin family from a beetle, *Allomyrina dichotoma*. *Biochem. Biophys. Res. Commun.* **1996**, *220*, 526–531. [CrossRef] [PubMed]

6. Suh, H.J.; Kim, S.R.; Lee, K.S.; Park, S.; Kang, S.C. Antioxidant activity of various solvent extracts from *Allomyrina dichotoma* (Arthropoda: Insecta) larvae. *J. Photochem. Photobiol. B Biol.* **2010**, *99*, 67–73. [CrossRef] [PubMed]

7. Yoon, Y.I.; Chung, M.Y.; Hwang, J.S.; Han, M.S.; Goo, T.W.; Yun, E.Y. *Allomyrina dichotoma* (Arthropoda: Insecta) larvae confer resistance to obesity in mice fed a high-fat diet. *Nutrients* **2015**, *7*, 1978–1991. [CrossRef] [PubMed]

8. Yoshikawa, K.; Umetsu, K.; Shinzawa, H.; Yuasa, I.; Maruyama, K.; Ohkura, T.; Yamashita, K.; Suzuki, T. Determination of carbohydrate-deficient transferrin separated by lectin affinity chromatography for detecting chronic alcohol abuse. *FEBS Lett.* **1999**, *458*, 112–116. [CrossRef]

9. Chung, M.Y.; Yoon, Y.I.; Hwang, J.S.; Goo, T.W.; Yun, E.Y. Anti-obesity effect of *Allomyrina dichotoma* (Arthropoda: Insecta) larvae ethanol extract on 3T3-L1 adipocyte differentiation. *Entomol. Res.* **2014**, *44*, 9–16. [CrossRef]

10. Morton, G.J.; Cummings, D.E.; Baskin, D.G.; Barsh, G.S.; Schwartz, M.W. Central nervous system control of food intake and body weight. *Nature* **2006**, *443*, 289–295. [CrossRef] [PubMed]

11. Elmquist, J.K.; Coppari, R.; Balthasar, N.; Ichinose, M.; Lowell, B.B. Identifying hypothalamic pathways controlling food intake, body weight, and glucose homeostasis. *J. Comp. Neurol.* **2005**, *493*, 63–71. [CrossRef] [PubMed]

12. Lupachyk, S.; Watcho, P.; Obrosov, A.A.; Stavniichuk, R.; Obrosova, I.G. Endoplasmic reticulum stress contributes to prediabetic peripheral neuropathy. *Exp. Neurol.* **2013**, *247*, 342–348. [CrossRef] [PubMed]

13. Cnop, M.; Foufelle, F.; Velloso, L.A. Endoplasmic reticulum stress, obesity and diabetes. *Trends Mol. Med.* **2012**, *18*, 59–68. [CrossRef] [PubMed]

14. Denis, R.G.; Arruda, A.P.; Romanatto, T.; Milanski, M.; Coope, A.; Solon, C.; Razolli, D.S.; Velloso, L.A. TNF-α transiently induces endoplasmic reticulum stress and an incomplete unfolded protein response in the hypothalamus. *Neuroscience* **2010**, *170*, 1035–1044. [CrossRef] [PubMed]

15. Hotamisligil, G.S. Endoplasmic reticulum stress and the inflammatory basis of metabolic disease. *Cell* **2010**, *140*, 900–917. [CrossRef] [PubMed]

16. Won, J.C.; Jang, P.G.; Namkoong, C.; Koh, E.H.; Kim, S.K.; Park, J.Y.; Lee, K.U.; Kim, M.S. Central administration of an endoplasmic reticulum stress inducer inhibits the anorexigenic effects of leptin and insulin. *Obesity* **2009**, *17*, 1861–1865. [CrossRef] [PubMed]

17. Noh, J.H.; Yun, E.Y.; Park, H.; Jung, K.J.; Hwang, J.S.; Jeong, E.J.; Moon, K.S. Subchronic oral dose toxicity of freeze-dried powder of *Allomyrina dichotoma* larvae. *Toxicol. Res.* **2015**, *31*, 69–75. [CrossRef] [PubMed]

18. Cakir, I.; Cyr, N.E.; Perello, M.; Litvinov, B.P.; Romero, A.; Stuart, R.C.; Nillni, E.A. Obesity induces hypothalamic endoplasmic reticulum stress and impairs proopiomelanocortin (POMC) post-translational processing. *J. Biol. Chem.* **2013**, *288*, 17675–17688. [CrossRef] [PubMed]

19. Cao, Z.P.; Wang, F.; Xiang, X.S.; Cao, R.; Zhang, W.B.; Gao, S.B. Intracerebroventricular administration of conjugated linoleic acid (CLA) inhibits food intake by decreasing gene expression of NPY and AgRP. *Neurosci. Lett.* **2007**, *418*, 217–221. [CrossRef] [PubMed]

20. Kalra, S.P.; Dube, M.G.; Pu, S.; Xu, B.; Horvath, T.L.; Kalra, P.S. Interacting appetite-regulating pathways in the hypothalamic regulation of body weight. *Endocr. Rev.* **1999**, *20*, 68–100. [CrossRef] [PubMed]

21. Wullschleger, S.; Loewith, R.; Hall, M.N. TOR signaling in growth and metabolism. *Cell* **2006**, *124*, 471–484. [CrossRef] [PubMed]

22. Padmanabhan, R. Electron-microscopic studies on the pathogenesis of exencephaly and cranioschisis induced in the rat after neural tube closure: Role of the neuroepithelium and choroid plexus. *Acta Anat.* **1990**, *137*, 5–18. [CrossRef] [PubMed]

23. Klok, M.D.; Jakobsdottir, S.; Drent, M.L. The role of leptin and ghrelin in the regulation of food intake and body weight in humans: A Review. *Obes. Rev.* **2007**, *8*, 21–34. [CrossRef] [PubMed]

24. Sahu, A. Minireview: A hypothalamic role in energy balance with special emphasis on leptin. *Endocrinology* **2004**, *145*, 2613–2620. [CrossRef] [PubMed]

25. Sahu, A. Leptin signaling in the hypothalamus: Emphasis on energy homeostasis and leptin resistance. *Front. Neuroendocrinol.* **2003**, *24*, 225–253. [CrossRef] [PubMed]

26. Schwartz, M.W. Brain pathways controlling food intake and body weight. *Exp. Biol. Med.* **2001**, *226*, 978–981.

27. Stevanovic, D.; Trajkovic, V.; Muller-Luhlhoff, S.; Brandt, E.; Abplanalp, W.; Bumke-Vogt, C.; Liehl, B.; Wiedmer, P.; Janjetovic, K.; Starcevic, V.; *et al.* Ghrelin-induced food intake and adiposity depend on central mtorc1/s6k1 signaling. *Mol. Cell. Endocrinol.* **2013**, *381*, 280–290. [CrossRef] [PubMed]

28. Martins, L.; Fernandez-Mallo, D.; Novelle, M.G.; Vazquez, M.J.; Tena-Sempere, M.; Nogueiras, R.; Lopez, M.; Dieguez, C. Hypothalamic mtor signaling mediates the orexigenic action of ghrelin. *PLoS ONE* **2012**, *7*, e46923. [CrossRef] [PubMed]

29. Stevanovic, D.; Starcevic, V.; Vilimanovich, U.; Nesic, D.; Vucicevic, L.; Misirkic, M.; Janjetovic, K.; Savic, E.; Popadic, D.; Sudar, E.; *et al.* Immunomodulatory actions of central ghrelin in diet-induced energy imbalance. *Brain Behav. Immun.* **2012**, *26*, 150–158. [CrossRef] [PubMed]

30. Lee, J.Y.; Oh, T.H.; Yune, T.Y. Ghrelin inhibits hydrogen peroxide-induced apoptotic cell death of oligodendrocytes via erk and p38MAPK signaling. *Endocrinology* **2011**, *152*, 2377–2386. [CrossRef] [PubMed]

31. Hu, C.Z.; Cao, Y.L.; Huo, H.Y.; Zhao, W.H.; Hu, J. Inhibitory effect of ghrelin on nicotine-induced VCAM-1 expression in human umbilical vein endothelial cells. *J. Cardiovasc. Pharmacol.* **2009**, *53*, 241–245. [CrossRef] [PubMed]

32. Kim, H.K.; Youn, B.S.; Shin, M.S.; Namkoong, C.; Park, K.H.; Baik, J.H.; Kim, J.B.; Park, J.Y.; Lee, K.U.; Kim, Y.B.; *et al.* Hypothalamic angptl4/fiaf is a novel regulator of food intake and body weight. *Diabetes* **2010**, *59*, 2772–2780. [CrossRef] [PubMed]

33. Cai, D.; Liu, T. Hypothalamic inflammation: A double-edged sword to nutritional diseases. *Ann. N. Y. Acad. Sci.* **2011**, *1243*, E1–E39. [CrossRef] [PubMed]

34. Purkayastha, S.; Zhang, H.; Zhang, G.; Ahmed, Z.; Wang, Y.; Cai, D. Neural dysregulation of peripheral insulin action and blood pressure by brain endoplasmic reticulum stress. *Proc. Natl. Acad. Sci. USA* **2011**, *108*, 2939–2944. [CrossRef] [PubMed]

35. Dobrin, P.; Canfield, T. Cuffed endotracheal tubes: Mucosal pressures and tracheal wall blood flow. *Am. J. Surg.* **1977**, *133*, 562–568. [CrossRef]

36. Youn, K.; Kim, J.Y.; Yeo, H.; Yun, E.Y.; Hwang, J.S.; Jun, M. Fatty acid and volatile oil compositions of *Allomyrina dichotoma* larvae. *Prev. Nutr. Food Sci.* **2012**, *17*, 310–314. [CrossRef] [PubMed]

37. Chung, M.Y.; Hwang, J.S.; Goo, T.W.; Yun, E.Y. Analysis of general composition and harmful material of Protaetia breviatarsis. *J. Life Sci.* **2013**, *23*, 664–668. [CrossRef]

38. Yoo, J.M.; Hwang, J.S.; Goo, T.W.; Yun, E.Y. Comparative analysis of nutritional and harmful components in Korean and Chinese meal worms (Tenebrio molitor). *J. Korean Soc. Food Sci. Nutr.* **2013**, *42*, 249–254. [CrossRef]

39. Chung, M.Y.; Kown, E.Y.; Hwang, J.S.; Goo, T.W.; Yun, E.Y. Establishment of food processing methods for larvae of *Allomyrina dichotoma*, Korean horn beetle. *J. Life Sci.* **2013**, *23*, 426–431. [CrossRef]

40. Moesgaard, S.G.; Ahren, B.; Carr, R.D.; Gram, D.X.; Brand, C.L.; Sundler, F. Effects of high-fat feeding and fasting on ghrelin expression in the mouse stomach. *Regul. Pept.* **2004**, *120*, 261–267. [CrossRef] [PubMed]

41. Ariyasu, H.; Takaya, K.; Hosoda, H.; Iwakura, H.; Ebihara, K.; Mori, K.; Ogawa, Y.; Hosoda, K.; Akamizu, T.; Kojima, M.; et al. Delayed short-term secretory regulation of ghrelin in obese animals: Evidenced by a specific ria for the active form of ghrelin. *Endocrinology* **2002**, *143*, 3341–3350. [CrossRef] [PubMed]

42. Toshinai, K.; Mondal, M.S.; Nakazato, M.; Date, Y.; Murakami, N.; Kojima, M.; Kangawa, K.; Matsukura, S. Upregulation of ghrelin expression in the stomach upon fasting, insulin-induced hypoglycemia, and leptin administration. *Biochem. Biophys. Res. Commun.* **2001**, *281*, 1220–1225. [CrossRef] [PubMed]

43. Komori, T.; Doi, A.; Nosaka, T.; Furuta, H.; Akamizu, T.; Kitamura, T.; Senba, E.; Morikawa, Y. Regulation of AMP-activated protein kinase signaling by AFF4 protein, member of AF4 (ALL1-fused gene from chromosome 4) family of transcription factors, in hypothalamic neurons. *J. Biol. Chem.* **2012**, *287*, 19985–19996. [CrossRef] [PubMed]

44. Mousseaux, D.; Le Gallic, L.; Ryan, J.; Oiry, C.; Gagne, D.; Fehrentz, J.A.; Galleyrand, J.C.; Martinez, J. Regulation of ERK1/2 activity by ghrelin-activated growth hormone secretagogue receptor 1a involves a PLC/PKCε pathway. *Br. J. Pharmacol.* **2006**, *148*, 350–365. [PubMed]

45. Ozcan, L.; Tabas, I. Role of endoplasmic reticulum stress in metabolic disease and other disorders. *Ann. Rev. Med.* **2012**, *63*, 317–328. [CrossRef] [PubMed]

46. Yoshida, H. ER stress and diseases. *FEBS J.* **2007**, *274*, 630–658. [CrossRef] [PubMed]

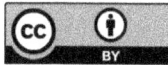

nutrients

MDPI

Article

Anti-Obesity Effect of 6,8-Diprenylgenistein, an Isoflavonoid of *Cudrania tricuspidata* Fruits in High-Fat Diet-Induced Obese Mice

Yang Hee Jo [1], Kyeong-Mi Choi [1], Qing Liu [1], Seon Beom Kim [1], Hyeong-Jin Ji [2], Myounghwan Kim [2], Sang-Kyung Shin [2], Seon-Gil Do [3], Eunju Shin [3], Gayoung Jung [3], Hwan-Soo Yoo [1], Bang Yeon Hwang [1] and Mi Kyeong Lee [1,*]

[1]   College of Pharmacy, Chungbuk National University, Cheongju, Chungbuk 28644, Korea; qow0125@naver.com (Y.H.J.); mirine0101@hanmail.net (K.-M.C.); liuqing7115@hotmail.com (Q.L.); suntiger85@hanmail.net (S.B.K.); yoohs@chungbuk.ac.kr (H.-S.Y.); byhwang@chungbuk.ac.kr (B.Y.H.)
[2]   Laboratory Animal Research Center, Chungbuk National University, Cheongju, Chungbuk 28644, Korea; jihjin@chungbuk.ac.kr (H.-J.J.); mhkim3340@naver.com (M.K.); skshin@chungbuk.ac.kr (S.-K.S.)
[3]   Wellness R&D Center, Univera, Inc., Seoul 05014, Korea; sgildo@univera.com (S.-G.D.); Ejayshin@univera.com (E.S.); gayoung@univera.com (G.J.)
*   Correspondence: mklee@chungbuk.ac.kr; Tel.: +82-43-261-2818

Received: 13 October 2015; Accepted: 10 December 2015; Published: 15 December 2015

Abstract: Obesity, which is characterized by excessive fat accumulation, is associated with several pathological disorders, including metabolic diseases. In this study, the anti-obesity effect of 6,8-diprenylgenistein (DPG), a major isoflavonoid of *Cudrania tricuspidata* fruits was investigated using high fat-diet (HFD)-induced obese mice at the doses of 10 and 30 mg/kg for six week. The body weight of the DPG-treated groups was significantly lower compared to the HFD-treated group. In addition, fat accumulation in epididymal adipose tissue and liver was dramatically decreased in the HFD + DPG groups. The food efficiency ratios of the HFD + DPG groups were also lower compared to the HFD group with the same food intake. Metabolic parameters that had increased in the HFD group were decreased in the HFD + DPG groups. Further studies demonstrate that DPG efficiently reduces lipogenic genes by regulation of transcription factors, such as peroxisome proliferator-activated receptor γ (PPARγ) and CCAAT/enhancer-binding protein α (C/EBPα), and hormones, such as leptin and adiponection. DPG also regulates acetyl-CoA carboxylase (ACC) and hydroxy-3-methylglutaryl coenzyme A reductase (HMGCR) by AMP-activated protein kinase (AMPK) activation. Taken together, DPG is beneficial for the regulation of obesity, especially resulting from high fat intake.

Keywords: 6,8-Diprenylgenistein (DPG); *Cudrania tricuspidata*; high-fat diet-induced obesity; lipid profile; AMPK

---

1. Introduction

The prevalence of obesity has increased continuously and became one of the major threats to global health due to the association with several pathological disorders, including diabetes, hypertension, atherosclerosis and cancer [1,2]. In the development of obesity, genetic and environmental factors are known to play important roles. In particular, a diet high in saturated fats is considered to be one of main contributors to obesity, particularly in the Western diet. Fat is digested into monoglycerides and fatty acids by lipase and absorbed fat is accumulated in adipose tissue through excessive adipocyte differentiation [3]. Adipocyte differentiation is an organized process regulated by various transcriptional factors depending on differentiation stages. CCAAT/enhancer-binding protein (C/EBP) β and δ are expressed in early stages of adipocyte differentiation. C/EBPs β and δ regulate the expression of peroxisome proliferator-activated receptor γ (PPARγ) and CCAAT/enhancer-binding protein α (C/EBPα), the most crucial transcriptional factors in adipogenesis [4]. Obesity is also closely related to the levels of leptin and adiponectin, adipose specific hormones. Leptin amount is proportionally correlated with obesity, while adiponection amount is inversely related to obesity [5]. Therefore, inhibition of adipogenesis by the regulation of transcription factors and hormones are one of the targets of anti-obesity strategies. AMPK is another regulator of cellular energy homeostasis. Phosphorylation by AMPK inactivates metabolic enzymes, such as acetyl CoA carboxylase (ACC) and hydroxy-3-methylglutaryl coenzyme A reductase (HMGCR), which results in fatty acid oxidation and reduced biosynthesis of fatty acid and cholesterol [6,7].

Phytochemicals are defined as the substances found in edible fruits and vegetables. Various phytochemicals are known to exhibit a potential for human health. In addition, favorable role of phytochemicals on the prevention and treatment of obesity have been reported. Epigallocatechin gallate of green tea is well known for its beneficial effect on obesity [8]. Xanthigen, a mixture of brown seaweed and pomegranate seed extract, showed anti-obesity activity in animal model [9]. Sulforaphane, an isothicyanate of broccoli and alkaloids of lotus leaves, showed beneficial effects on obesity [10,11].

Fruits are good sources of diverse phytochemicals. Especially, polyphenols, such as flavonoids, are considered as major functional components of fruit. They possess diverse biological activities (e.g., antioxidant, estrogenic, anti-inflammatory and anti-cancer activity [12–14]. As a result, the utility of this fruit as an ingredient in dietary supplements and functional foods ingredients is being actively investigated in many fields.

Cudrania tricuspidata, which belongs to the Moraceae family, is a thorny tree cultivated in East Asia including Korea. The fruits of *C. tricuspidata* are widely consumed as fresh fruits, jams, and processed products, such as wine and vinegar. They are known for its diverse biological activities such as antioxidant, anti-inflammatory and immunomodulatory activity [15–17]. We previously reported the pancreatic lipase inhibitory activity of *C. tricuspidata* fruits. 6,8-diprenylgenistein (DPG), a major isoflavonoid of *C. tricuspidata* fruits (Figure 1) was suggested as an active constituent [18]. Moreover, the inhibitory activity of DPG on diacylglycerol acyltransferase (DGAT), a key enzyme in triglyceride synthesis, has been reported [19]. Therefore, further studies have been attempted to elucidate anti-obesity effect in high fat diet (HFD)-induced animal model and its potential mechanisms, to verify the anti-obesity activity of DPG.

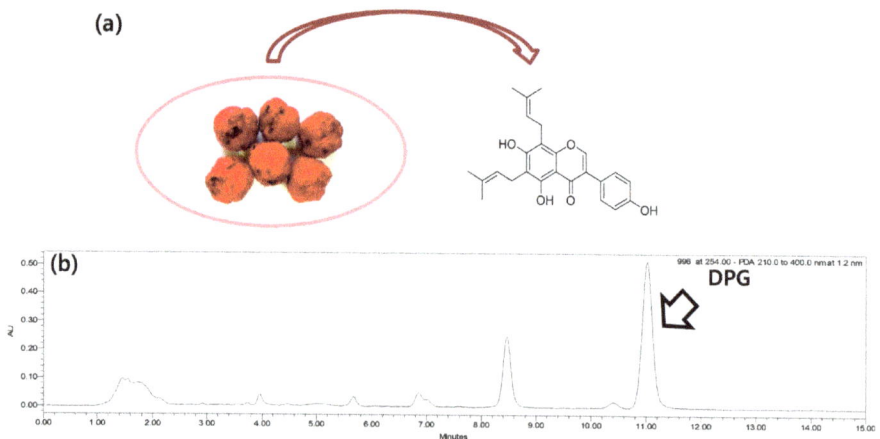

Figure 1. (**a**) Structure of 6,8-diprenylgenistein (DPG) from *C. tricuspidata* fruits; (**b**) High performance liquid chromatography (HPLC) chromatogram of the extract of *C. tricuspidata* fruits.

2. Experimental Section

2.1. Chemicals

Antibodies against peroxisome proliferator-activated receptor γ (PPARγ) and hydroxy-3-methylglutaryl coenzyme A reductase (HMGCR) were purchased from Santa Cruz Biotechnology, Inc. (Santa Cruz, CA, USA). Antibodies against CCAAT/enhancer-binding protein α (C/EBPα), adiponectin, phospho-AMP-activated protein kinase alpha (p-AMPKα), phospho-AMP-activated protein kinase β1 (p-AMPKβ), phospho-acetyl-CoA carboxylase (p-ACC), and β-actin were obtained from Cell Signaling Technology (Beverly, MA, USA). The antibody against leptin was obtained from GeneTex, Inc. (Irvine, CA, USA).

2.2. Preparation of DPG

DPG, a major isoflavonoid of *C. tricuspidata* fruits was isolated, as previously reported [18] (Figure 1a,b). The purity was higher than 95%, as measured HPLC analysis.

2.3. Animal Treatment

Male C57BL/6J mice (n = 60, 4 weeks old, 15% ± 10% g) were purchased from Central Lab. Animal Inc., Seoul, Korea. All mice were housed in a room with controlled temperature (21–23 °C), humidity (55%–60%), and lighting (12-h light/dark cycle) and given water *ad libitum*. After acclimation for 1 week, the mice were randomly divided into the following four groups (n = 15/group): ND (normal diet), HFD, HFD + DPG10 (10 mg DPG/kg mice) and HFD + DPG30 (30 mg DPG/kg mice). ND group was fed with a normal diet (4.3% fat of diet, 7% of kcal from fat). The HFD, HFD + DPG10 and HFD + DPG30 groups were fed HFD (24% fat including 0.5% cholesterol of diet, 45% of kcal from fat) (Table S1). DPG samples were prepared in distilled water (DW) at the concentrations of 10 mg/mL or 30 mg/mL. DPG samples were administered orally (10 mL/kg) to HFD + DPG groups, and DW (10 mL/kg) was administered orally to the ND and HFD groups for 6 weeks. At the end of experiment, the mice were sacrificed and their blood and organs were collected. The protocol for this study was approved by the Animal Care and Use Committee of Chungbuk National University (Approval No. CBNUA-644-13-01).

2.4. Serum Biochemical Parameters

All mice were fasted for 12 h before they were sacrificed. Blood was collected and serum was obtained by the centrifugation at 3500 g for 10 min at 4 °C. The content of triglyceride, total cholesterol, low-density lipoprotein (LDL) cholesterol, high-density lipoprotein (HDL) cholesterol, alanine transaminase (ALT) and aspartate transaminase (AST) were determined using Hitachi7080 analyzer.

2.5. Histopathology

Histological photograph of adipose tissue was analyzed based on the paraffin method using a light microscope. Epididymal adipose tissue was fixed with 10% neutral buffered formalin and embedded in paraffin block. Six μm sections were cut and mounted on glass slide. Paraffin was removed with xylen and alcohol. The sections were then stained with hematoxylin and eosin (H&E). After dehydration by alcohol, the photograph was taken with light microscope. The size of epididymal adipocyte was calculated by Image analysis system (IPKR-1003, Saramsoft Co., Ltd., Seoul, Korea). For the detection of lipid deposition in liver, liver section were prepared from frozen liver and stained with Oil Red O, as previously reported [20].

2.6. Western Blot Analysis

Epididymal adipose tissues were homogenized in lysis buffer containing 50 mM Tris-HCl (pH 7.4), 1% Triton X-100, 0.2% sodium deoxycholate, 0.2% sodium dodecylsulfate, 1 mM phenylmethylsulfonyl fluoride, and a protease inhibitor cocktail tablet. The homogenate was centrifuged at 18,300 g for 30 min at 4 °C, and the supernatant was collected. The total protein concentration of each lysate was measured using bicinchoninic acid (BCA) Protein Assay Reagent. Proteins in the lysates were electrophoretically separated in 7.5% to 15% SDS polyacrylamide gel and then transferred to polyvinylidene difluoride membranes. The membranes were blocked in 5% bovine serum albumin overnight at 4 °C and then incubated overnight at 4 °C with the following primary antibodies: PPARγ, C/EBPα, leptin, adiponectin, p-AMPKα, p-AMPKβ, p-ACC, HMGCR, and β-actin. Membranes were next incubated with horseradish peroxidase-conjugated secondary antibodies overnight at 4 °C. Bands were visualized with enhanced chemiluminescence, and the intensities of the bands were quantified in WCIF Image J (University Health Network Research, Toronto, ON, Canada) for Windows.

2.7. Statistical Analysis

Values are expressed as the mean ± standard error (SE). The evaluation of statistical significance was determined by Levene's test followed by one-way ANOVA or Turkey HSD-test with a value of $p < 0.05$ considered to be statistically significant.

3. Results

3.1. Effects of DPG on Body Weight and Food Efficiency Ratio

The effect of DPG on obesity was investigated using HFD-induced male C58BL/6J mice. DPG was administered to HFD-induced obese mice at doses of 10 mg/kg (DPG10) and 30 mg/kg (DPG30), respectively, for 6 weeks. In our study, the body weights was increased in the HFD group, whereas the body weight of HFD + DPG10 and HFD + DPG30 groups were significantly lower compared to HFD groups (Figure 2). On day 42, at the end of the experiment, the body-weight gains of the ND and HFD group were 3.39 g and 7.81 g, respectively. However, the body weight gains of HFD + DPG10 and HFD + DPG30-treated group were significantly lower compared to the HFD group as 5.25 g and 5.13 g, respectively (Table 1).

The food efficiency ratio (FER) of HFD was much higher compared to that of ND group. The FERs of the HFD + DPG10 and HFD + DPG30 groups were also significantly lower compared to the HFD group with no differences in food intake (Table 1).

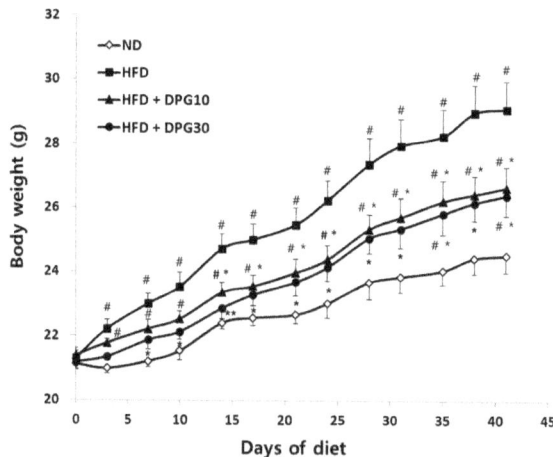

Figure 2. Effect of DPG10 and DPG30 on body weight in high fat-diet (HFD)-induced obese mice. Results are expressed as the mean ± SE (*n* = 12–15). [#] $p < 0.05$ compared with ND (normal diet) group, [*] $p < 0.05$, [**] $p < 0.01$ compared with HFD group.

Table 1. Effect of DPG on body weight gain, food intake and FER.

Group	Body Weight Gain (g/Mice/6 Weeks)	Food Intake (g/Day/Mice)	FER [1]
ND	3.39 ± 0.48	3.49 ± 0.03	0.023 ± 0.003
HFD	7.81 ± 0.98 [##]	2.71 ± 0.03 [##]	0.069 ± 0.008 [##]
HFD + DPG10	5.25 ± 0.65 [#,*]	2.73 ± 0.04 [##]	0.046 ± 0.005 [##,*]
HFD + DPG30	5.13 ± 0.50 [#*]	2.74 ± 0.09 [##]	0.044 ± 0.004 [##,*]

DPG: 6,8-Diprenylgenistein; FER: the food efficiency ratio; ND: normal diet; HFD: high fat diet. [1] Food efficiency ratio was calculated as the body weight gain/food intake. [#] $p < 0.05$, [##] $p < 0.01$ compared with ND group, [*] $p < 0.05$ compared with HFD group.

3.2. Effect of DPG on Fat Accumulation

The effect of DPG on fat accumulation was examined. The relative ratio of epididymal fat per body weight was significantly higher in the HFD group compared to the ND group. The amount of epididymal fat was significantly lower in the HFD + DPG10 and HFD + DPG30 groups (Figure 3a). The epididymal adipocyte size in HFD group was markedly enlarged compared to that in ND groups. However, adipocyte sizes of HFD + DPG10 and HFD + DPG30 groups were significantly smaller than those of HFD group (Figure 3b). Fat accumulation in liver was increased in HFD group, whereas decreased in HFD + DPG10 and HFD + DPG30 groups (Figure 4a). In addition, the increase of liver weight in HFD group was also significantly reduced in HFD + DPG10 and HFD + DPG30 groups (Figure 4b).

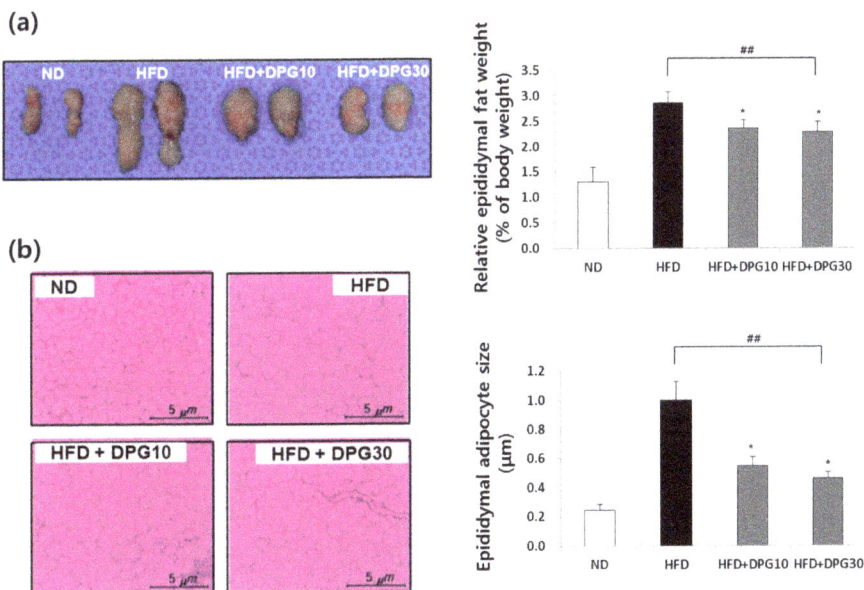

Figure 3. Effect of DPG10 and DPG30 on weight and size of adipocyte tissues in HFD-induced obese mice. (**a**) Epididymal adipose tissue; (**b**) sections of epididymal adipose tissue stained with hematoxylin and eosin (H&E). [##] $p < 0.01$ compared with ND group, [*] $p < 0.05$ compared with HFD group.

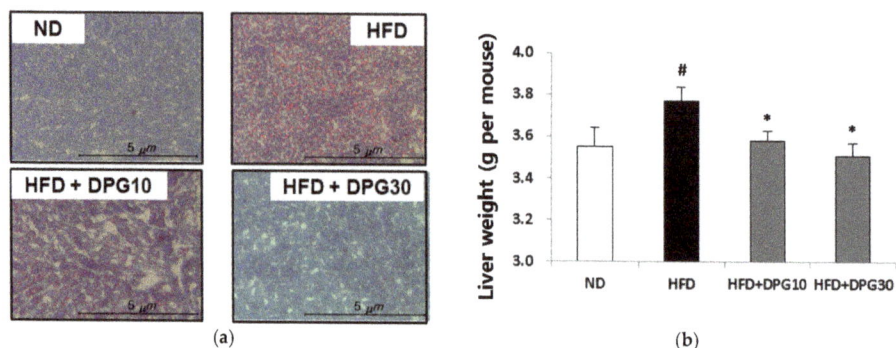

Figure 4. Effect of DPG10 and DPG30 on fat accumulation in liver and liver weight in HFD-induced obese mice. (a) Liver sections stained with Oil Red O; (b) liver weight per mouse. [#] $p < 0.05$ compared with ND group, * $p < 0.05$ compared with HFD group.

3.3. Effect of DPG on Serum Lipid Profiles

Regular high fat and high cholesterol diet leads to the changes in enzyme and lipid profiles. The HFD caused elevation of the serum levels of ALT and AST which were lower in the HFD + DPG10 and HFD + DPG30 groups. Administration of DPG also significantly reduced the levels of lipid metabolic parameters including LDL, HDL and total cholesterol, and triglyceride. In particular, the HFD-induced increase of triglyceride was markedly decreased in the DPG-treated groups (Table 2).

Table 2. Effect of DPG on biochemical parameters of serum in HFD-induced obese mice.

Group	ND	HFD	HFD + DPG10	HFD + DPG30
AST [1]	46.54 ± 5.55	58.85 ± 8.83	53.22 ± 5.21	50.48 ± 4.02 **
ALT [1]	20.13 ± 2.85	24.25 ± 3.35	21.18 ± 2.14 *	20.54 ± 2.98 **
Total cholesterol [2]	101.95 ± 10.46	151.25 ± 14.02	135.78 ± 13.44 *	130.15 ± 15.20 **
HDL cholesterol [2]	62.61 ± 7.41	83.03 ± 6.63	76.19 ± 6.75 *	75.75 ± 6.87 *
LDL cholesterol [2]	4.60 ± 0.82	8.17 ± 1.31	6.77 ± 1.41 *	6.45 ± 1.38 *
Triglyceride [2]	30.71 ± 10.13	50.55 ± 13.71	35.19 ± 10.65 *	33.72 ± 7.48 **

AST: aspartate transaminase; ALT: alanine transaminase. [1] IU/L, [2] mg/dL. * $p < 0.05$, ** $p < 0.01$ compared with HFD group.

3.4. Effect of DPG on Adipogenesis in Adipose Tissue

Adipogenesis includes increase in expression transcription factors such as PPARγ and C/EBPα [4,21]. As shown in Figure 5, the expression of PPARγ and C/EBPα in epididymal adipose tissue of HFD group was elevated up to 2-fold and 5-fold, respectively, compared to ND group. DPG markedly suppressed the HFD-induced elevation in the expression of PPARγ and C/EBPα as comparable to ND group (Figure 5a).

Adipose tissue secretes adipokines such as leptin and adiponectin. HFD cause differential effects on these adipokines [22,23]. The leptin expression was increased in HFD group, whereas adiponection expression was decreased in HFD group. DPG reversed the HFD-induced increase in leptin expression and decrease in adiponection expression (Figure 5b).

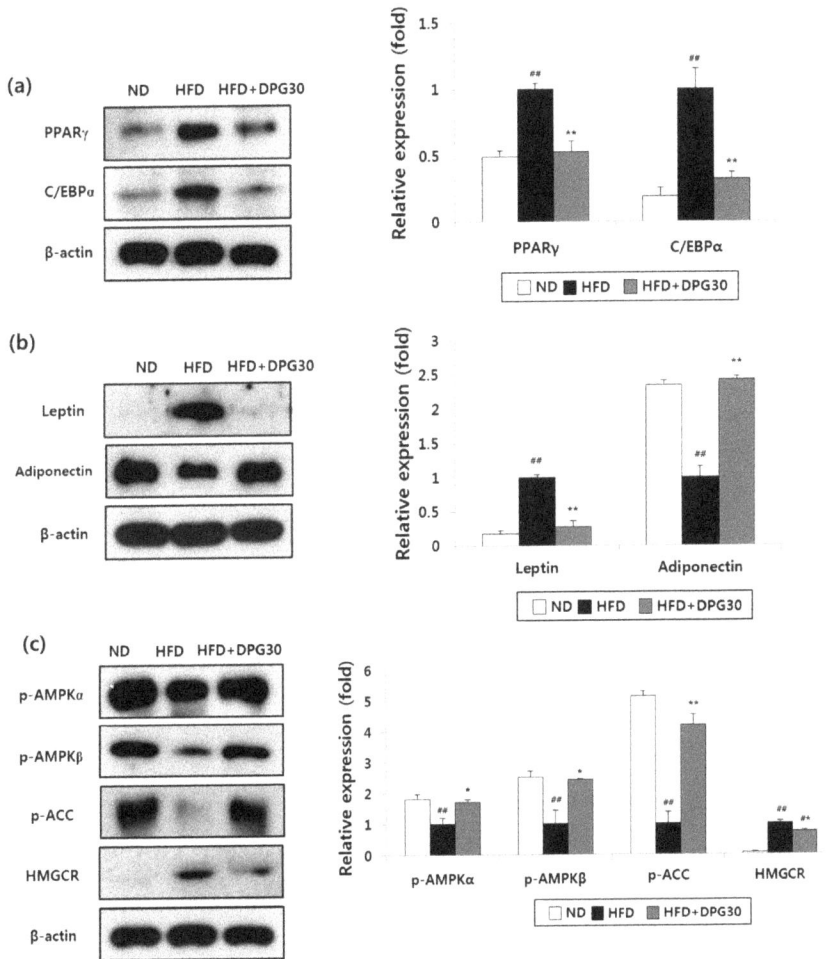

Figure 5. Effect of DPG on the expression of adipogenesis-related proteins in adipose tissue. (**a**) PPARγ and C/EBP α; (**b**) leptin and adiponectin; (**c**) p-AMPKα, p-AMPKβ, p-ACC, and HMBCR. Values are expressed as mean ± SE. [#] $p < 0.05$, [##] $p < 0.01$ compared with ND group, [*] $p < 0.05$, [**] $p < 0.01$ compared with HFD group.

3.5. Effect of DPG on AMPK Pathway

AMPK is a heterotrimer consisting of a catalytic subunit (α) and 2 regulatory subunits (β and γ). AMPK, a regulator of energy homeostasis, plays a major role in lipid metabolism. AMPK activation via phosphorylation promotes phosphorylation and inactivation of acetyl CoA carboxylase (ACC), which results in reduced biosynthesis of fatty acids and stimulation of fatty acid oxidation [6,7]. As expected, phosphorylation of AMPK and ACC was reduced in HFD group and DPG promoted phorphorylation of AMPK and ACC (Figure 5c).

HMG-CoA reductase (HMGCR) is another key enzyme that control cholesterol synthesis [24]. The expression of HMGCR was increased in epididymal adipose tissue of HFD groups and was lower in HFD + DPG groups compared to that of HFD controls (Figure 5c).

4. Discussion

Due to the harmful effect of obesity on human health, investigations for anti-obesity therapeutics have been actively conducted in many fields. Especially, food and food ingredients are considered as good targets for anti-obesity agents to prevent obesity and obesity-associated disorders [4,25–28]. In our previous study, we suggested anti-obesity activity of *C. tricuspidata* fruits and its major isoflavonoid, DPG [18]. In this study, we investigated the anti-obesity potential of DPG in HFD-induced obese mice.

Diet-induced obesity in rodents has been used as an animal model to investigate environmental effect. Rodents fed HFD become obese and show distinctive symptoms such as increase of adipose tissue, disturbance of lipid metabolism, hyperinsulinemia and fatty liver, which are typically associated with human obesity [29]. In our present study, HFD-induced obesity was clearly confirmed by many factors such as increase of body weight, adipocyte size, fat accumulation and liver weight, and disturbance of lipid metabolism. However, oral administration of DPG, at doses of 10 and 30 mg/kg, dramatically improved HFD-induced obesity in many parameters.

First, the body weight in HFD + DPG groups were significantly lower than HFD groups (Figure 2). Food intake was higher in the ND group than in HFD groups, but did not significantly differ among the HFD, HFD + DPG10 and HFD + DPG30 groups. However, FERs of HFD + DPG10 and HFD + DPG30 groups were significantly reduced compared to HFD group (Table 1). Therefore, decrease of body weight in HFD + DPG10 and HFD +DPG30 group was achieved partially by decrease of FER not by loss of appetite. Consistent with FER, DPG inhibits pancreatic lipase, which plays key roles in fat digestion [18]. Therefore, DPG inhibited fat absorption by pancreatic lipase inhibition without any effect on appetite, which leaded the reduction of body weight gain.

Increase of fat accumulation and abnormal lipid metabolism were also observed in HFD group, which was improved in HFD + DPG10 and HFD + DPG30 groups. Especially, the epididymal fat weight and adipocyte size were greatly increased in HFD groups, which were reduced in HFD + DPG10 and HFD + DPG30 (Figure 3a,b). HFD-induced increase of the liver weight and fat accumulation in liver also improved in HFD + DPG10 and HFD + DPG30 groups (Figure 4a,b). Therefore, DPG inhibited fat accumulation into liver, which resulted in decrease of liver weight. In addition, biochemical parameters related to lipid metabolism, such as HDL, LDL, total cholesterol and triglyceride were also recovered in HFD + DPG10 and HFD + DPG30 (Table 2). Taken together, DPG mainly act on inhibition of fat accumulation, which further resulted in decrease in liver weight and lipid profiles in blood. Therefore, DPG might be effective in liver dysfunction induced by HFD, which was supported by the improvement of ALT and AST parameters in HFD + DPG10 and HFD + DPG30 groups.

Excessively absorbed fat is accumulated as adipose tissue through adipocyte differentiation. Adipogenic differentiation is a well-organized process tightly regulated by sequential activation of many transcriptional factors. PPARγ and C/EBPα play pivotal roles in adipogenesis by regulating gene expression for fat accumulation [30,31]. Adipogenesis is also regulated by leptin and adiponection, specific hormones secreted from adipose tissue [32,33]. Leptin amount is proportionally correlated with obesity, while adiponection amount is inversely related to obesity [29]. DPG effectively reduced the expression of PPARγ and C/EBPα, which were increased by HFD (Figure 5a). In addition, DPG significantly reduced leptin expression increased by HFD and restored the adiponection expression reduced by HFD (Figure 5b). Therefore, DPG efficiently reduced lipogenic genes by regulation of transcription factors and hormones, eventually leading to the suppression of lipogenesis.

To better understand the signal pathway for lipogenesis, effect of DPG on AMPK signaling was investigated. AMPK acts as an energy sensor and maintain energy homeostasis [34]. AMPK regulates fatty acid oxidation and cholesterol synthesis via ACC and HMGCR, thus has become an attractive therapeutic target in the treatment of metabolic disorders including obesity [35]. Consistent with reduced parameters of fat in epididymal, liver and serum, the levels of phosphorylation of AMPKs and ACC were higher in HFD + DPG group compared to those of HFD group. DPG also reduced expression of HMGCR (Figure 5c). In addition, DPG is a pancreatic lipase inhibitor [18]. Taken together, it is persuasive that DPG inhibited fat absorption by the inhibition of pancreatic lipase, and reduced lipogenesis via AMPK activation and followed by fatty acid oxidation and inhibition of cholesterol synthesis, which might contribute the improvement of metabolic parameters and eventually leading to the anti-obesity effect *in vivo*.

DPG is 6,8-diprenylgenistein, which means that the chemical structure of DPG is similar to genistein except for two additional prenyl moieties. Genestein, is also reported to be efficient for metabolic diseases including obesity [36]. However, DPG showed stronger inhibition on pancreatic lipase than genistein in our assay system [18], which suggested the importance of prenyl moieties of DPG. HPLC analysis showed the high content of DPG in *C. tricuspidata* fruits (Figure 1b). The extract of *C. tricuspidata* fruits contains as much as 5.4% of DPG when extracted with 70% ethanol [18]. Our present study shows that administration of 10 mg/kg is sufficient for maximum efficacy of DPG in HFD-induced obesity. Therefore, daily intake of 10–15 g *C. tricuspidata* fruits corresponds to 10 mg/kg DPG for man, which will be beneficial in regulation of obesity. In addition, *C. tricuspidata* fruits also contain diverse isoflavonoids including DPG and genistein [16,18]. Therefore, we suggest that DPG and *C. tricuspidata* fruits might be beneficial for the regulation of obesity, especially obesity resulting from high fat intake.

5. Conclusions

DPG, a major isoflavonoid of *C. tricuspidata* fruits improved many parameters of HFD-induced obesity. In particular, DPG significantly reduced epididymal fat and the serum triglyceride content, which had increased due to the HFD. Administration of DPG also improved liver dysfunction as suggested by reduced fat accumulation and the levels of ALT and AST increased by HFD. Further study suggests that DPG efficiently reduces lipogenic genes by regulation of transcription factors and hormones, and regulates ACC and HMGCR by AMPK activation. Taken together, DPG are beneficial for the regulation of obesity, especially obesity resulting from high fat intake.

Supplementary Materials: The following are available online at http://www.mdpi.com/2072-6643/7/12/5544/s1, Table S1: Composition of experimental diets.

Acknowledgments: This study was supported by a grant from the Eco-Innovation Project (grant No. 416-111-006) of the Ministry of Environment, Korea.

Author Contributions: S.-G.D., E.S., G.J. and M.K.L. conceived and designed the experiments; Y.H.J., K.-M.C., Q.L., S.B.K., H.-J.J. and S.-K.S. performed the experiments; M.K., H.-S.Y., B.Y.H. and M.K.L. analyzed the data; M.K.L. wrote the paper.

Conflicts of Interest: The authors declare no conflict of interest.

References

1. Kopelman, P.G. Obesity as a medical problem. *Nature* **2000**, *404*, 635–643. [PubMed]
2. Visscher, T.L.; Seidell, J.C. The public health impact of obesity. *Ann. Rev. Public Health* **2001**, *22*, 355–375. [CrossRef] [PubMed]
3. Yun, J.W. Possible anti-obesity therapeutics from nature—A review. *Phytochemistry* **2010**, *71*, 1625–1641. [CrossRef] [PubMed]
4. Farmer, S.R. Transcriptional control of adipocyte formation. *Cell Metab.* **2006**, *4*, 263–273. [CrossRef] [PubMed]
5. Maffei, M.; Halaas, J.; Ravussin, E.; Pratley, R.E.; Lee, G.H.; Zhang, Y. Leptin levels in human and rodent: Measurement of plasma leptin and ob RNA in obese and weight-reduced subjects. *Nat. Med.* **1995**, *1*, 1155–1161. [CrossRef] [PubMed]
6. Ruderman, N.B.; Carling, D.; Prentki, M.; Cacicedo, J.M. AMPK, insulin resistance, and the metabolic syndrome. *J. Clin. Investig.* **2013**, *123*, 2764–2772. [CrossRef] [PubMed]
7. Hardie, D.G. Regulation of fatty acid and cholesterol metabolism by the AMP-activated protein kinase. *Biochim. Biophys. Acta* **1992**, *1123*, 231–238. [CrossRef]
8. Legeay, S.; Rodier, M.; Fillon, L.; Faure, S.; Clere, N. Epigallocatechin gallate: A review of its beneficial properties to prevent metabolic syndrome. *Nutrients* **2015**, *7*, 5443–5468. [CrossRef] [PubMed]

9. Choi, K.M.; Jeon, Y.S.; Kim, W.; Lee, A.; Kim, Y.G.; Lee, J.H.; Kang, Y.E.; Jung, J.C.; Lee, J.; Min, B.; *et al.* Xanthigen attenuates high-fat diet-induced obesity through down-regulation of PPARγ and activation of the AMPK pathway. *Food Sci. Biotechnol.* **2014**, *23*, 931–935. [CrossRef]
10. Choi, K.M.; Lee, Y.S.; Kim, W.; Kim, S.J.; Shin, K.O.; Yu, J.Y.; Lee, M.K.; Lee, Y.M.; Hong, J.T.; Yun, Y.P.; *et al.* Sulforaphane attenuates obesity by inhibiting adipogenesis and activating the AMPK pathway in obese mice. *J. Nutr. Biochem.* **2014**, *25*, 201–207. [CrossRef] [PubMed]
11. Ahn, J.H.; Kim, E.S.; Lee, C.; Kim, S.; Cho, S.H.; Hwang, B.Y.; Lee, M.K. Chemical constituents from *Nelumbo nucifera* leaves and their anti-obesity effects. *Bioorg. Med. Chem. Lett.* **2013**, *23*, 3604–3608. [CrossRef] [PubMed]
12. Buchholz, T.; Melzig, M.F. Polyphenolic compounds as pancreatic lipase inhibitors. *Planta Med.* **2015**, *81*, 771–783. [CrossRef] [PubMed]
13. Senaphan, K.; Kukongviriyapan, U.; Sangartit, W.; Pakdeechote, P.; Pannangpetch, P.; Prachaney, P.; Greenwald, S.E.; Kukongviriyapan, V. Ferulic acid alleviates changes in a rat model of metabolic syndrome induced by high-carbohydrate, high-fat diet. *Nutrients* **2015**, *7*, 6446–6464. [CrossRef] [PubMed]
14. Kawakami, Y.; Kiyosawa, T.; Nakamura, S.; Osada, K. Effects of isoflavone supplementation on disturbances in lipid metabolism and antioxidant system due to exogenous cholesterol oxidation products in rats. *J. Funct. Foods* **2014**, *7*, 212–218. [CrossRef]
15. Lee, H.; Ha, H.; Lee, J.K.; Seo, C.S.; Lee, N.H.; Jung, D.Y.; Park, S.J.; Shin, H.K. The fruits of *Cudrania tricuspidata* suppress development of atopic dermatitis in NC/Nga mice. *Phytother. Res.* **2012**, *26*, 594–599. [CrossRef] [PubMed]
16. Han, X.H.; Hong, S.S.; Jin, Q.; Li, D.; Kim, H.K.; Lee, J.; Kwon, S.H.; Lee, D.; Lee, C.K.; Lee, M.K.; *et al.* Prenylated and benzylated flavonoids from the fruits of *Cudrania tricuspidata*. *J. Nat. Prod.* **2009**, *72*, 164–167. [CrossRef] [PubMed]
17. Cho, E.J.; Yokozawa, T.; Rhyu, D.Y.; Kim, S.C.; Shibahara, N.; Park, J.C. Study on the inhibitory effects of Korean medicinal plants and their main compounds on the 1,1-diphenyl-2-picrylhydrazyl radical. *Phytomedicine* **2003**, *10*, 544–551. [CrossRef] [PubMed]
18. Jeong, J.Y.; Jo, Y.H.; Lee, K.Y.; Do, S.G.; Hwang, B.Y.; Lee, M.K. Optimization of pancreatic lipase inhibition by *Cudrania tricuspidata* fruits using response surface methodology. *Bioorg. Med. Chem. Lett.* **2014**, *24*, 2329–2333. [CrossRef] [PubMed]
19. Oh, W.K.; Lee, C.H.; Seo, J.H.; Chung, M.Y.; Cui, L.; Fomum, Z.T.; Kang, J.S.; Lee, H.S. Diacylglycerol acyltransferase-inhibitory compounds from *Erythrina senegalensis*. *Arch. Pharm. Res.* **2009**, *32*, 43–47. [CrossRef] [PubMed]
20. Fowler, S.D.; Greenspan, P. Application of Nile red, a fluorescent hydrophobic probe, for the detection of neutral lipid deposits in tissue sections: Comparison with oil red O. *J. Histochem. Cytochem.* **1985**, *33*, 833–836. [CrossRef] [PubMed]
21. White, U.A.; Stephens, J.M. Transcriptional factors that promote formation of white adipose tissue. *Mol. Cell Endocrinol.* **2010**, *318*, 10–14. [CrossRef] [PubMed]
22. Ouchi, N.; Parker, J.L.; Lugus, J.J.; Walsh, K. Adipokines in inflammation and metabolic disease. *Nat. Rev. Immunol.* **2011**, *11*, 85–97. [CrossRef] [PubMed]
23. Rajala, M.W.; Scherer, P.E. Minireview: The adipocyte-at the crossroads of energy homeostasis, inflammation, and atherosclerosis. *Endocrinology* **2003**, *144*, 3765–3773. [CrossRef] [PubMed]
24. Tobert, J.A. Lovastatin and beyond: The history of the HMG-CoA reductase inhibitors. *Nat. Rev. Drug Discov.* **2003**, *2*, 517–526. [CrossRef] [PubMed]
25. Choi, K.M.; Lee, Y.S.; Shin, D.M.; Lee, S.; Yoo, K.S.; Lee, M.K.; Lee, J.H.; Kim, S.Y.; Lee, Y.M.; Hong, J.T.; *et al.* Green tomato extract attenuates high-fat-diet-induced obesity through activation of the AMPK pathway in C57BL/6 mice. *J. Nutr. Biochem.* **2013**, *24*, 335–342. [CrossRef] [PubMed]
26. Bhaswant, M.; Poudyal, H.; Mathai, M.L.; Ward, L.C.; Mouatt, P.; Brown, L. Green and black cardamom in a diet-induced rat model of metabolic syndrome. *Nutrients* **2015**, *7*, 7691–7707. [CrossRef] [PubMed]
27. Aguirre, L.; Fernández-Quintela, A.; Arias, N.; Portillo, P.P. Resveratrol: Anti-obesity mechanisms of action. *Molecules* **2014**, *19*, 18632–18655. [CrossRef] [PubMed]

28. Okuda, M.H.; Zemdegs, J.C.S.; Santana, A.A.; Santamarina, A.B.; Moreno, M.F.; Hachul, A.C.L.; Santos, B.; Nascimento, O.; Ribeiro, E.B.; Oyama, L.M. Green tea extract improves high fat diet-induced hypothalamic inflammation, without affecting serotoninergic system. *J. Nutr. Biochem.* **2014**, *25*, 1084–1089. [CrossRef] [PubMed]

29. Sclafani, A.; Springer, D. Dietary obesity in adult rats: Similarities to hypothalamic and human obesity syndromes. *Physiol. Behav.* **1976**, *17*, 461–471. [CrossRef]

30. Ntambi, J.M.; Young-Cheul, K. Adipocyte differentiation and gene expression. *J. Nutr.* **2000**, *130*, 3122S–3126S. [PubMed]

31. Tong, Q.; Hotamisligil, G.S. Molecular mechanisms of adipocyte differentiation. *Rev. Endocr. Metab. Disord.* **2001**, *2*, 349–355. [CrossRef] [PubMed]

32. Nedvidkova, J.; Smitka, K.; Kopsky, V.; Hainer, V. Adiponectin, an adipocyte-derived protein. *Physiol. Res.* **2005**, *54*, 133–140. [PubMed]

33. Diez, J.J.; Iglesias, P. The role of the novel adipocyte-derived hormone adiponectin in human disease. *Eur. J. Endocrinol.* **2003**, *148*, 293–300. [CrossRef] [PubMed]

34. Carling, D.; Zammit, V.A.; Hardie, D.G. A common bicyclic protein kinase cascade inactivates the regulatory enzymes of fatty acid and cholesterol biosynthesis. *FEBS Lett.* **1987**, *223*, 217–222. [CrossRef]

35. Steinberg, G.R.; Kemp, B.E. AMPK in health and disease. *Physiol. Rev.* **2008**, *89*, 1025–1078. [CrossRef] [PubMed]

36. Behloul, N.; Wu, G. Genistein: A promising therapeutic agent for obesity and diabetes treatment. *Eur. J. Pharmacol.* **2013**, *698*, 31–38. [CrossRef] [PubMed]

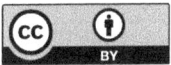

nutrients

Article

Moderately Low Magnesium Intake Impairs Growth of Lean Body Mass in Obese-Prone and Obese-Resistant Rats Fed a High-Energy Diet

Jesse Bertinato [1,2,*], Christopher Lavergne [1,3], Sophia Rahimi [1,2], Hiba Rachid [1,4], Nina A. Vu [1,2], Louise J. Plouffe [1] and Eleonora Swist [1]

1   Nutrition Research Division, Health Products and Food Branch, Health Canada,
    Sir Frederick G. Banting Research Centre, 251 Sir Frederick Banting Driveway, Ottawa, ON K1A 0K9,
    Canada; clave024@uottawa.ca (C.L.); sophia.rahimi@mail.mcgill.ca (S.R.);
    hiba-rachid-92@hotmail.com (H.R.); nvu008@uottawa.ca (N.A.V.); louise.j.plouffe@hc-sc.gc.ca (L.J.P.);
    eleonora.swist@hc-sc.gc.ca (E.S.)
2   Department of Biochemistry, Microbiology, and Immunology, University of Ottawa, Ottawa,
    ON K1H 8M5, Canada
3   Department of Biology, University of Ottawa, Ottawa, ON K1N 6N5, Canada
4   Food Science and Nutrition Program, Carleton University, Ottawa, ON K1S 5B6, Canada
*   Correspondence: jesse.bertinato@hc-sc.gc.ca; Tel.: +1-613-957-0924; Fax: +1-613-946-6212

Received: 24 November 2015; Accepted: 22 April 2016; Published: 28 April 2016

Abstract: The physical and biochemical changes resulting from moderately low magnesium (Mg) intake are not fully understood. Obesity and associated co-morbidities affect Mg metabolism and may exacerbate Mg deficiency and physiological effects. Male rats selectively bred for diet-induced obesity (OP, obese-prone) or resistance (OR, obese-resistant) were fed a high-fat, high-energy diet containing moderately low (LMg, 0.116 ± 0.001 g/kg) or normal (NMg, 0.516 ± 0.007 g/kg) Mg for 13 weeks. The growth, body composition, mineral homeostasis, bone development, and glucose metabolism of the rats were examined. OP and OR rats showed differences ($p < 0.05$) in many physical and biochemical measures regardless of diet. OP and OR rats fed the LMg diet had decreased body weight, lean body mass, decreased femoral size (width, weight, and volume), and serum Mg and potassium concentrations compared to rats fed the NMg diet. The LMg diet increased serum calcium (Ca) concentration in both rat strains with a concomitant decrease in serum parathyroid hormone concentration only in the OR strain. In the femur, Mg concentration was reduced, whereas concentrations of Ca and sodium were increased in both strains fed the LMg diet. Plasma glucose and insulin concentrations in an oral glucose tolerance test were similar in rats fed the LMg or NMg diets. These results show that a moderately low Mg diet impairs the growth of lean body mass and alters femoral geometry and mineral metabolism in OP and OR rats fed a high-energy diet.

Keywords: bone; diet; glucose; growth; lean body mass; magnesium deficiency; obesity; rat

1. Introduction

Magnesium (Mg) is an essential nutrient and co-factor in hundreds of metabolic reactions in the body. Mg is required for cell proliferation, cellular energy production, mineral metabolism, bone development, and glucose homeostasis [1–4]. Nutrition surveys in North America indicate that Mg consumption is below recommended intakes for a large segment of the population [5,6]. Furthermore, diseases such as type 2 diabetes [7] and use of certain medications [8] can increase Mg loss and predispose individuals to Mg deficiency. The low Mg intakes in comparison to current recommendations combined with the high prevalence of factors that can increase Mg requirements raise concern about widespread Mg deficiency. Biochemical data lend further support.

Hypomagnesemia (low serum Mg) exists in the general population and the incidence is high in certain subpopulations [7,9,10].

Despite evidence suggesting Mg deficiency in the general population, the health implications are unclear. Several factors account for this, including concerns that dietary recommendations for Mg [11] may be set too high [12] and that much of the evidence relating lower Mg intake or serum Mg with diseases and health conditions is based on observational studies. In addition, overt symptoms of Mg deficiency (e.g., hypocalcemia) are rarely observed in the general population and there is uncertainty regarding the serum Mg concentration needed for optimal health.

Since Mg is required for many enzymatic reactions, Mg deficiency can presumably affect numerous physiological processes. Some studies have reported changes in body composition with dietary Mg restriction. In rats, maternal and postnatal feeding of a Mg-deficient diet decreased body weight, lean body mass, and fat free mass and increased percentage body fat in the offspring [13,14]. In contrast, body weight, fat mass, and lean mass were similar in rats fed a high-fat diet containing normal or low Mg beginning after weaning [15].

Studies in rats and mice have shown that dietary Mg restriction impairs bone growth, changes bone architecture, and increases bone fragility [16–21]. An uncoupling of bone formation and bone resorption was observed in rats fed a very low Mg diet [22]. Mg-depleted rats showed greater bone resorption with an increase in the number of tartrate-resistant acid phosphatase-positive osteoclasts and a decrease in the number of osteoblasts per area of bone surface [22]. With less severe dietary Mg restriction (diets containing 10%–50% of nutritional requirement), the number of osteoblasts per bone surface were not affected in the distal femur of rats [16–18,23]. However, rats fed a Mg-deficient diet containing as high as 50% of nutritional requirement showed a greater number of osteoclasts per bone surface, reduced bone mineral content, and lower percentage of trabecular bone volume in the distal femur [16].

The effects of Mg deficiency on parathyroid hormone (PTH) secretion/action and calcium (Ca) homeostasis may partly account for the observed effects on bone [23]. In humans, severe Mg deficiency impairs PTH secretion, causing hypocalcemia [24]. In rats, severe Mg deficiency increases serum Ca and decreases serum PTH [18,20]. With severe dietary Mg restriction, competition between Mg and Ca for intestinal absorption and reabsorption in the kidney may be diminished in rats, causing a rise in serum Ca concentration [23]. The observed decrease in serum PTH may be a consequence of the rise in serum Ca or direct impairment of PTH secretion [23]. Under conditions of milder dietary Mg restriction, a decrease in serum Ca and an increase in serum PTH have been reported in rats [16]. With less severe Mg restriction, competition between Mg and Ca may still exist and the small reduction in serum Mg may affect the Ca-sensing receptor in a similar way as Ca, thus increasing PTH secretion [23]. It is only when the degree of Mg deficiency becomes more pronounced that PTH secretion is reduced.

There is evidence to suggest that Mg deficiency may contribute to insulin resistance and glucose intolerance [13]. Maternal and perinatal Mg restriction in rats induced insulin resistance and decreased insulin response to a glucose challenge [13]. A recent study showed decreased phosphorylation of proteins involved in the insulin-signaling pathway in rats fed a Mg-deficient, high-fat diet, suggesting decreased insulin sensitivity, but blood glucose and insulin concentrations did not differ compared to rats fed a normal Mg diet [15]. In human studies, lower Mg intakes or serum Mg concentrations have been associated with reduced bone mineral density [25], type 2 diabetes [26–29], and poorer insulin sensitivity and glucose control [9,30].

At present the physiological effects of moderately low Mg intakes are incompletely understood. The objective of this study was to examine physical and biochemical changes in rats fed moderately low Mg in the context of a high-fat, high-energy diet. Effects on body weight, body composition, mineral metabolism, bone development, and glucose homeostasis were investigated. Given that obesity and associated co-morbidities (e.g., type 2 diabetes) can affect Mg metabolism, effects were examined in rat strains selectively bred for susceptibility or resistance to diet-induced obesity. We report that a moderate decrease in dietary Mg impairs growth of lean body mass, alters femoral geometry, and induces changes in serum and bone mineral concentrations in these rat strains.

2. Materials and Methods

2.1. Animal Protocol and Diets

Fifty Crl:OP (CD) (OP, obese-prone) and 50 Crl:OR (CD) (OR, obese-resistant) male rats (Charles River Canada, St. Constant, QC, Canada) of six weeks of age were used in this study. OP ($n = 25$/diet group) and OR ($n = 25$/diet group) rats were fed high-fat, high-energy diets (Dyets, Inc., Bethlehem, PA, USA) containing moderately low (LMg, 0.116 ± 0.001 g/kg diet) or normal (NMg, 0.516 ± 0.007 g/kg diet) Mg. Compositions and energy densities of the diets are shown in Table S1. Diets were formulated using the AIN-93G mineral mix [31] without Mg and supplemented with either 0.100 (LMg) or 0.500 (NMg) g of Mg (as Mg oxide) per kg diet. Mg concentrations in the final diets were slightly higher than expected based on the amount of Mg oxide added. The additional Mg comes from other diet ingredients. Diets were a modified version of the Research Diets, Inc. D12266B formulation used previously to induce obesity in rats [32–34]. Diets were pelleted for more accurate measurement of food consumption.

OP and OR rats were assigned to diet groups based on initial body weight so that mean body weights in each diet group were similar at the start of the study. Rats were housed individually in solid-bottom cages held in vented racks. Cages had a wire-grille insert on the bottom and contained a stainless steel platform and shelter. Rats were put on a 12:12-h light-dark cycle and had free access to food and demineralized water throughout the study. Food consumption and body weight for each rat was measured twice a week. Food consumption was determined by measuring food missing from the feeder. Results for body weight measurements and parameters related to food consumption were not reported between days 46–64 and 78–81 because some rats were fasted on the selected days of measurements. The body composition of each rat was measured at the beginning (week 0), middle (weeks 8 and 9), and end (week 14) of the study using an EchoMRI-4in1™ system (EchoMRI, Houston, TX, USA).

After 13 weeks of feeding the diets, rats were fasted overnight (~12 h) in metabolic cages for collection of urine. Rats were then killed by exsanguination under general isoflurane anesthesia. Blood was collected from the abdominal aorta by syringe and dispensed into a Trace Element Serum tube (14-816-154, Thermo Fisher Scientific, Ottawa, ON, Canada) for isolation of serum. Hind legs and adipose depots were extracted and immediately frozen on dry ice and then stored at −80 °C until analysis. The experimental protocol was approved by the Health Products and Food Branch Animal Care Committee of Health Canada (Protocol No.: 2014-007).

During the study, five OR rats fed the LMg diet and two OR rats fed the NMg diet died unexpectedly without symptoms. The number of deaths did not differ ($p \geqslant 0.05$, Fisher's exact test) among diet groups. Serology reports from sentinel rats were negative, suggesting that an infectious agent was not responsible. Post-mortem examination did not reveal significant lesions suggestive of infection, toxicity, or lymphoma and the final judgment was sudden death of undetermined cause. Results from an additional four rats were excluded from the analyses. These rats were euthanized following unintentional gavage of solution into the lungs during a practice ($n = 3$) and the experimental ($n = 1$) oral glucose tolerance test (OGTT).

2.2. OGTT

During week 13 of the study an OGTT was performed on subgroups ($n = 10$/group) of OP and OR rats with the highest and lowest percentage body fat measurements at weeks 8–9 of the study, respectively. Following an overnight fast (~12 h), a 0.4 g/mL dextrose solution was orally administered to the rats by gavage (2 g dextrose/kg body weight). Blood samples (~250 µL) were drawn from the tail vein before dextrose dosing (0 min) and 30, 60, and 120 min after dosing. Blood samples were dispensed into BD Microtainer™ tubes with lithium heparin (13-680-62, Thermo Fisher Scientific) for isolation of plasma. Plasma samples were immediately frozen at $-80\ ^\circ$C until analysis.

2.3. Femur Isolation and Physical Measurements

Femurs were isolated from the right leg. Skin and flesh was removed using a scalpel and forceps. Wet and dry femur weights were measured using a Mettler Toledo AT261 delta range analytical balance (Mettler Toledo, Mississauga, ON, Canada). Femur length and width were measured using a dial caliper (Mitutoyo Canada Inc., Toronto, ON, Canada). Femur length corresponds to the distance from the greater trochanter to the lateral condyle. Femur width was the distance between medial and lateral surfaces at midshaft. Femur volume was determined using a PYREX™ specific gravity bottle (01-716, Thermo Fisher Scientific). Femur volume was calculated as the mass of water displaced by the femur in grams divided by the density of water ($0.99997\ \text{g}/\text{cm}^3$). Femur density was calculated as the wet weight in grams divided by the volume in cubic centimeters.

2.4. Mineral Analyses

Diets (~1 g samples) and femurs were placed in preweighted quartz beakers and dried overnight at $100\ ^\circ$C in an Isotemp® oven (Thermo Fisher Scientific). Samples were cooled, placed in a desiccator for 1 h and then weighed to obtain dry weights. Diets and femurs were ashed using a combination of dry ashing using an Isotemp® Programmable Forced Draft Furnace (Thermo Fisher Scientific) and wet ashing using concentrated trace metal grade nitric acid (Thermo Fisher Scientific). Ashes were solubilized in dilute nitric acid. Solubilized ashes and urine samples were analyzed for mineral concentrations using a 700 Series inductively coupled plasma optical emission spectrometer (Agilent Technologies Canada Inc., Mississauga, ON, Canada). Operating conditions have been described previously [35]. Concentrations of minerals were derived from a standard calibration curve prepared using the CALEDON-88 multi-element standard (Inorganic Ventures, Christiansburg, VA, USA). Analytical accuracy was verified using National Institute of Standards and Technology traceable reference material™ (SCP Science, Baie D'Urfé, QC, Canada).

2.5. Assays

Mineral concentrations in serum and urine creatinine were measured using the ABX Pentra 400 chemistry analyzer (HORIBA Instruments Inc., Irvine, CA, USA). Plasma insulin and glucose were measure using the Rat Ultrasensitive Insulin ELISA (80-INSRTU-E01, Alpco Diagnostics, Salem, NH, USA) and Glucose Colorimetric Assay Kit (10009582, Cayman Chemical, Ann Arbor, MI, USA), respectively. Serum PTH and osteocalcin were measured using the Rat BioActive Intact PTH ELISA Kit (60-2700, Immutopics, Inc., San Clemente, CA, USA) and Osteocalcin Rat Enzyme Immunoassay Kit (BT-490, Alfa Aesar, Ward Hill, MA, USA), respectively. Urine deoxypyridinoline (DPD) was determined using the MicroVue™ DPD EIA Kit (8007, Quidel Corporation®, San Diego, CA, USA).

2.6. Statistical Analyses

Results are reported as means $\pm$ SD. Two-way ANOVA was used for analysis of parameters measured at a single time point to examine the overall effects of strain and diet. Fisher's least significant difference *post hoc* test was performed for parameters with a significant ($p < 0.05$) strain $\times$ diet interaction. Mixed-design ANOVA was used for analysis of parameters measured at multiple time points to determine the effects and interactions of time, strain, and diet. For parameters with a significant time $\times$ strain or time $\times$ diet interaction, univariate results are presented for the effect of strain or diet at each time point, respectively. Homogeneity of variances was assessed using Levene's test. Data that showed unequal variances were transformed prior to analysis. Fisher's exact test was used to determine differences in proportions. The area under the glucose and insulin curves was calculated using the trapezoidal rule with the Area below Curves function in SigmaPlot 12.5 (Systat

Software Inc., Chicago, IL, USA). Statistical analyses were performed using Statistica 7 (StatSoft, Tulsa, OK, USA). Statistical significance was set at $p < 0.05$.

3. Results

This study examined the effects of a moderately low Mg diet high in fat and energy on growth, body composition, energy intake, energy efficiency, mineral homeostasis, bone development, and glucose metabolism in OP and OR rats. The effect of rat strain and diet on each parameter is presented. Body weights differed between rat strains and between rats fed the low or normal Mg diets (Figure 1). Body weights at the start of the study were higher for OR than OP rats. From day 25 to the end of the study, OP rats were heavier than OR rats and rats fed the low Mg diet were lighter than rats fed the normal Mg diet.

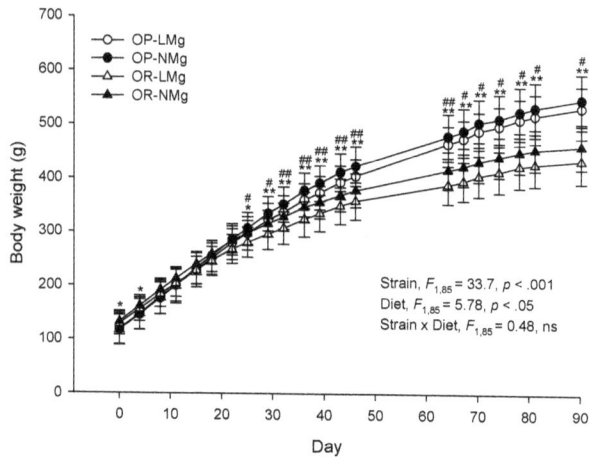

Figure 1. Body weights of rats. Results are presented as means $\pm$ SD, $n = 18$–25. Results were analyzed by mixed-design ANOVA to determine effects and interactions of time, strain, and diet. Time $\times$ strain and time $\times$ diet interactions ($p < 0.05$) were observed and univariate results are shown for effects of strain (*, $p < 0.05$; **, $p < 0.001$) and diet (#, $p < 0.05$; ##, $p < 0.01$). ns, $p \geqslant 0.05$.

Percentage lean body mass was higher, but total lean body mass was lower in OR compared to OP rats at weeks 8–9 and week 14 (Table 1). Rats fed the low Mg diet had lower total lean body mass at weeks 8–9 and week 14. Percentage body fat, total body fat, and weight of four distinct fat depots were higher in OP compared to OR rats at week 14 (Table 1). Percentage and total body fat did not differ between rats fed the low or normal Mg diets. Weight of mesenteric fat was lower in rats fed the low Mg diet.

Energy intakes did not differ between rat strains (Figure 2A). Rats fed the low Mg diet had lower energy intakes compared to rats fed the normal Mg diet. OP rats had superior energy efficiency compared to OR rats (Figure 2B). Energy efficiency was similar for rats fed the low or normal Mg diets. Food consumption did not differ between rat strains, but was lower for rats fed the low Mg diet (Figure S1). Similarly, Mg intake was comparable between rat strains, but was lower for rats fed the low Mg diet (Figure S2).

Concentrations of minerals and markers of bone metabolism were examined in the serum (Table 2) and urine (Table 3) of the rats. Concentrations of minerals and bone markers in serum and urine differed between rat strains. Serum and urine Mg concentrations were lower in rats fed the low Mg diet. Serum Ca concentrations were higher and serum potassium (K) concentrations were lower in rats fed the low Mg diet. The low Mg diet decreased serum PTH concentration only in OR rats (Table 2). Serum osteocalcin and urine DPD concentrations were similar in rats fed the low or normal Mg diets (Tables 2 and 3).

Table 1. Body composition of rats.

Parameter	OP-LMg (n = 25)	OP-NMg (n = 23)	OR-LMg (n = 18)	OR-NMg (n = 23)	Strain	Diet	Strain × Diet
Lean (%) [1]					$F_{1,85} = 9.4, p < 0.01$	$F_{1,85} = 0.9$, ns	$F_{1,85} = 0.0$, ns
wk 0	85.5 ± 1.8	85.4 ± 1.4	85.2 ± 1.5	85.3 ± 1.7	$F_{1,85} = 0.3$, ns		
wk 8–9	77.2 ± 3.4	76.1 ± 3.6	79.0 ± 2.3	78.2 ± 2.7	$F_{1,85} = 8.68, p < 0.01$		
wk 14	72.2 ± 3.5	72.1 ± 4.2	75.2 ± 2.5	74.5 ± 2.8	$F_{1,85} = 13.5, p < 0.001$		
Lean (g) [1]					$F_{1,85} = 34.7, p < 0.001$	$F_{1,85} = 4.19, p < 0.05$	$F_{1,85} = 0.32$, ns
wk 0	83.9 ± 22.1	83.4 ± 23.3	92.1 ± 18.4	95.1 ± 17.3	$F_{1,85} = 5.11, p < 0.05$	$F_{1,85} = 0.085$, ns	
wk 8–9	333 ± 24	344 ± 33	297 ± 28	312 ± 21	$F_{1,85} = 35.1, p < 0.001$	$F_{1,85} = 5.29, p < 0.05$	
wk 14	387 ± 29	396 ± 29	331 ± 26	346 ± 21	$F_{1,85} = 89.3, p < 0.001$	$F_{1,85} = 4.83, p < 0.05$	
Fat (%) [1]					$F_{1,85} = 23.8, p < 0.001$	$F_{1,85} = 1.36$, ns	$F_{1,85} = 0.061$, ns
wk 0	10.6 ± 1.1	10.6 ± 1.2	10.0 ± 1.2	10.1 ± 0.8	$F_{1,85} = 4.74, p < 0.05$		
wk 8–9	17.9 ± 3.3	18.9 ± 3.3	14.9 ± 2.2	15.9 ± 2.6	$F_{1,85} = 22.6, p < 0.001$		
wk 14	22.6 ± 3.4	22.9 ± 4.2	18.6 ± 2.7	19.7 ± 2.9	$F_{1,85} = 25.0, p < 0.001$		
Fat (g) [1]					$F_{1,85} = 44.5, p < 0.001$	$F_{1,85} = 3.24$, ns	$F_{1,85} = 0.079$, ns
wk 0	10.4 ± 3.1	10.3 ± 3.0	10.9 ± 2.7	11.4 ± 2.7	$F_{1,85} = 1.42$, ns		
wk 8–9	78.0 ± 19.7	86.2 ± 19.6	56.6 ± 12.2	64.3 ± 15.0	$F_{1,85} = 34.8, p < 0.001$		
wk 14	122 ± 24	127 ± 30	83 ± 18	93 ± 21	$F_{1,85} = 52.6, p < 0.001$		
Ing fat (g) [2]	11.2 ± 2.5	11.8 ± 3.2	6.4 ± 1.5	7.3 ± 2.0	$F_{1,85} = 85.3, p < 0.001$	$F_{1,85} = 2.04$, ns	$F_{1,85} = 0.566$, ns
Retro fat (g) [2]	21.7 ± 3.7	22.2 ± 4.7	13.9 ± 3.2	15.3 ± 3.7	$F_{1,85} = 77.3, p < 0.001$	$F_{1,85} = 1.48$, ns	$F_{1,85} = 0.259$, ns
Mes fat (g) [2]	10.0 ± 2.5	10.7 ± 2.8	6.0 ± 1.4	7.0 ± 1.6	$F_{1,85} = 70.4, p < 0.001$	$F_{1,85} = 4.29, p < 0.05$	$F_{1,85} = 0.666$, ns
Epi fat (g) [2]	15.8 ± 2.9	15.9 ± 4.1	9.2 ± 2.7	10.9 ± 2.6	$F_{1,85} = 74.1, p < 0.001$	$F_{1,85} = 2.02$, ns	$F_{1,85} = 1.37$, ns

Values are means ± SD; [1] Analyzed by mixed-design ANOVA to determine the effects and interactions of time, strain, and diet. Univariate results are shown for each time point for parameters with significant ($p < 0.05$) time × strain or time × diet interaction; [2] Analyzed by two-way ANOVA; ns, $p \geq 0.05$. Epi, epididymal; Ing, inguinal; Mes, mesenteric; Retro, retroperitoneal; wk, week.

Table 2. Serum minerals and bone markers.

Parameter	Groups				ANOVA [1]		
	OP-LMg (n = 25)	OP-NMg (n = 23)	OR-LMg (n = 18)	OR-NMg (n = 23)	Strain	Diet	Strain × Diet
Mg (mmol/L)	0.52 ± 0.11	0.74 ± 0.12	0.63 ± 0.10	0.85 ± 0.13	$F_{1,85} = 20.0, p < 0.001$	$F_{1,85} = 75.0, p < 0.001$	$F_{1,85} = 0.017$, ns
Ca (mmol/L)	2.67 ± 0.10	2.58 ± 0.11	2.78 ± 0.11	2.70 ± 0.12	$F_{1,85} = 23.2, p < 0.001$	$F_{1,85} = 12.4, p < 0.001$	$F_{1,85} = 0.090$, ns
P (mmol/L)	1.77 ± 0.24	1.83 ± 0.22	1.68 ± 0.17	1.75 ± 0.12	$F_{1,85} = 4.05, p < 0.05$	$F_{1,85} = 2.84$, ns	$F_{1,85} = 0.007$, ns
K (mmol/L)	3.99 ± 0.33	4.20 ± 0.25	4.32 ± 0.31	4.44 ± 0.21	$F_{1,85} = 23.1, p < 0.001$	$F_{1,85} = 7.43, p < 0.01$	$F_{1,85} = 0.54$, ns
Na (mmol/L)	143 ± 1	143 ± 1	143 ± 1	143 ± 2	$F_{1,85} = 0.6$, ns	$F_{1,85} = 0.8$, ns	$F_{1,85} = 0.9$, ns
PTH (ng/L)	152 ± 75 [c]	125 ± 34 [c]	221 ± 81 [b]	306 ± 165 [a]	$F_{1,85} = 48.2, p < 0.001$	$F_{1,85} = 0.89$, ns	$F_{1,85} = 5.30, p < 0.05$
OC (µg/L)	25.6 ± 8.2	24.8 ± 6.5	19.9 ± 6.5	21.3 ± 4.0	$F_{1,85} = 11.1, p < 0.01$	$F_{1,85} = 0.042$, ns	$F_{1,85} = 0.628$, ns

Values are means ± SD; [1] Analyzed by two-way ANOVA. Fisher's least significant difference *post hoc* test was performed for the parameter with a significant ($p < 0.05$) strain × diet interaction. Values within the row without a common superscript letter differ, $p < 0.05$. ns, $p \geq 0.05$. Ca, calcium; K, potassium; Mg, magnesium; Na, sodium; OC, osteocalcin; P, phosphorus; PTH, parathyroid hormone.

Table 3. Urine minerals and deoxypyridinoline.

Parameter	Groups				ANOVA [1]		
	OP-LMg (n = 25)	OP-NMg (n = 23)	OR-LMg (n = 18)	OR-NMg (n = 23)	Strain	Diet	Strain × Diet
Mg (mg/g Cr)	27 ± 10	92 ± 25	26 ± 11	100 ± 31	$F_{1,85} = 0.01$, ns	$F_{1,85} = 308$, $p < 0.001$	$F_{1,85} = 0.84$, ns
Ca (mg/g Cr)	14 ± 2	14 ± 2	17 ± 3	16 ± 3	$F_{1,85} = 26.8$, $p < 0.001$	$F_{1,85} = 0.348$, ns	$F_{1,85} = 0.058$, ns
P (mg/g Cr)	885 ± 302	960 ± 415	1323 ± 276	1261 ± 252	$F_{1,85} = 29.4$, $p < 0.001$	$F_{1,85} = 0.009$, ns	$F_{1,85} = 1.01$, ns
K (mg/g Cr)	2160 ± 430	2190 ± 610	2530 ± 550	2560 ± 550	$F_{1,85} = 10.7$, $p < 0.01$	$F_{1,85} = 0.076$, ns	$F_{1,85} = 0.00$, ns
Na (mg/g Cr)	367 ± 199	371 ± 171	198 ± 99	227 ± 110	$F_{1,85} = 22.4$, $p < 0.001$	$F_{1,85} = 0.244$, ns	$F_{1,85} = 0.148$, ns
DPD (nmol/mmol Cr)	93 ± 21	103 ± 24	159 ± 36	171 ± 49	$F_{1,85} = 85.9$, $p < 0.001$	$F_{1,85} = 2.35$, ns	$F_{1,85} = 0.037$, ns

Values are means ± SD; [1] Analyzed by two-way ANOVA; ns, $p \geqslant 0.05$; Ca, calcium; Cr, creatinine; DPD, deoxypyridinoline; K, potassium; Mg, magnesium; Na, sodium; P, phosphorus.

A

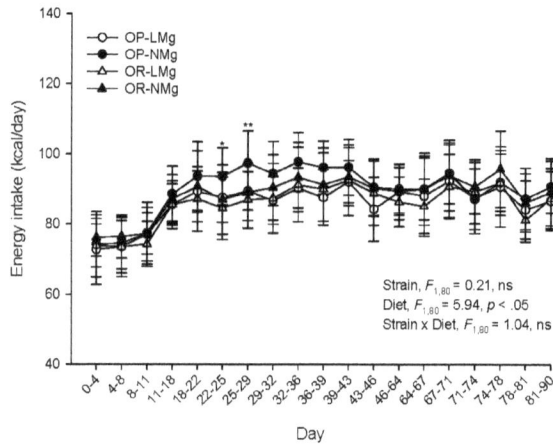

B

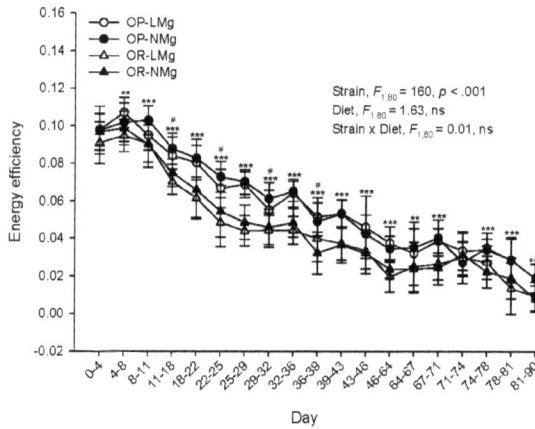

Figure 2. Energy intake and energy efficiency of rats. Results are presented as means ± SD, n = 17–25. Results for energy intake (**A**); and energy efficiency (**B**) were analyzed by mixed-design ANOVA to determine effects and interactions of time, strain, and diet. Univariate results are shown for effects of strain (*, $p < 0.05$; **, $p < 0.01$; ***, $p < 0.001$) or diet (#, $p < 0.05$) when a significant ($p < 0.05$) time × strain or time × diet interaction was observed, respectively. Energy efficiency = (body weight gain (g/day)/energy intake (kcal/day)). ns, $p \geqslant 0.05$.

Femoral mineral concentrations and physical measurements were assessed in the rats. OP and OR rats showed differences in Mg, K, and sodium (Na) concentrations in femur (Table 4). Concentration of Mg was lower and concentrations of Ca and Na were higher in femurs of rats fed the low Mg diet.

Measurements for femur width, dry weight, and density were higher, whereas femur length:width ratio was lower in OP compared to OR rats (Table 5). Measurements for femur width, wet weight, dry weight, and volume were lower in rats fed the low Mg diet. The low Mg diet increased femur length:width ratio only in OR rats.

Table 4. Concentrations of minerals in femur.

Parameter	Groups				ANOVA [1]		
	OP-LMg (n = 25)	OP-NMg (n = 22)	OR-LMg (n = 18)	OR-NMg (n = 23)	Strain	Diet	Strain × Diet
Mg (mg/g DW)	2.88 ± 0.26	4.55 ± 0.15	3.61 ± 0.25	4.94 ± 0.15	$F_{1,84}$ = 164, p < 0.001	$F_{1,84}$ = 1266, p < 0.001	$F_{1,84}$ = 3.50, ns
Ca (mg/g DW)	282 ± 8	279 ± 5	283 ± 11	275 ± 9	$F_{1,84}$ = 0.71, ns	$F_{1,84}$ = 9.77, p < 0.01	$F_{1,84}$ = 2.08, ns
P (mg/g DW)	137 ± 4	139 ± 4	138 ± 5	136 ± 5	$F_{1,84}$ = 0.53, ns	$F_{1,84}$ = 0.03, ns	$F_{1,84}$ = 2.36, ns
K (mg/g DW)	1.91 ± 0.11	1.96 ± 0.11	2.18 ± 0.17	2.17 ± 0.09	$F_{1,84}$ = 86.8, p < 0.001	$F_{1,84}$ = 0.45, ns	$F_{1,84}$ = 1.33, ns
Na (mg/g DW)	9.18 ± 0.29	8.75 ± 0.21	8.94 ± 0.45	8.50 ± 0.22	$F_{1,84}$ = 14.9, p < 0.001	$F_{1,84}$ = 45.6, p < 0.001	$F_{1,84}$ = 0.00, ns

Values are means ± SD; [1] Analyzed by two-way ANOVA; ns, $p \geqslant 0.05$; Ca, calcium; DW, dry weight; K, potassium; Mg, magnesium; Na, sodium; P, phosphorus.

Table 5. Physical measurements of femur.

Parameter	Groups				ANOVA [1]		
	OP-LMg (n = 25)	OP-NMg (n = 23)	OR-LMg (n = 18)	OR-NMg (n = 23)	Strain	Diet	Strain × Diet
Length (mm) [2]	38.8 ± 0.6	39.0 ± 1.0 [4]	38.8 ± 0.7	39.1 ± 0.6	$F_{1,84}$ = 0.0, ns	$F_{1,84}$ = 2.4, ns	$F_{1,84}$ = 0.1, ns
Width (mm) [3]	4.59 ± 0.12	4.63 ± 0.28	4.16 ± 0.21	4.32 ± 0.17	$F_{1,85}$ = 76.2, p < 0.001	$F_{1,85}$ = 5.65, p < 0.05	$F_{1,85}$ = 2.78, ns
Length:width ratio	8.46 ± 0.19 [c]	8.49 ± 0.48 [4,c]	9.35 ± 0.42 [a]	9.05 ± 0.32 [b]	$F_{1,84}$ = 87.8, p < 0.001	$F_{1,84}$ = 2.96, ns	$F_{1,84}$ = 4.36, p < 0.05
Wet weight (g)	0.933 ± 0.050	0.951 ± 0.082 [4]	0.899 ± 0.064	0.944 ± 0.057	$F_{1,84}$ = 2.21, ns	$F_{1,84}$ = 5.35, p < 0.05	$F_{1,84}$ = 0.89, ns
Dry weight (g)	0.686 ± 0.035	0.693 ± 0.055 [4]	0.640 ± 0.050	0.672 ± 0.041	$F_{1,84}$ = 12.0, p < 0.001	$F_{1,84}$ = 4.04, p < 0.05	$F_{1,84}$ = 1.71, ns
Volume (cm³)	0.596 ± 0.032	0.611 ± 0.058 [4]	0.584 ± 0.042	0.618 ± 0.038	$F_{1,84}$ = 0.06, ns	$F_{1,84}$ = 6.73, p < 0.05	$F_{1,84}$ = 0.99, ns
Density (g/cm³)	1.57 ± 0.02	1.56 ± 0.03 [4]	1.54 ± 0.02	1.53 ± 0.02	$F_{1,84}$ = 30.3, p < 0.001	$F_{1,84}$ = 2.9, ns	$F_{1,84}$ = 0.3, ns

Values are means ± SD; [1] Analyzed by two-way ANOVA; Fisher's least significant difference post hoc test was performed for the parameter with a significant ($p < 0.05$) strain × diet interaction; Values within the row without a common superscript letter differ, $p < 0.05$; ns, $p \geqslant 0.05$; [2] Length from the greater trochanter to the lateral condyle; [3] Midshaft mediolateral width; [4] $n = 22$.

An OGTT was performed on a subgroup of rats in each group to investigate the effect of the low Mg diet on glucose homeostasis. Mean percentage body fat for these rats at the end of the study were 25.9% ± 2.5% (OP-LMg), 26.6% ± 2.1% (OP-NMg), 16.7% ± 1.4% (OR-LMg), and 17.3% ± 1.6% (OR-NMg). At the 30 min time point, plasma glucose concentration was higher in OR rats compared to OP rats regardless of diet (Figure 3A). Plasma glucose concentrations were similar for OP and OR rats fed the low or normal Mg diets at each time point (Figure 3A). The area under the glucose curve did not differ between rat strains or rats fed the low or normal Mg diets (Figure 3C). OP rats had higher plasma insulin concentrations at each time point compared to OR rats (Figure 3B). Area under the insulin curve was also greater for OP rats (Figure 3D). Plasma insulin concentrations at each time point and area under the insulin curve were similar in OP and OR rats fed the low or normal Mg diets.

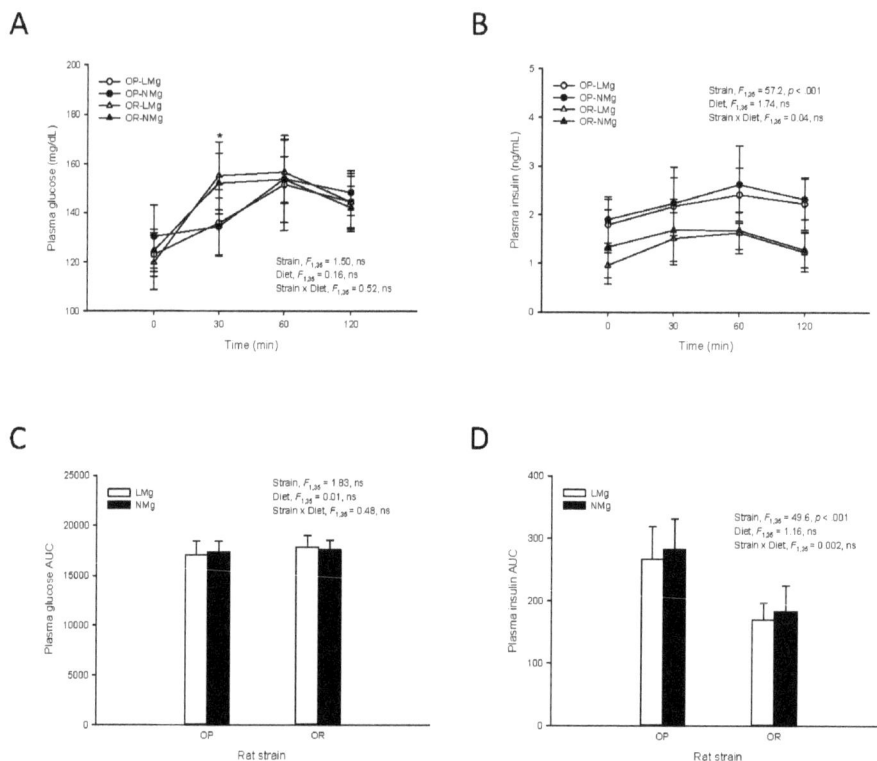

Figure 3. Plasma glucose and insulin during an oral glucose tolerance test conducted at week 13 of the study. Plasma glucose and insulin concentrations (**A,B**) and the respective area under the curve (AUC) (**C,D**); Dextrose solution (0.4 g/mL) was orally administered to the rats (2 g dextrose/kg body weight) after an overnight fast. Blood was collected from the tail vein before dosing (0 min) and 30, 60, and 120 min after dosing. Results are displayed as means ± SD, $n = 9$–10. Results were analyzed by mixed-design ANOVA to determine the effects and interactions of time, strain, and diet (**A,B**); For glucose a significant ($p < 0.05$) time × strain interaction was observed and univariate results are shown for effect of strain (*, $p < 0.001$). AUC results were analyzed by two-way ANOVA (**C,D**). ns, $p \geqslant 0.05$.

4. Discussion

This study examined physical and biochemical changes in rats fed a moderately low Mg diet with the aim of identifying physiological processes sensitive to reduction in Mg intake. Obesity and associated co-morbidities such as type 2 diabetes affect Mg metabolism [7] and may increase vulnerability to Mg deficiency and adverse health outcomes. For this reason effects were investigated in rats selectively bred for susceptibility or resistance to diet-induced obesity. The high-fat, high-energy diets used in this study induced differences in adiposity between OP and OR rats validating our experimental model. OP rats had greater fat mass and percentage body fat at weeks 8–9 and at the end of the study.

The low Mg diet contained 23% of nutritional requirement for growing rats [31]. This degree of deficiency may exist in some individuals in the extreme lower percentiles of usual Mg intakes [11] (pp. 392–393). The low Mg diet depressed Mg status in both rat strains as evidenced by reductions in Mg concentrations in serum, urine, and femur.

Some evidence suggests that Mg status may affect body composition. In a placebo-controlled, randomized trial, supplementation of overweight women with 250 mg of Mg daily for eight weeks resulted in an increase in lean body mass and decrease in fat mass compared to baseline values [36]. In rats, maternal and postnatal Mg restriction caused a decrease in lean body mass and increase in percentage body fat in the offspring [13,14]. In the present study the low Mg diet decreased body weight and lean body mass in both rat strains, demonstrating that dietary Mg restriction after weaning impairs the growth of lean body mass. The low Mg diet did not affect percentage or total fat mass, indicating a greater effect on growth of lean mass as opposed to accumulation of fat. Energy efficiency of rats fed the low or normal Mg diets was similar, meaning that rats consumed a similar amount of energy from food for a similar amount of body weight gain. These results indicate that metabolic inefficiency was not the cause of the lower body weight and lean mass. The data also do not support a repartitioning of dietary energy from lean body mass to adipose tissue in rats fed low Mg since fat mass did not increase. The lower energy intake (and food consumption) observed for rats fed the low Mg diet is likely explained by the impaired growth and smaller size of the rats. Together, these results demonstrate that growth of lean body mass is sensitive to decreases in Mg intake and a moderately low Mg diet does not promote adiposity in rats selectively bred for susceptibility or resistance to diet-induced obesity.

There is compelling evidence indicating that Mg plays an important role in the control of cell proliferation [3,4] and protein synthesis [37]. Impaired cell growth and/or downregulation of protein synthesis may have contributed to the observed decrease in growth of lean body mass of rats fed the low Mg diet. Effects on the secretion or action of anabolic hormones such as insulin-like growth factor 1 or testosterone could also explain the impaired growth of lean body mass [38,39].

The low Mg diet reduced femur size (width, weight, and volume) in both rat strains and increased femoral length:width ratio in OR rats. These findings are noteworthy since the physical characteristics of a bone (shape and size) influence its mechanical strength [40]. Femoral structural geometry has been shown to adapt to mechanical loading [41], and therefore these femoral changes may be a consequence of a lesser mechanical load because of the lower body weight of rats fed the low Mg diet. Even though bone density and markers of bone formation (serum osteocalcin) and resorption (urine DPD:creatinine ratio) were unaffected by diet, specific effects on processes that influence bone development cannot be excluded. Bone development in rats is sensitive to reduction in Mg intake [16–19]. A low Mg diet containing 50% of nutritional requirement decreased the percentage of trabecular bone volume and bone mineral content of the distal femur in rats [16]. It has been proposed that increased release of substance P and inflammatory cytokines in response to Mg depletion may contribute to bone loss [16,17]. The increase in femur Ca and Na concentrations observed in this study for rats fed the low Mg diet may be a result of the lower amount of Mg incorporated into the bone.

Serum Ca has been shown to increase in rats and mice in response to moderate or severe Mg deficiency [18,20,21]. Serum Ca increased in both rat strains fed the low Mg diet. In OR rats there was an associated decrease in serum PTH, which excludes hyperactivity of the parathyroid gland as the cause. Ca and Mg compete for intestinal absorption and reabsorption in the kidney [42,43]. Increased Ca absorption and/or reabsorption resulting from diminished Mg antagonism may account for the observed rise in serum Ca. The associated decrease in PTH in OR rats may be explained by hypoactivity of the parathyroid gland in response to the rise in serum Ca. This is supported by experiments in Mg-deficient rats demonstrating increased blood Ca and hypoactivity of the parathyroid gland determined by histologic and morphometric analyses [20]. OP rats fed the low Mg diet did not show a reduction in PTH despite a rise in serum Ca. The higher basal serum Ca (and perhaps PTH) in OR rats may have sensitized the parathyroid gland to an additional rise in serum Ca.

A decrease in serum K concentration was observed for rats fed the low Mg diet. A reduction in serum K is often associated with Mg deficiency [44]. It has been proposed that Mg deficiency causes K wasting by increasing renal K excretion [44]. In this study, urine K concentration was not elevated in rats fed low Mg; however, urine minerals were only measured at the end of the study and thus we cannot comment on urinary excretion of minerals at earlier time points in the study.

Lower Mg intakes and serum Mg concentrations have been associated with type 2 diabetes [26–29]. A number of mechanisms have been proposed to explain the negative effect of diabetes on Mg status including increased renal Mg loss from glycosuria [7]. Whether moderately low Mg intakes adversely affect glucose homeostasis is less clear. In this study, the effects of the low Mg diet on plasma insulin and glucose concentrations were examined during an OGTT. OP rats with the highest percentage body fat and OR rats with the lowest percentage body fat were selected to allow for investigation of any modifying effect of adiposity. Plasma insulin concentrations were higher in OP than OR rats, which is in agreement with the greater insulin resistance previously described for obese-prone rats [45–47]. Plasma glucose and insulin concentrations were unaffected by diet, indicating that any effects of the low Mg diet on glucose control and insulin resistance were minor. The results also indicate that the differences in adiposity and insulin resistance between OP and OR rats did not influence the outcome. At the 30 min time point, OR rats showed higher plasma glucose compared to OP rats, irrespective of diet. This may be explained by slower intestinal glucose absorption and reduced entry of glucose into the bloodstream in OP rats. Delayed and lower glucose absorption has been reported for obese compared to lean rats [48]. The results of this study differ from the results of an earlier study that showed greater insulin resistance, impaired glucose tolerance, and lower insulin response to a glucose challenge in Mg-restricted rats [13]. An important distinction, however, is that rats in that study were born to dams that were deprived of Mg before conception and during pregnancy.

OP and OR rats showed differences in body composition, femoral physical measurements, markers of bone metabolism, plasma insulin, and serum and femur mineral concentrations. Despite these differences, for most parameters examined, an interaction between diet and strain was not observed, indicating that the low Mg diet had a similar effect in both rat strains. The exceptions were a decrease in serum PTH concentration and an increase in the femur length:width ratio, which was only observed in OR rats fed the low Mg diet. These results indicate that the greater adiposity in OP rats did not exacerbate the physical and biochemical changes induced by the low Mg diet.

The results from this study should be interpreted in the context of the experimental design. Rats were fed low Mg in the background of a high-fat, high-energy diet and therefore the effects may not be generalizable to lower fat and energy diets. It should be noted, however, that the low and normal Mg diets only differed in Mg content and therefore the reported physical and biochemical differences can be attributed to differences in Mg intake. It should also be mentioned that rats in this study were selectively bred for susceptibility or resistance to diet-induced obesity. Peculiarities in genetic makeup may have predisposed these rats to the effects of a low Mg diet. Caution is also warranted when extending these findings to humans, in particular effects on the Ca–PTH axis. Rats develop hypercalcemia in response to a moderate Mg deficiency, whereas humans develop hypocalcemia secondary to hypoparathyroidism and reduced circulating PTH concentration [24,49–51].

5. Conclusions

This study has shown that moderately low Mg intake when consuming a high-fat, high-energy diet causes prominent physiological changes in both OP and OR rats. The low Mg diet reduced body weight gain and growth of lean body mass and bone (femur) of the rats. In addition, serum and bone mineral concentrations were altered. These results underscore the importance of evaluating these physiological parameters in future studies exploring the public health risks from low Mg consumption.

Supplementary Materials: The following are available online at http://www.mdpi.com/2072-6643/8/5/253/s1.

Acknowledgments: We thank Dominique Patry for help with the serum mineral and urine creatinine measurements. We are also grateful to Julie Todd, Cina Aghazadeh Sanaei, Kevin Kittle, Karine Chamberland, Don Caldwell, Martha Navarro, and Philip Griffin for care of the rats and assistance with the necropsies. This research was funded by the Bureau of Nutritional Sciences, Health Canada.

Author Contributions: J.B. conceived and designed the experiments; C.L., S.R., H.R., N.A.V., and L.J.P. performed the experiments; J.B., C.L., S.R., H.R., and E.S. analyzed the data; J.B. wrote the paper.

Conflicts of Interest: The authors declare no conflict of interest. The founding sponsors had no role in the design of the study; in the collection, analyses, or interpretation of the data; in the writing of the manuscript, and in the decision to publish the results.

References

1. Volpe, S.L. Magnesium in disease prevention and overall health. *Adv. Nutr.* **2013**, *4*, 378S–383S. [CrossRef] [PubMed]

2. Elin, R.J. Magnesium: The fifth but forgotten electrolyte. *Am. J. Clin. Pathol.* **1994**, *102*, 616–622. [CrossRef] [PubMed]

3. Wolf, F.I.; Cittadini, A. Magnesium in cell proliferation and differentiation. *Front. Biosci.* **1999**, *4*, D607–D617. [CrossRef] [PubMed]

4. Cittadini, A.; Wolf, F.I.; Bossi, D.; Calviello, G. Magnesium in normal and neoplastic cell proliferation: State of the art on *in vitro* data. *Magnes. Res.* **1991**, *4*, 23–33. [PubMed]

5. Ford, E.S.; Mokdad, A.H. Dietary magnesium intake in a national sample of US adults. *J. Nutr.* **2003**, *133*, 2879–2882. [PubMed]

6. Health Canada. Do Canadian Adults Meet Their Nutrient Requirements through Food Intake Alone? Available online: http://www.hc-sc.gc.ca/fn-an/surveill/nutrition/commun/art-nutr-adult-eng.php (accessed on 23 September 2015).

7. Pham, P.C.; Pham, P.M.; Pham, S.V.; Miller, J.M.; Pham, P.T. Hypomagnesemia in patients with type 2 diabetes. *Clin. J. Am. Soc. Nephrol.* **2007**, *2*, 366–373. [CrossRef] [PubMed]

8. De Baaij, J.H.; Hoenderop, J.G.; Bindels, R.J. Magnesium in man: Implications for health and disease. *Physiol. Rev.* **2015**, *95*, 1–46. [CrossRef] [PubMed]

9. Bertinato, J.; Xiao, C.W.; Ratnayake, W.M.; Fernandez, L.; Lavergne, C.; Wood, C.; Swist, E. Lower serum magnesium concentration is associated with diabetes, insulin resistance, and obesity in South Asian and white Canadian women but not men. *Food Nutr. Res.* **2015**, *59*, 25974. [CrossRef] [PubMed]

10. Whang, R.; Hampton, E.M.; Whang, D.D. Magnesium homeostasis and clinical disorders of magnesium deficiency. *Ann. Pharmacother.* **1994**, *28*, 220–226. [PubMed]

11. Institute of Medicine. *Dietary Reference Intakes for Calcium, Phosphorus, Magnesium, Vitamin D, and Fluoride*; National Academy Press: Washington, DC, USA, 1997; pp. 190–249.

12. Hunt, C.D.; Johnson, L.K. Magnesium requirements: New estimations for men and women by cross-sectional statistical analyses of metabolic magnesium balance data. *Am. J. Clin. Nutr.* **2006**, *84*, 843–852. [PubMed]

13. Venu, L.; Kishore, Y.D.; Raghunath, M. Maternal and perinatal magnesium restriction predisposes rat pups to insulin resistance and glucose intolerance. *J. Nutr.* **2005**, *135*, 1353–1358. [PubMed]

14. Venu, L.; Padmavathi, I.J.; Kishore, Y.D.; Bhanu, N.V.; Rao, K.R.; Sainath, P.B.; Ganeshan, M.; Raghunath, M. Long-term effects of maternal magnesium restriction on adiposity and insulin resistance in rat pups. *Obesity* **2008**, *16*, 1270–1276. [CrossRef] [PubMed]

15. Sales, C.H.; Santos, A.R.; Cintra, D.E.; Colli, C. Magnesium-deficient high-fat diet: Effects on adiposity, lipid profile and insulin sensitivity in growing rats. *Clin. Nutr.* **2014**, *33*, 879–888. [CrossRef] [PubMed]

16. Rude, R.K.; Gruber, H.E.; Norton, H.J.; Wei, L.Y.; Frausto, A.; Kilburn, J. Reduction of dietary magnesium by only 50% in the rat disrupts bone and mineral metabolism. *Osteoporos. Int.* **2006**, *17*, 1022–1032. [CrossRef] [PubMed]

17. Rude, R.K.; Gruber, H.E.; Norton, H.J.; Wei, L.Y.; Frausto, A.; Kilburn, J. Dietary magnesium reduction to 25% of nutrient requirement disrupts bone and mineral metabolism in the rat. *Bone* **2005**, *37*, 211–219. [CrossRef] [PubMed]
18. Rude, R.K.; Gruber, H.E.; Norton, H.J.; Wei, L.Y.; Frausto, A.; Mills, B.G. Bone loss induced by dietary magnesium reduction to 10% of the nutrient requirement in rats is associated with increased release of substance P and tumor necrosis factor-alpha. *J. Nutr.* **2004**, *134*, 79–85. [PubMed]
19. Stendig-Lindberg, G.; Koeller, W.; Bauer, A.; Rob, P.M. Experimentally induced prolonged magnesium deficiency causes osteoporosis in the rat. *Eur. J. Intern. Med.* **2004**, *15*, 97–107. [CrossRef] [PubMed]
20. Jones, J.E.; Schwartz, R.; Krook, L. Calcium homeostasis and bone pathology in magnesium deficient rats. *Calcif. Tissue Int.* **1980**, *31*, 231–238. [CrossRef] [PubMed]
21. Rude, R.K.; Gruber, H.E.; Wei, L.Y.; Frausto, A.; Mills, B.G. Magnesium deficiency: Effect on bone and mineral metabolism in the mouse. *Calcif. Tissue Int.* **2003**, *72*, 32–41. [CrossRef] [PubMed]
22. Rude, R.K.; Kirchen, M.E.; Gruber, H.E.; Meyer, M.H.; Luck, J.S.; Crawford, D.L. Magnesium deficiency-induced osteoporosis in the rat: Uncoupling of bone formation and bone resorption. *Magnes. Res.* **1999**, *12*, 257–267. [PubMed]
23. Rude, R.K.; Singer, F.R.; Gruber, H.E. Skeletal and hormonal effects of magnesium deficiency. *J. Am. Coll. Nutr.* **2009**, *28*, 131–141. [CrossRef] [PubMed]
24. Rude, R.K.; Oldham, S.B.; Sharp, C.F., Jr.; Singer, F.R. Parathyroid hormone secretion in magnesium deficiency. *J. Clin. Endocrinol. Metab.* **1978**, *47*, 800–806. [CrossRef] [PubMed]
25. Orchard, T.S.; Larson, J.C.; Alghothani, N.; Bout-Tabaku, S.; Cauley, J.A.; Chen, Z.; LaCroix, A.Z.; Wactawski-Wende, J.; Jackson, R.D. Magnesium intake, bone mineral density, and fractures: Results from the women's health initiative observational study. *Am. J. Clin. Nutr.* **2014**, *99*, 926–933. [CrossRef] [PubMed]
26. Kao, W.H.; Folsom, A.R.; Nieto, F.J.; Mo, J.P.; Watson, R.L.; Brancati, F.L. Serum and dietary magnesium and the risk for type 2 diabetes mellitus: The atherosclerosis risk in communities study. *Arch. Intern. Med.* **1999**, *159*, 2151–2159. [CrossRef] [PubMed]
27. Larsson, S.C.; Wolk, A. Magnesium intake and risk of type 2 diabetes: A meta-analysis. *J. Intern. Med.* **2007**, *262*, 208–214. [CrossRef] [PubMed]
28. Ma, J.; Folsom, A.R.; Melnick, S.L.; Eckfeldt, J.H.; Sharrett, A.R.; Nabulsi, A.A.; Hutchinson, R.G.; Metcalf, P.A. Associations of serum and dietary magnesium with cardiovascular disease, hypertension, diabetes, insulin, and carotid arterial wall thickness: The ARIC study. Atherosclerosis risk in communities study. *J. Clin. Epidemiol.* **1995**, *48*, 927–940. [CrossRef]
29. Villegas, R.; Gao, Y.T.; Dai, Q.; Yang, G.; Cai, H.; Li, H.; Zheng, W.; Shu, X.O. Dietary calcium and magnesium intakes and the risk of type 2 diabetes: The Shanghai women's health study. *Am. J. Clin. Nutr.* **2009**, *89*, 1059–1067. [CrossRef] [PubMed]
30. Cahill, F.; Shahidi, M.; Shea, J.; Wadden, D.; Gulliver, W.; Randell, E.; Vasdev, S.; Sun, G. High dietary magnesium intake is associated with low insulin resistance in the Newfoundland population. *PLoS ONE* **2013**, *8*, e58278. [CrossRef] [PubMed]
31. Reeves, P.G.; Nielsen, F.H.; Fahey, G.C., Jr. AIN-93 purified diets for laboratory rodents: Final report of the American Institute of Nutrition ad hoc writing committee on the reformulation of the AIN-76A rodent diet. *J. Nutr.* **1993**, *123*, 1939–1951. [PubMed]
32. Aziz, A.A.; Kenney, L.S.; Goulet, B.; Abdel-Aal, E. Dietary starch type affects body weight and glycemic control in freely fed but not energy-restricted obese rats. *J. Nutr.* **2009**, *139*, 1881–1889. [CrossRef] [PubMed]
33. Boustany, C.M.; Bharadwaj, K.; Daugherty, A.; Brown, D.R.; Randall, D.C.; Cassis, L.A. Activation of the systemic and adipose renin-angiotensin system in rats with diet-induced obesity and hypertension. *Am. J. Physiol. Regul. Integr. Comp. Physiol.* **2004**, *287*, R943–R949. [CrossRef] [PubMed]
34. Bertinato, J.; Aroche, C.; Plouffe, L.J.; Lee, M.; Murtaza, Z.; Kenney, L.; Lavergne, C.; Aziz, A. Diet-induced obese rats have higher iron requirements and are more vulnerable to iron deficiency. *Eur. J. Nutr.* **2014**, *53*, 885–895. [CrossRef] [PubMed]
35. Bertinato, J.; Lavergne, C.; Vu, N.A.; Plouffe, L.J.; Wood, C.; Griffin, P.; Xiao, C.W. l-Lysine supplementation does not affect the bioavailability of copper or iron in rats. *J. Trace Elem. Med. Biol.* **2016**. [CrossRef] [PubMed]
36. Moslehi, N.; Vafa, M.; Sarrafzadeh, J.; Rahimi-Foroushani, A. Does magnesium supplementation improve body composition and muscle strength in middle-aged overweight women? A double-blind, placebo-controlled, randomized clinical trial. *Biol. Trace Elem. Res.* **2013**, *153*, 111–118. [CrossRef] [PubMed]

37. Dørup, I.; Clausen, T. Effects of magnesium and zinc deficiencies on growth and protein synthesis in skeletal muscle and the heart. *Br. J. Nutr.* **1991**, *66*, 493–504. [CrossRef] [PubMed]

38. Dørup, I.; Flyvbjerg, A.; Everts, M.E.; Clausen, T. Role of insulin-like growth factor-1 and growth hormone in growth inhibition induced by magnesium and zinc deficiencies. *Br. J. Nutr.* **1991**, *66*, 505–521. [CrossRef] [PubMed]

39. Maggio, M.; Ceda, G.P.; Lauretani, F.; Cattabiani, C.; Avantaggiato, E.; Morganti, S.; Ablondi, F.; Bandinelli, S.; Dominguez, L.J.; Barbagallo, M.; *et al.* Magnesium and anabolic hormones in older men. *Int. J. Androl.* **2011**, *34*, e594–e600. [CrossRef] [PubMed]

40. Bouxsein, M.L.; Karasik, D. Bone geometry and skeletal fragility. *Curr. Osteoporos. Rep.* **2006**, *4*, 49–56. [CrossRef] [PubMed]

41. Petit, M.A.; Beck, T.J.; Lin, H.M.; Bentley, C.; Legro, R.S.; Lloyd, T. Femoral bone structural geometry adapts to mechanical loading and is influenced by sex steroids: The Penn State young women's health study. *Bone* **2004**, *35*, 750–759. [CrossRef] [PubMed]

42. Alcock, N.; Macintyre, I. Inter-relation of calcium and magnesium absorption. *Clin. Sci.* **1962**, *22*, 185–193. [PubMed]

43. Bertinato, J.; Lavergne, C.; Plouffe, L.J.; El Niaj, H.A. Small increases in dietary calcium above normal requirements exacerbate magnesium deficiency in rats fed a low magnesium diet. *Mag. Res.* **2014**, *27*, 35–47.

44. Huang, C.-L.; Kuo, E. Mechanism of hypokalemia in magnesium deficiency. *J. Am. Soc. Nephrol.* **2007**, *18*, 2649–2652. [CrossRef] [PubMed]

45. Chang, S.; Graham, B.; Yakubu, F.; Lin, D.; Peters, J.C.; Hill, J.O. Metabolic differences between obesity-prone and obesity-resistant rats. *Am. J. Physiol.* **1990**, *259*, R1103–R1110. [PubMed]

46. Madsen, A.N.; Hansen, G.; Paulsen, S.J.; Lykkegaard, K.; Tang-Christensen, M.; Hansen, H.S.; Levin, B.E.; Larsen, P.J.; Knudsen, L.B.; Fosgerau, K.; *et al.* Long-term characterization of the diet-induced obese and diet-resistant rat model: A polygenetic rat model mimicking the human obesity syndrome. *J. Endocrinol.* **2010**, *206*, 287–296. [CrossRef] [PubMed]

47. Paulsen, S.J.; Jelsing, J.; Madsen, A.N.; Hansen, G.; Lykkegaard, K.; Larsen, L.K.; Larsen, P.J.; Levin, B.E.; Vrang, N. Characterization of beta-cell mass and insulin resistance in diet-induced obese and diet-resistant rats. *Obesity* **2010**, *18*, 266–273. [CrossRef] [PubMed]

48. Garcia-Martinez, C.; Lopez-Soriano, F.J.; Argiles, J.M. Intestinal glucose absorption is lower in obese than in lean zucker rats. *J. Nutr.* **1993**, *123*, 1062–1067. [PubMed]

49. Chiba, T.; Okimura, Y.; Inatome, T.; Inoh, T.; Watanabe, M.; Fujita, T. Hypocalcemic crisis in alcoholic fatty liver: Transient hypoparathyroidism due to magnesium deficiency. *Am. J. Gastroenterol.* **1987**, *82*, 1084–1087. [PubMed]

50. Mukai, A.; Yamamoto, S.; Matsumura, K. Hypocalcemia secondary to hypomagnesemia in a patient with Crohn's disease. *Clin. J. Gastroenterol.* **2015**, *8*, 22–25. [CrossRef] [PubMed]

51. Shah, B.R.; Santucci, K.; Finberg, L. Magnesium deficiency as a cause of hypocalcemia in the CHARGE association. *Arch. Pediatr. Adolesc. Med.* **1994**, *148*, 486–489. [CrossRef] [PubMed]

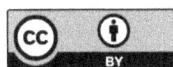

MDPI AG

St. Alban-Anlage 66

4052 Basel, Switzerland

Tel. +41 61 683 77 34

Fax +41 61 302 89 18

http://www.mdpi.com

Nutrients Editorial Office

E-mail: nutrients@mdpi.com

http://www.mdpi.com/journal/nutrients

www.ingramcontent.com/pod-product-compliance
Lightning Source LLC
Chambersburg PA
CBHW051313020426
42333CB00028B/3318